Pharmacology in Anesthesia Practice

Anita Gupta, DO, PharmD

Associate Professor, Medical Director
Division of Pain Medicine and Regional Anesthesiology
Department of Anesthesiology and Perioperative Medicine
Drexel University College of Medicine
Philadelphia, PA

Nina Singh-Radcliff, MD

Private Practice Anesthesiologist
New Jersey

OXFORD

UNIVERSITY PRESS

OXFORD
UNIVERSITY PRESS

Oxford University Press is a department of the University of Oxford.
It furthers the University's objective of excellence in research, scholarship,
and education by publishing worldwide.

Oxford   New York
Auckland   Cape Town   Dar es Salaam   Hong Kong   Karachi
Kuala Lumpur   Madrid   Melbourne   Mexico City   Nairobi
New Delhi   Shanghai   Taipei   Toronto

With offices in
Argentina   Austria   Brazil   Chile   Czech Republic   France   Greece
Guatemala   Hungary   Italy   Japan   Poland   Portugal   Singapore
South Korea   Switzerland   Thailand   Turkey   Ukraine   Vietnam

Oxford is a registered trade mark of Oxford University Press in the UK and
certain other countries.

Published in the United States of America by
Oxford University Press
198 Madison Avenue, New York, NY 10016

© Oxford University Press 2013

Library of Congress Cataloging-in-Publication Data
Pharmacology in anesthesia practice / [edited by] Anita Gupta, Nina Singh-Radcliff.
p. ; cm.
Includes bibliographical references and index.

Summary: "In anesthesia practice and treatment, pharmacology and therapeutics are intimately related,
synergistic, and mutually reinforcing. Rapid advances in pharmacotherapy often offer myriad treatment
options for clinicians to sort through when developing patient management strategies. In turn, the principles
of clinical therapeutics are rooted in fundamental pharmacology. Clinicians must understand pharmacologic
principles in order to formulate and implement therapeutic algorithms that maximize patient benefit.
Pharmacology in Anesthesia Practice provides clinicians with a rapid and easy review of the most commonly
utilized pharmacologic agents during perioperative care. Clinical application is emphasized throughout.
It aims to offer clinicians point-of-care guidance from internationally recognized authors and centers of
excellence"—Provided by publisher.

ISBN 978-0-19-978267-3 (pbk. : alk. paper)

I. Gupta, Anita. II. Singh-Radcliff, Nina.

[DNLM: 1. Anesthetics—pharmacology.   2. Analgesics—pharmacology.   3. Anesthesia—
methods.   4. Drug Therapy—methods.   5. Perioperative Care—methods. QV 81]

RD82.2

615.7'81—dc23

2013003208

ISBN-13: 978-0-19-978267-3

9 8 7 6 5 4 3 2 1
Printed in the United States of America
on acid-free paper

Pharmacology
Anesth   Practi

Preface

The perioperative care of patients requires a unique knowledge base and skill set that differs widely. The practice of medicine has encompassed patient management through intervention to prevention and ultimately to treatment of disease. Particularly in the field of anesthesiology, there are rapid advances in pharmacotherapy, which often offers a myriad of treatment options for patients and clinicians. This handbook on pharmacology in anesthesia practice provides a concise reference for clinicians in anesthesiology. This handbook will provide rapid and easy review for clinicians for the most commonly utilized medications in anesthesia practice with an emphasis on the clinical application of the medication. Students, scholars, and educators in anesthesiology approach the field from divergent practice perspectives; therefore, this book provides a resource to bring these practices together. Clinicians apply the principles of basic pharmacology, and an understanding of the principles and practice of clinical pharmacology to formulate and implement therapeutic algorithms that maximize patient benefit. The aim of this work is to provide in one source authoritative information from leaders in anesthesiology on the use of pharmacologic agents during perioperative care. The work is an indispensable resource for a variety of clinicians and provides a point of care guide utilizing contributions of nationally and internationally recognized authors from institutions with advanced practices and centers of excellence.

There are many who deserve acknowledgment, without whose efforts this textbook would not have been possible. These individuals have given their time to prepare and revise their chapters to realize vision for this textbook, and we take this opportunity to express our foremost gratitude for their scholarly contributions. We sincerely hope that their contributions will benefit students and practitioners of pharmacology and therapeutics in the ever-growing field of anesthesiology.

Contents

Contributors

John G. Augoustides, MD
Department of Anesthesiology and
Critical Care
Hospital of the University of
Pennsylvania
Philadelphia, PA

Emily Baird, MD
Department of Anesthesiology and
Critical Care
Hospital of the University of
Pennsylvania
Philadelphia, PA

Jane C. Ballantyne, MD
Professor
Division of Pain Medicine
University of Washington
Seattle, Washington

Gaurav Bhatia, MD
Department of Anesthesiology and
Critical Care
Hospital of the University of
Pennsylvania
Philadelphia, PA

Shannon Bianchi, MD
Department of Anesthesiology and
Critical Care
Hospital of the University of
Pennsylvania
Philadelphia, PA

Shanique Brown, MD
Department of Anesthesiology and
Critical Care
Hospital of the University of
Pennsylvania
Philadelphia, PA

Maurizio Cereda, MD
Department of Anesthesiology and
Critical Care
Hospital of the University of
Pennsylvania
Philadelphia, PA

Jason Choi, MD
Department of Anesthesiology and
Critical Care
Hospital of the University of
Pennsylvania
Philadelphia, PA

Katherine Chuy, MD
Department of Anesthesiology and
Critical Care
Hospital of the University of
Pennsylvania
Philadelphia, PA

Matt N. Decker, BS
Department of Anesthesiology and
Critical Care
Hospital of the University of
Pennsylvania
Philadelphia, PA

Elizabeth W. Duggan, MD
Department of Anesthesiology and
Critical Care
Jefferson Health System
Philadelphia, PA

Michael J. Duggan, MD
Department of Anesthesiology and
Critical Care
Jefferson Health System
Philadelphia, PA

Nabil Elkassabany, MD
Department of Anesthesiology and
Critical Care
Hospital of the University of
Pennsylvania
Philadelphia, PA

Jared Feinman, MD
Department of Anesthesiology and
Critical Care
Hospital of the University of
Pennsylvania
Philadelphia, PA

Robert Gaiser, MD
Department of Anesthesiology and
Critical Care
Hospital of the University of
Pennsylvania
Philadelphia, PA

Philip Gallegos, MD
Attending Anesthesiologist,
Contributor

William Gao, MD
Attending Anesthesiologist,
Contributor

Anita Gupta, DO, PharmD
Associate Professor, Medical Director
University Pain Institute
Division of Pain Medicine & Regional
Anesthesiology
Department of Anesthesiology and
Perioperative Medicine
Drexel University College of
Medicine
Philadelphia, PA

Jiri Horak, MD
Department of Anesthesiology and
Critical Care
Hospital of the University of
Pennsylvania
Philadelphia, PA

Peter Killoran, MD
Attending Anesthesiologist,
Contributor

Meghan Lane-Fall, MD
Department of Anesthesiology and
Critical Care
Hospital of the University of
Pennsylvania
Philadelphia, PA

Matthew Lesneski, MD
Department of Anesthesiology and
Critical Care
Hospital of the University of
Pennsylvania
Philadelphia, PA

Gaurav Malhotra, MD
Department of Anesthesiology and
Critical Care
Hospital of the University of
Pennsylvania
Philadelphia, PA

Amna Mehdi, BS
Department of Public Health
Rutgers University
New Brunswick, NJ

Todd Miano, PharmD, BCPS
Contributor

Gregory Moy, MD
Department of Anesthesiology and
Critical Care
Hospital of the University of
Pennsylvania
Philadelphia, PA

Jonas A. Nelson, MD
Department of Anesthesiology and
Critical Care
Hospital of the University of
Pennsylvania
Philadelphia, PA

Priscilla Nelson, MD
Department of Anesthesiology and
Critical Care
Hospital of the University of
Pennsylvania
Philadelphia, PA

Katherine C. Normand, MD
Attending Anesthesiologist,
Contributor

Onyi Onuoha, MD
Department of Anesthesiology and
Critical Care
Hospital of the University of
Pennsylvania
Philadelphia, PA

Mona Patel, MD
Department of Anesthesiology and
Critical Care
Hospital of the University of
Pennsylvania
Philadelphia, PA

Emily E. Peoples, MD
Department of Anesthesiology and
Critical Care
University of Michigan
Ann Arbor, MI

Jesse Raiten, MD
Department of Anesthesiology and
Critical Care
Hospital of the University of
Pennsylvania
Philadelphia, PA

Chitra Ramasubbu, MD
Department of Anesthesiology and
Critical Care Medicine
Division of Pain Medicine
Johns Hopkins University
Baltimore, MD

Kris E. Radcliff, MD
Attending Physician, Contributor

Sander Schlichter, MD
Department of Anesthesiology and
Critical Care
Hospital of the University of
Pennsylvania
Philadelphia, PA

Thomas H. Scott. MD
Department of Anesthesiology and
Critical Care
Hospital of the University of
Pennsylvania
Philadelphia, PA

Nina Singh-Radcliff, MD
Contributor and Co-Editor

Devin Tang, MD
Department of Anesthesiology and
Critical Care
Hospital of the University of
Pennsylvania
Philadelphia, PA

Elizabeth Valentine, MD
Department of Anesthesiology and
Critical Care
Hospital of the University of
Pennsylvania
Philadelphia, PA

Cristianna Vallera, MD
Attending Anesthesiologist,
Contributor

Ellen Wang, MD
Attending Anesthesiologist,
Contributor

Alissa Wilmot, MD
Department of Anesthesiology and
Critical Care
Hospital of the University of
Pennsylvania
Philadelphia, PA

Lisa Witkin, MD
Department of Anesthesiology and
Critical Care
Hospital of the University of
Pennsylvania
Philadelphia, PA

Crystal C. Wright, MD
Attending Anesthesiologist,
Contributor

Tygh Wycoff, MD
Department of Anesthesiology and
Critical Care
Hospital of the University of
Pennsylvania
Philadelphia, PA

Peter Yi, MD
Department of Anesthesiology and
Critical Care
Hospital of the University of
Pennsylvania
Philadelphia, PA

Chapter 1

Inhalational Agents

Chapter 1.1

Volatile Anesthetics

Philip Gallegos, MD and Nina Singh-Radcliff, MD

Clinical Uses/Indications

- Induction and maintenance of general anesthesia
- Bronchodilation during status asthmaticus

Pharmacodynamics

- Halogenated hydrocarbons, hydrophobic; "volatile" agents
- An "ideal" volatile agent is odorless, not metabolized, poorly soluble in blood, tissue, and the breathing circuit (allows for quick onset/offset), cheap, can be stored for long periods, nontoxic, nonflammable, noncombustible; does not affect cardiac, pulmonary, or other organs
- Loss of consciousness, amnesia, and immobility; mechanism unknown!! Believed to act on multiple areas (unlike IV meds that act on single receptor), disrupt electrical transmission (via proteins, membrane receptors, intracellular enzyme systems), block excitatory transmission (can also enhance) and synapses at a lower concentration than axonal synapses.
- Minimum Alveolar Concentration (MAC). The alveolar concentration of volatile agent, at 1 atm, that is required to produce immobility in 50% of patients at skin incision; termed 1MAC. Allows an assessment of potency; standardization of doses for different agents; an index of depth, induction, and recovery (measurement of expired gases can be extrapolated to alveolar MAC and hence brain tissue levels after equilibration); consistent across species; and are additive (coadministration with N_2O or other volatile agent). However, does *not* reflect an individual's response, is indirectly measured by end-tidal monitors to reflect *alveolar* concentration, and does not guarantee amnesia. MAC is ↓ by benzodiazepines, opioids, sedatives (dexmedetomidine, propofol, ketamine, barbiturates, clonidine) increasing age (↓ ~6% per decade), lidocaine, acute alcohol intoxication, hypothermia (↓ 50% for every 10° C), hypotension (MAP < 40 mm Hg), hyponatremia, metabolic acidosis, anemia (Hct < 10%), hypercarbia ($paCO_2$ > 95 mmHg), hypoxia (paO_2 < 38 mm Hg), and pregnancy (after ~8 wks). MAC is ↑ with chronic alcoholism, sympathetics (acute cocaine and amphetamine intoxication, ephedrine, levodopa), infants (greatest

at 6 months), hyperthermia, thyrotoxicosis, hypernatremia, genetic factors (redheads have ~19% ↑ requirement).

- MAC awake (~0.35 for iso-, sevo-, desflurane; ~0.5 N_2O, halothane): alve- olar agent concentration where 50% of patients (pts) voluntarily respond (eye opening) to commands. *Not* equivalent to MAC aware/recall.
- MAC95 (MAC = 1.3): alveolar concentration where 95% of pts do not respond to skin incision
- MAC BAR (MAC ~1.6): alveolar concentration where 50% of pts have a block of sympathetic response (HR, BP, noradrenaline levels) to surgical stimulation
- MAC BAR95: alveolar concentration where 95% of pts have a block of adren- ergic response
- MAC EI (~1.3): alveolar concentration to prevent laryngeal response to ETT intubation
- MAC-hr: MAC time for exposure to the volatile agent (MAC multiplied by hour increments; eg, 1.25 MAC for 2 h represents 2.5 MAC-hr). Used as a comparative measure of exposure when calculating adverse effects and set- ting dose-limits. Does not account for differences in metabolism, effects at different concentrations, or fresh gas flow.

Pharmacokinetics

- Liquid at room temperature (vaporized for inhalational administration).
- Partial pressures are denoted as $P_{location}$. (P_{brain}, P_A, P_a, etc; units are mm Hg). However, volatile agents are denoted as *fractions*: $F_{location}$ (F_{brain}, F_A, F_a, etc; units are %). Sevoflurane 2% indicates that it constitutes 2% of the total inspired gas
- Tissue groups. The vessel-rich group (brain, heart, liver, kidney, endocrine organs) receives significant blood flow (hence volatile agent delivery) and concentrations quickly rise; however, has *small* overall capacity. The muscle (skin, muscle), fat, and vessel-poor group (bone, ligaments, teeth, hair, and cartilage) receives less blood flow (hence volatile agent delivery) and con- centrations take longer to rise; however has *large* capacity and functions as a "depot." When volatile agent is stored in a "depot" it is essentially diverted from the brain (site of action) and ↓ induction and emergence, par- ticularly with volatiles that have ↑ blood:gas solubility or with ↑ duration of administration (MAC-hr)
- Partition coefficients. Ratio of the amount of substance present in one phase compared with another (assumes 2 phases at equal volume and specified tem- perature). Allows assessment of relative solubilities between blood and gas, brain, muscle, or fat (provides a means to assess and compare the quantity and time needed for uptake and saturation of a tissue). Halothane's blood:gas par- tition coefficient = 2.4; at equilibrium, the concentration of halothane in blood is 2.4 times that of halothane in a gas in contact with the blood.
- Fi: Inspired concentration of volatile agent. Affected by fresh gas flow rates, concentration of agent delivered, ventilation (rate, TV), volume of the

breathing system (circuit length and diameter), and absorption (circuit, machine). Fi is increased with ↑ fresh gas flow rates, ↑ concentration delivered, and ↑ ventilation as well as ↓ breathing circuit volume and absorption.

- F_A: Alveolar concentration of volatile agent. F_A is affected by F_i (input) as well as factors affecting uptake from the lungs (output): blood:gas solubility, CO, and venous-arterial partial pressure difference. Because $F_A \sim F_{blood} \sim F_{brain}$ at equilibrium, an assessment of anesthetic depth (induction, maintenance, and recovery) can be extrapolated from F_A. F_A (and rate of induction) is ↑ with poorly soluble gases, ↓ CO/alveolar blood flow, and ↓ venous-arterial partial pressure differences. Note that F_A is indirectly measured by end tidal monitors that reflect alveolar concentrations ($F_{ETagent}$).

- F_A/F_i ratio. Less than 1 due to uptake of anesthetic agent by the pulmonary circulation (if no uptake, could equal 1, but not possible to exceed on induction). F_A/F_i nears 1 when ↑ F_A and/or ↑ Fi, and is a method of assessing speed of onset.

- Elimination. Recovery from anesthesia depends on lowering anesthetic concentration in brain tissue; F_A is used as a surrogate indicator of F_{brain} ($F_{ETagent} \sim F_A \sim F_a \sim F_{brain}$). Volatile agents are eliminated by exhalation, biotransformation, and transcutaneous loss. Factors that speed induction also speed recovery: ↑fresh gas flow, ↓anesthesia machine-circuit volume and absorption, ↓solubility, ↑CBF, and ↑ventilation.

- Variable-bypass vaporizers are utilized for halothane, sevoflurane, isoflurane. Fresh gas flow from the machine passes through the vaporizer and gets divided into a bypass chamber and a sump chamber (dial determines ratio of flow between the chambers). The sump chamber functions as a liquid reservoir where fresh gas flow becomes saturated with agent (thus, ↑ sump flow occurs with ↑ dial concentration or ↑ fresh gas flow; results in ↑ F_i and ↑ F_A/F_i).

- Heated vaporizers are utilized for desflurane due to its ↑ vapor pressure (see desflurane)

Cautions/Adverse Reactions

- CNS. Not an analgesic. Cerebral vasodilator; uncouples cerebral autoregulation (however, hyperventilation can offset the ↑ blood flow since vasculature remains responsive to CO_2 levels). Affects SSEP and MEP monitoring (↑ latency, ↓ amplitude) in a dose-dependent manner; affects EEG monitoring.

- Cardiac. Main effect is ↓ SVR with isoflurane, sevoflurane, and desflurane; halothane ↓ CO to a greater extent than SVR. More profound effects when advanced age, ↑ vascular tone, ↓ cardiac function, coadministration of medications (eg, propofol), and hypovolemia. May be blunted by coadministration of N_2O, adequate volume status, narcotic-based technique. Prolongs QT interval.

- Pulmonary. ↓ TV, ↑ RR. Minute ventilation in a SV patient is roughly maintained, however is less efficient (↑ dead space ventilation). Hypoxic and hypercarbic respiratory responses are blunted. ↓ FRC due to effects on diaphragm, chest wall, and blood flow to abdomen and pulmonary cavity. Blunts hypoxic pulmonary vasoconstriction, which may ↑ shunting (minimal).

- Hepatic. Direct and indirect hepatoxicity from metabolism and degradation that result in the formation of reactive intermediates. These intermediates can attach to native hepatic proteins, and the body may interpret these "new" protein compounds as foreign and mount an immune response (form antibodies). Antibodies to trifluoroacylated proteins have been detected, suggesting this mechanism. Although halothane is the usual culprit, it has also been reported in the other volatile agents.
- Malignant hyperthermia triggers.

Halothane

Clinical Uses/Relevance to Anesthesiology

- Oldest of all modern anesthetics; available and in use today (low cost, in developing countries, certain congenital heart defects, not pungent)

Pharmacodynamics

- Most potent volatile agent; MAC 0.76
- CNS. Cerebral vasodilator with ↑ CBF throughout all parts of the brain. At concentrations >1%, ↑ CBF up to 200% (compared to 20% with isoflurane); nearly abolishes cerebral autoregulation (uncouples $CMRO_2$ and CBF). Vascular tone response to CO_2 is maintained (however, hyperventilation needs to be instituted *prior* to halothane administration; other volatiles can be done *concurrently*). Dose-dependent ↓ in $CMRO_2$ (up to 25% ↓; lowest of all volatiles). Impedes CSF absorption, minimally ↓ formation. EEG shows a biphasic pattern: initial activation at subanesthetic doses followed by dose-dependent ↓.
- Cardiac. ↓ cardiac contractility (greater than other volatiles) and ↓ SVR (less than other volatiles). Myocardial depression results from interference of Na^+/Ca^{++} exchange and intracellular Ca^{++} utilization. Sensitizes the heart to arrhythmias (greater than other volatiles). Depresses SA node and ↓ conduction velocity; mildly affects AV node (prolongs conduction velocity, ↑ refractoriness); the combination results in a junctional rhythm or bradycardia. Junctional tachycardia may occur when anticholinergics are administered to treat sinus bradycardia (due to greater depression of the SA node compared with the AV node). Also sensitizes the heart to the arrhythmogenic effects of epinephrine (not to exceed 0.45 mL/kg of a 1:100 000 solution per hour) and other sympathomimetics (terbutaline, aminophylline, theophylline); likely the result of interfering with slow calcium channel conductance. Blunts the baroreceptor reflex (impairs compensatory tachycardia), compounding halothane's effects on myocardial contractility; functions as a "beta-blocker." This effect, however, may be useful in idiopathic hypertrophic subaortic stenosis and infundibular pulmonic stenosis. Myocardial depression is exacerbated by beta-blockers and calcium channel blockers.

- Respiratory. Bronchodilator (most potent) via inhibition of intracellular calcium immobilization; makes it useful in the treatment of status asthmaticus. Hypoxic and hypercarbic respiratory drives are depressed for a longer period of time than other volatiles after discontinuation.
- Neuromuscular. Skeletal muscle relaxant; potentiates nondepolarizing neuromuscular-blocking agents. MH trigger.
- Hepatic. ↓ hepatic blood flow to the portal vein and hepatic artery. "Halothane hepatitis" has an incidence of 1:35 000 cases; and is ↑ with middle-aged obese women, familial predisposition to toxicity, personal history of toxicity, or multiple halothane anesthetics at short intervals. Halothane is oxidatively metabolized by cytochrome P450 2E1, and metabolites, particularly trifluoroacetyl moieties, can covalently attach to native hepatic proteins. The "new," altered hepatic proteins may mount an antibody response. ↑ AST, ALT, bilirubin; jaundice and encephalopathy. Diagnosis of exclusion; therefore, need to rule out other causes such as surgical complications, perioperative hypotension, viral causes (CMV, EBV), other drug reactions
- Renal. ↓ RBF, GFR, and UOP from ↓ BP, CO. Filtration fraction ↑ due to ↓ RBF:GFR ratio. May be ↓ with preoperative hydration

Pharmacokinetics

- Relatively nonflammable. Vapor pressure 244 mm Hg
- Blood:gas coefficient 2.54 (greatest) and tissue:blood coefficient results in slow induction and recovery (dissolves in blood and stored in tissues or "depots" instead of attaining adequate brain concentrations; "diverted").
- Not pungent, making useful for inhalation induction
- Metabolized by the liver up to 40% (greatest of all modern volatiles); Compound A formation
- Unstable in hydrated and dessicated carbon dioxide absorbent

Desflurane

Clinical Uses/Relevance to Anesthesiology

- Maintenance of GA; pungency and airway irritation make less ideal for inhalation inductions.
- Expensive (and less potent, requiring more), however may be administered with low flows (compared to sevoflurane)

Pharmacodynamics

- Differs from isoflurane only in the substitution of a single fluorine for a single chlorine. Least potent volatile anesthetic; MAC 6.2 (however, 17 times more potent than N_2O)

- CNS. ↓ blood:gas solubility facilitates quick onset and offset; 50% quicker wake-up time than isoflurane. Uncouples cerebral autoregulation (dose-related ↓ in CMRO$_2$ however ↑ CBF from cerebral vasodilation; less profound than with other agents). The ↑ CBF, CBV, and ICP can be offset by hyperventilation instituted concurrently with halothane.
- Cardiac. ↑ HR and BP seen when depressed vagal tone or dose is rapidly ↑ (transient, and due to ↑ catecholamine levels; more profound in pts with cardiovascular disease)
- Respiratory. Potent bronchodilator. However, pungent and can evoke coughing, breath-holding, laryngospasm, and salivation, particularly at induction and emergence.
- Neuromuscular. Relaxes smooth muscle and potentiates the effects of nondepolarizing neuromuscular blocking agents. Dose-dependent ↓ in response to TOF, tetanic peripheral nerve stimulation.

Pharmacokinetics

- Chlorine substitution results in a ↑ vapor density; 669 mm Hg (at room temperature, near 1 atm). At sea level it is close to its boiling point and at ↑ altitudes such as Denver, Colorado, desflurane will boil at room temperature. As a result, it requires a specialized vaporizer that electrically heats the agent in order to pressurize it to 2 atm and keep it in liquid form.
- Blood:Gas partition coefficient = 0.45 at 37°C; low solubility in both blood and tissue ↑ wash-in and wash-out of anesthetic. May cause emergence delirium, particularly in pediatric patients.
- Minimal metabolism in humans and resistant to defluorination (does not ↑ fluoride concentrations); very resistant to degradation during storage
- Degraded by hydrated CO$_2$ absorbent (greater than other agents) and forms carbon monoxide in dessicated CO$_2$ absorbent.

Isoflurane

Clinical Uses/Relevance to Anesthesiology

- Maintenance of GA; pungency and airway irritation make less ideal for inhalation inductions.
- Cheap, potent, can be administered with ↓ fresh gas flows
- Status asthmaticus (not as potent as halothane)

Pharmacodynamics

- CNS. ↓ CMRO$_2$ and able to produce an electrically silent EEG at 2 MAC. Vasodilation (↑ CBF, ICP) when concentration > 1 MAC; however can be reversed when hypoventilation is concurrently instituted

- Cardiac. Minimal depression of cardiac contractility. ↓ SVR (vasodilation), causes ↓ BP. Similar to desflurane, rapid ↑ in concentration leads to transient ↑ in HR, BP, and plasma levels of norepinephrine (↑ HR may result from the partial preservation of carotid baroreflexes, which respond to ↓ in BP). Coronary artery vasodilation may result in coronary artery steal syndrome (dilation of normal arteries diverts blood flow away from fixed stenotic lesions that are maximally dilated and flow-dependent; similar to how adenosine stresses the heart and unmasks myocardium at risk for ischemia during stress tests).
- Respiratory. Depressant effects resemble other volatile agents but with less pronounced tachypnea
- Neuromuscular. MH trigger. Relaxes smooth muscle and potentiates the effects of nondepolarizing NMBD. Mild beta-adrenergic stimulation ↑ skeletal muscle blood flow.
- Hepatic. ↑ total hepatic blood flow
- Renal. ↓ RBF, GFR, UOP

Pharmacokinetics

- Vapor pressure 240 mm Hg
- Not stable in hydrated CO_2 absorbent; carbon monoxide formation in dessicated CO_2 absorbent.
- Minimal metabolism, thus little potential risk of nephrotoxicity or hepatic dysfunction.

Sevoflurane

Clinical Uses/Relevance to Anesthesiology

- Inhalational induction; nonpungency allows for smooth induction. Sevoflurane 4–8% with 50% N_2O can be achieved in ~1–3 mins
- Maintenance of general anesthesia
- Status asthmaticus; potent bronchodilator

Pharmacodynamics

- MAC 2.2
- CNS. Uncouples cerebral autoregulation (↓ $CMRO_2$ however cerebral vasodilator). Vasodilation can be reversed with concurrent institution of hyperventilation. May evoke seizure activity on EEG. Rapid emergence may cause emergence delirium (particularly in pediatrics)
- Cardiac. Mild ↓ of myocardial contractility; ↓ SVR, BP (lesser degree than isoflurane, desflurane). Mild, if any, effect on HR (thus CO not as well maintained with ↓ BP). Does not sensitize heart to catecholamine-induced arrhythmias.

- Respiratory. Less irritating than desflurane and more $\uparrow$ onset/offset compared with isoflurane (smooth and rapid mask induction in pediatrics and adults). Respiratory depressant. Bronchodilator (similar potency as isoflurane)
- Neuromuscular. MH trigger. Relaxes smooth muscle and potentiates the effects of nondepolarizing NMBD (can provide adequate muscle relaxation for intubation following an inhalation induction).
- Hepatic. Blood flow maintained
- Renal. Slightly $\downarrow$ RBF. Potential for nephrotoxicity secondary to $\uparrow$ in inorganic fluoride (in vivo metabolism is 5–10 times greater than isoflurane). Additionally, Compound A is a nephrotoxic by-product that results from exposure to warm, moist soda lime. Production is $\uparrow$ with baralyme, $\downarrow$ fresh gas flows, $\uparrow$ CO_2, and $\uparrow$ MAC-hr

Pharmacokinetics

- Blood:gas solubility at 0.65 (low) results in $\uparrow$ wash-in and wash-out
- Fresh gas flows > 1 L/min; however, if exceeds 2 MAC-hr 2L/min is suggested
- Vapor pressure of 160 mm Hg at 20°C.

References

1. Sharp JH, Trudell JR, Cohen EN. Volatile metabolites and decomposition products of halothane in man. *Anesthesiology.* 1979;50:2–8.

2. Fang ZX, Eger EI II, Laster MJ, Chortkoff BS, Kandel L, Ionescu P. Carbon monoxide production from degradation of desflurane, enflurane, isoflurane, halothane, and sevoflurane by soda lime and Baralyme®. *Anesth Analg.* 1995;80:1187–1193.

3. Eger EI, Eisenkraft JB, Weiskopf RB. *The Pharmacology of Inhaled Anesthetics.* 3rd ed. Sponsored by the Dannemiller Memorial Educational Foundation; 2002.

4. Stoelting RK. *Pharmacology and Physiology in Anesthetic Practice.* 3rd ed. Philadelphia: Lippincott; 1999.

5. Shafer S. Principles of pharmacokinetics and pharamacodynamics. In: Longnecker DE, Tinker JH, Morgan GE, eds. *Principles and Practice of Anesthesiology.* 2nd ed. St. Louis, MO: Mosby-Year Book; 1997.

6. Eger EI II. Uptake of inhaled anesthetics: The alveolar to inspired anesthetic difference. In: *Anesthetic Uptake and Action.* Baltimore: Williams & Wilkins; 1974:77–96.

7. Lerman J, Schmitt-Bantel BI, Gregory GA, et al. Effect of age on the solubility of volatile anesthetics in human tissues. *Anesthesiology.* 1986;65:307–311.

8. Yasuda N, Lockhart SH, Eger EI II, et al. Kinetics of desflurane, isoflurane, and halothane in humans. *Anesthesiology.* 1991;74:489–498.

9. Carpenter RL, Eger EI II, Johnson BH, et al. The extent of metabolism of inhaled anesthetics in humans. *Anesthesiology.* 1986;65:201–205.

10. Eger EI II: *Desflurane (Suprane): A Compendium and Reference.* Rutherford, NJ: Healthpress Publishing Group; 1993:1–119.

Chapter 1.2

Nitrous Oxide

Philip Gallegos, MD and Nina Singh-Radcliff, MD

Clinical Uses/Anesthetic Implications

- Unconsciousness; adjuvant inhaled anesthetic that must be coadministered with volatiles, opioids, and sedatives to provide general anesthesia. Cheap, with fast onset/offset, provides hemodynamic stability, and capable of providing up to 0.7 MAC. However, not potent (MAC 104%), precluding its use as a complete general anesthetic.
- Analgesia; only inhaled agent with this capability. Dentistry procedures; IV line placement; cesarean sections for "patchy" epidural or spinal; anesthetic maintenance (adjuvant)
- Mask induction; children and adults (often coadministered with volatile agent), not pungent, fast onset
- End of case; quick onset/offset allows downward titration of volatiles to hasten wake-up (can avoid compromising awareness for expediency)
- Cesarean sections under GA; does not affect uterine tone (unlike volatiles) and is often coadministered in high concentrations with volatiles after the fetus is delivered (allows maintenance of GA, reduction of volatile agent concentration)
- Schools of thought vary....Long track record of use, and relatively inexpensive; however, in the absence of specific situations contraindicating its use, it can be favorably recommended after individual patient's risks and benefits are weighed.

Pharmacodynamics

- Colorless, odorless, sweet-smelling gas; inorganic
- Anesthetic properties: mechanism unknown. Likely affects several receptors including ion channels, NMDA, GABA, 5-HT3, and glycine. Although N_2O is a nonvolatile, nonhalogenated, and nonvapor inhalational agent, it provides measurable amnestic and unconsciousness characteristics similar to volatile agents (MAC units). Its low potency (MAC 104%), precludes it from providing general anesthesia as a sole agent (O_2 must also be provided). Therefore, it needs to be coadministered with volatile and/or other sedatives as part of a

balanced technique (implementation of more than one agent in order to maximize benefits, while minimizing disadvantages). Its MAC contribution is additive with volatile agents (0.5 MAC volatile agent + 0.5 MAC N_2O = 1 MAC).

- Analgesic properties. Mechanism likely involves direct intraspinal antinociception by stimulating enkephalin release. Enkephalins bind to opioid receptors in the brain stem that trigger descending noradrenergic pathways (rather than depression of limbic function); abolished by naloxone. Estimated analgesic efficacy equivalent to 10–15 mg of morphine at an Fi_{N2O} of 30%. Referred to as "laughing gas" due to the euphoric feeling that ensues upon inhalation (possible effect at the thalamic nuclei).
- CNS. Anesthetic and analgesic effects in brain stem, brain, and spinal cord as mentioned above. ↑ $CMRO_2$, thus ↑ CBF and ↑ CBV (resultant mild ↑ ICP). ↓ amplitude and ↑ latency in SSEPs to a greater extent than volatile agents). Potentially antineuroprotective (↑ tissue damage and worsened neurological outcomes).
- Cardiac. Minimal or negligible clinical effects on BP, HR, CO; although a direct myocardial depressant in vitro, its depressant effects are surpassed by its augmentation of sympathetic tone in vivo. ↑ venous tone results in ↑ preload to the heart, and also may contribute to its cardiostability profile (may facilitate difficult venipuncture). When combined with a volatile agent, typically less circulatory depression than if either agent is used alone, providing an improved hemodynamic profile (KEY BENEFIT!!). However, N_2O may unmask myocardial depression in patients with cardiac disease or severe hypovolemia, leading to significant ↓ in BP, CO, and the potential for myocardial ischemia. Coadministration with opioids (depresses sympathetic outflow) may profoundly ↓ BP, CO
- Respiratory. ↓ TV (direct depression of medullary ventilator centers), ↑ RR (CNS stimulation). Unlike volatiles, does not ↓ MV (may actually ↑ MV and ↓ $ETCO_2$). ↓ FRC from altered lung mechanics (cephalad movement of stomach contents, ↓ chest wall expansion, ↑ thoracic blood volume result in atelectasis and shunting). Relaxes bronchial smooth muscle (direct effect, and ↓ afferent tone) and activates pulmonary stretch receptors. Hypoxic drive is markedly ↓ (as little as 0.1 MAC N_2O can ↓ hypoxemic drive by 50%). Coadministered with respiratory depressants may have greater than expected pulmonary depression.
- Neuromuscular. No significant skeletal muscle relaxation (unlike volatile agents). Not a malignant hyperthermia trigger
- Hepatic. ↓ blood flow (lesser extent than volatiles)
- Gastrointestinal. May cause nausea and vomiting in susceptible patients
- Renal. ↑ RVR, and may ↓ RBF, GFR, UOP

Pharmacokinetics

- Not a vapor; true gas by definition. Molecular weight = 44; Boiling Point = −88 degrees Celsius @ 760 mm Hg; Vapor Pressure = 39 000 mm Hg @ 20 degrees Celsius. Nonflammable, nonexplosive, but will support combustion.

- Gas at room temperature and ambient pressure. Critical temperature > room temperature; therefore, pressurization allows maintenance in liquid form within the cylinder. Remains as a liquid until a pressure of 750 psi, then converts to gas form (Boyle's law is applicable only in gas form; in liquid form, or pressure >750 psi, amount present can be calculated by weight). When ↑ flows, may notice significant cooling of the cylinder; heat/energy is consumed when liquid is converted to gas
- Onset of action, peak effect, and duration of action are determined by Fi and ventilator settings
- Blood:gas partition value: 0.47; responsible for rapid onset and offset (able to quickly reach high brain concentrations since does not get sequestered into blood or other tissues)
- Transported in blood as free gas; does not combine with hemoglobin.
- Concentration effect is most pronounced with N_2O. The ↓ low potency results in ↑ Fi (and hence ↑ FA) combined with the ↓ blood:gas coefficient further ↑ FA; the result is a rapid rate of rise of Fi/FA. Upon initial administration, the ↑ FA results in large amounts of N_2O being taken up from the alveoli, leaving behind the other atmospheric gases and volatile agents. This results in a concentration effect of the remaining gases and agents and in turn a faster rate of rise of arterial and brain concentrations (see second gas effect below). Furthermore, the large, rapid alveolar uptake of N_2O causes a negative pressure within the alveoli, analogous to a "partial pressure vacuum," and is referred to as the "augmented gas inflow effect" (gases in the breathing circuit are taken up into the lungs at a faster rate). Despite desflurane's lower blood/gas coefficient, N_2O has a faster rate of rise for FA/Fi.…concentration outweighs solubility.
- Second gas effect is a concept that builds on the concentration effect discussed above. When a volatile agent is coadministered (second gas), its rate of rise of arterial tension is enhanced as well. In turn, the brain concentration is attained more quickly as well, enhancing induction. This concept by comparing administration of 0.5% halothane with 70% N_2O or 10% N_2O; the rate of rise of FA/Fi is ↑ at ↑ N_2O concentrations. Despite its occurrence, the second gas effect lacks significant clinical effects.
- Elimination occurs primarily via the pulmonary route (expiration); reverse of uptake and distribution.
- ↓ blood/gas solubility results in rapid offset (brain concentration is reached quickly since not absorbed and diverted into "depots" of fat, muscle, etc).
- Biotransformation is limited to 0.4%; reduced to N_2 in the GI tract by anaerobic bacteria.
- Stable in hydrated and dessicated CO_2 absorbent

Side Effects/Cautions

- May ↑ the incidence of PONV. Recent meta-analysis shows ↑ risk only in high-risk pts (low-risk pts did not demonstrate ↑ PONV); antiemetic prophylaxis may be sufficient to negate this factor. Risks vs benefits need to be weighed for the particular pt however, since both volatile agents and opioids contribute to PONV (N_2O may allow for ↓ administration of both particularly for self-limited stimuli).

- Inactivation of vitamin B12, which hinders methionone sythetase and hence folate metabolism. Folate deficiency may result in bone marrow depression (megaloblastic anemia) and neurological deficiencies (peripheral neuropathies and pernicious anemia). Requires significant exposure of >24 hrs.

- Embryonic development. Animal models suggest mild teratogenic effects, however, no evidence in humans. Randomized controlled studies have not been conducted due to ethical issues; retrospective studies in nearly 6000 pregnant pts have failed to reveal any adverse outcomes for pt or fetus.

- Expansion of air-filled structures and bubbles. Air-filled spaces contain FIO_2 at 21% and N_2 at ~70%. N_2O's ↓ potency results in ↑ Fi (inspired concentration), combined with its ↓ blood:gas partition coefficient (stays in gas phase, does not dissolve extensively in the blood). This results in ↑ amounts of N_2O in the blood (in gas form) that will enter air-filled spaces in order to attain partial pressure equilibrium. Expansion of air-spaces is further exacerbated by N_2's blood:gas partition coefficient being 30 times < N_2O. It hinders N_2 reaching the new partial pressure equilibrium with N_2O since it cannot easily leave the air-space to enter into the blood; gets "stuck" and results in expansion of the air space. Effect is determined by blood flow and duration of administration. Avoid in PTX, pneumocephalus, VAE (or pts at high risk), emphysema with blebs, bowel obstruction, tympanic surgery grafts, retinal surgery where gas bubbles are utilized, and abdominal procedures where bowel distention will hinder visualization. Air-filled cuffs such as PACs or ETT cuffs may result in tissue damage or tracheal damage respectively.

- Arrhythmias. ↑ endogenous catecholamine levels from SNS stimulation; arrhythmia threshold with epinephrine, halothane, sympathomimetics may be ↓.

- ↑ PVR. Constricts pulmonary vasculature and ↑ RVEDP. May be more pronounced with preexisting pulmonary hypertension.

- Diffusion hypoxia. Results from principles of the concentration and second gas effect, but in reverse and at emergence. The "wash-out" of ↑ concentrations of N_2O from the blood into the alveoli can dilute alveolar concentrations of O_2 and CO_2 (alveolar hypoxemia and hypocarbia can ↓ respiratory drive, and further exacerbate hypoxemia). May be avoided by instituting FIO_2 1.0 at the time of emergence

References

1. Becker DE Rosenberg M. Nitrous oxide and the inhalation anesthetics. *Anesth Prog.* 2008;55124–131.

2. Eger EI. Respiratory effects of nitrous oxide. In: Eger EI, ed. *Nitrous Oxide.* New York: Elsevier; 1985.

3. Eisele JH. Cardiovascular effects of nitrous oxide. In: Eger EI, ed. *Nitrous Oxide*. New York: Elsevier; 1985.

4. Eger EI. Pharmacokinetics. In: Eger EI, ed. *Nitrous Oxide*. New York: Elsevier; 1985.

5. Zhang C, Davies MF, Guo TZ, Maze M. The analgesic action of nitrous oxide is dependent on the release of norepinephrine in the dorsal horn of the spinal cord. *Anesthesiology*. 1999;91:1401–1407.

6. Nunn JF. Clinical aspects of the interaction between nitrous oxide and vitamin B12. *Br J Anaesth*. 1987;59:3–13.

7. Mazze RI, Kallen B. Reproductive outcome after anesthesia and operation during pregnancy: a registry study of 5405 cases. *Am J Obstet Gynecol*. 1989;161:1178–1185.

8. Hopkins PM. Nitrous oxide: a unique drug of continuing importance for anaesthesia. *Best Pract Res Clin Anaesthesiol*. 2005;19(3):381–389.

9. Eger EI II. Concentration and second gas effects. In: *Anesthetic Uptake and Action*, Baltimore, MD: Williams & Wilkins; 113–121.

10. Epstein RM, Rackow H, Salanitre E, Wolf GL. Influence of the concentration effect on the uptake of anesthetic mixtures: the second gas effect. *Anesthesiology*. 1964;25:364–371.

Chapter 2

Induction Agents

Chapter 2.1

Propofol

Ellen Wang, MD and Nina Singh-Radcliff, MD

Clinical Uses/Relevance to Anesthesiology

- Rapid acting intravenous hynoptic agent with faster psychomotor recovery than thiopental; utilized as a sole agent to produce differential levels of consciousness, from light sedation to induction and maintenance of general anesthesia
- Component of a balanced anesthetic technique. Useful to decrease concentrations of volatile agents/nitrous oxide during SSEP, MEP, and EEG monitoring; with opioids and benzodiazepines for MAC or TIVA techniques
- ICP treatment, neuroprotection, burst suppression
- Quick deepening of anesthetic, without prolonged effects (intraoperatively, end of case)
- Emergence delirium (benzodiazepines have longer duration, accumulate, and can have paradoxical reaction)
- Sedation for procedures, ventilated patients (quick onset, quick recovery)
- Does not trigger malignant hyperthermia
- Anticonvulsant
- Nausea and vomiting rescue; reduces incidence of PONV when used for maintenance
- Antipruritic effects, from opioids and cholestatic liver disease
- Chronic refractory headache

Pharmacology

- Phenol ring with two isopropyl groups attached (2,6-diisopropylphenol).
- Potentiates GABA receptor binding by attaching to the beta subunit of the $GABA_A$ receptor. GABA is an inhibitory neurotransmitter that hyperpolarizes the cell membrane (increases Cl^- conductance), preventing depolarization with resultant neurotransmission.
- Mechanism of action also involves inhibition of Ach release in the hippocampus and prefrontal cortex; inhibition of NMDA in CNS; direct depressant effect on neurons of the spinal cord; antiemetic effect by decreasing serotonin levels in the

area postrema; increase of dopamine concentrations in the nucleus accumbens (a phenomenon noted with drugs of abuse and pleasure-seeking behavior)

- CNS. Hypnotic (ranges from sedation to LOC depending on dose); no analgesia (not antianalgesic like barbiturates); reduces $CMRO_2$ with resultant decrease in CBF, ICP, and IOP (blunting of electrical activity and ability to achieve burst suppression reduces O_2 consumption and can provide neuroprotection during focal ischemia similar to thiopental); no change to cerebrovascular autoregulation (unlike volatiles, does not dilate cerebral vasculature and uncouple $CMRO_2$ and CBF; thus does not increase ICP); does not impair CO_2 effects on cerebral vessel tone. May impair CPP from drop in MAP (CPP = MAP − ICP) causing ischemia. Despite occurrence of twitching, spontaneous movement, hiccupping (likely due to subcortical glycine antagonism), has an anticonvulsant effect. Nonetheless, grand mal seizures seen in 1 in 50 000 (up to 6 d after anesthesia; usually prior history of seizures). Decreases amplitude and increases latency on SSEPs; does not affect BAEP. Does not potentiate neuromuscular blockade. Can produce euphoria, and may have abuse potential.
- CV. Profound decrease in SBP from vasodilation of arterial and venous systems, as well as myocardial depression. Dose-dependent reduction in preload, afterload, contractility, MAP (up to 40%), CO. More pronounced with hypovolemia, rapid injection, and elderly pts. Blocks arterial baroreceptor response to hypotension (preventing compensatory reflex tachycardia; reduced SV not met by increased HR to maintain CO). Additionally, profound bradycardia and asystole can occur in healthy adults, extremes of age, negative chronotropic medications, or surgical procedures associated with the oculocardiac reflex. Possible cardioprotective effects during cardiac surgery. Suppresses SVTs (may avoid in EP studies).
- Pulmonary. Potent respiratory depressant; reduces TV and hence MV. Blunts ventilatory response to hypoxia and hypercapnia; incidence and duration of apnea depend on dose, speed of injection, and concomitant premedication (~10% of GI cases with propofol have desaturation). Blunts upper airway reflexes and produces bronchodilation to greater extent than thiopental (but less than volatile agents); however can cause histamine release (less than barbiturates, etomidate). Attenuates magnitude of HPV. Potential benefits during ARDS (may reduce free radical mediators, cyclooxygenase-catalyzed lipid peroxidation).
- Endocrine. Does not affect cortisol synthesis or the response to ACTH stimulation; in vitro studies have shown propofol to reduce lymphocyte proliferation, inhibit phagocytosis and killing of bacteria

Pharmacokinetics

- pH 7, water insoluble; V_d 20–40 L; protein binding 97%
- Onset: 90–100 seconds ("one arm-brain circulation"); BP drop starts at ~200 seconds (quicker with increased age, hypovolemia)

- Offset: 2–8 minutes; terminated by redistribution from the brain to other compartments.
- Elimination: Rapid plasma clearance (20–30 mL/kg/min) results in rapid t-elimination ½ life of 3–24 h. This results from a rapid central compartment clearance by hepatic and extrahepatic metabolism (likely the reason for a more complete recovery compared to thiopental). The liver metabolizes propofol to inactive water-soluble compounds (glucuronide, sulfate) that are renally excreted; the lungs and kidneys are responsible for 30%-60% of elimination (thus metabolism still takes place during the anhepatic phase of liver transplant). 3% is excreted unchanged via urine and feces. Elderly have lower V_d, however with slower clearance rates; age <3 years have larger central compartment volume (50%) and a more rapid clearance (25%) requiring larger dosing. Hepatic disease increases V_d, reduces metabolism, and slightly prolongs elimination half-life and recovery (extrahepatic metabolism occurs).
- Stable at room temperature and not light sensitive
- Dilution with 5% dextrose in water; caution when diluting as may crack emulsion, degrade propofol, change pharmacological effects.
- Context-sensitive ½ life. Elimination ½ time after a continuous infusion is a function of infusion duration.
- CPB. Increased central volume and clearance necessitate higher initial infusion rates to maintain adequate propofol plasma concentration
- Concentration-dependent inhibition of cytochrome P-450 that may alter drugs metabolized by this enzyme (eg, opiates)

Formulations

- IV only
- Concentration typically 1% (10 mg/ml); 2% available in some countries to decrease volume and lipid load for long-term sedation
- Formulated in an emulsion containing 10% soybean oil, 2.25% glycerol, and 1.2% lecithin to facilitate solubility in aqueous solution; because these support bacterial growth, ethyl-endiamine-tetra-acetic acid, metabisulfite (sulfa allergic pts may have problem), or benzyl alcohol are added as retardants of bacterial growth

Adult Dose

- CP_{50} refers to the blood concentration needed for 50% of subjects to not respond to a defined stimulus; reduced by concurrent administration of other sedatives (similar concept as MAC)
- Induction: 1–2.5 mg/kg IV bolus; 50–200 mcg/kg/min infusion; reduce when elderly (smaller V_d), impaired cardiovascular reserve, premedication with benzodiazepines, opioids, lidocaine
- Sedation: 25–100 mcg/kg/min IV; titrate to effect

- TIVA maintenance (sole): 200–350 mcg/kg/min IV; reduced when coadministered with other anesthetics (75–120 mcg/kg/min IV + remifentanil 0.15–0.2 mcg/kg/min IV; 100–200 mcg/kg/min IV + N_2O)
- Long-term sedation: >30 mcg/kg/min IV usually amnestic; should not exceed 80 mcg/kg/min IV
- Women may require a higher dose than men; may awaken faster
- Nausea/vomiting: 10–20 mg IV or 10 mcg/kg/min as infusion
- Emergence delirium: 10–20 mg IV boluses
- Chronic headaches: 20–30 mg IV q 3–4 minutes up to 400 mg.

Pediatric Dose

- Induction: 2.5–3.5 mg/kg IV
- Sedation: 1 mg/kg IV bolus, followed by 25–100 mcg/kg/min IV infusion titrated to effect
- TIVA maintenance (sole): 200–350 mcg/kg/min IV infusion
- Adjunct with other drugs. Propofol infusion rates can be reduced when combined with remifentanil, ketamine, midazolam, volatile agents, nitrous.

Adverse Events

- Emulsions support bacterial growth despite additives; solutions should be used as soon as possible and < 6 h after opening the vial; sepsis and death have been reported
- Potential cross-allergenicity to soybeans and egg yolk; anaphylactoid reactions reported
- Propofol infusion syndrome. Rare, potentially fatal complication characterized by metabolic acidosis, rhabdomyolysis of cardiac and skeletal muscle, arrhythmias (bradycardia, atrial fibrillation, VT and SVT, BBB, and asystole), myocardial failure, renal failure, hepatomegaly, and death. Labs may reveal myoglobinuria, downsloping ST-segment elevation, increased CK, troponin, K+, Cr, azotaemia, malonylcarnitine, and C5-acylcarnitine. Seen in critically ill children and adults, and long-term anesthesia when doses exceed 4–5 mg/kg/h for long periods (>48 h), sepsis, serious cerebral injury. Possibly due to mitochondrial toxicity, mitochondrial defects, impaired tissue oxygenation, and carbohydrate deficiency. Tx by immediately discontinuing, cardiac support, and correction of metabolic acidosis.
- May increase serum triglycerides; has been associated with pancreatitis; usually seen in elderly, longer ICU stay, longer infusion duration.
- Caution in pregnancy as it decreases MAP and crosses placenta rapidly and can lead to neonatal depression
- Pain on injection; can be reduced by premedication with opioid or coadministration with lidocaine; dilution and use of larger veins can reduce pain

- Fentanyl and alfentanil concentrations may be increased by concomitant administration of propofol

Etomidate

Nina Singh-Radcliff, MD and Ellen Wang, MD

Clinical Uses/Indications

- Rapid acting intravenous hypnotic drug for induction of anesthesia when HD stability is desired (CAD, AS, carotid stenosis, increased intracranial pressure, floor/STAT intubations, hypovolemia); can be coadministered with propofol (reduces adverse effects of both drugs)
- Not typically utilized for continuous infusion to provide sedation or maintenance of GA due to adrenocortical suppression (may be considered during propofol shortages)
- Electroconvulsive therapy; capable of producing longer seizures compared with other hypnotics
- Seizure foci mapping
- Cardioversion in pts with low EF

Pharmacology

- Carboxylated imidazole derivative; hypnotic (sedation to LOC depending on dose)
- Binds to GABA receptor, and potentiates binding of GABA neurotransmitter to receptor. Results in Cl^- conduction (hyperpolarizes membrane), reducing depolarization, and inhibits neurotransmission
- CNS. Reduces $CMRO_2$, with resultant decrease in CBF, CBV, and ICP. Additionally, is a potent cerebral vasoconstrictor (further reduces CBF, CBV, and hence ICP). Does not disrupt CO_2's effect on cerebrovascular tone. Not analgesic. May maintain CPP better than other induction medications (maintenance of MAP; CPP = MAP − ICP). Increases amplitude and latency of SSEPs. Not neuroprotective. May have disinhibitory effects on extrapyramidal motor center, resulting in myoclonus (up to 50% incidence); may increase IOP, make DL or LMA insertion difficult (can be attenuated with propofol, NMBD, opioids). Can cause grand mal seizures and increased EEG activity in epileptics. Headaches.
- CV. Maintains HDs (key!!): contractility, CO, HR, PAOP, CVP, SV, CI, PVR (may be due to the unique lack of effect on the SNS, baroreceptor function, no histamine release). Mild decrease in MAP can occur from decreased SVR (hypovolemic states may see drop in BP). Sympathetic and baroreceptor reflexes remain intact; thus DL and intubation may cause marked increases in BP

- Pulmonary. Decreases TV and hence MV (less than propofol, thiopental). Right-shift in CO_2 response curve, decreased response to hypoxia (especially in pulmonary cripples). Apnea more likely with rapid injection, coadministration of opioids or volatiles. May see brief hyperventilation followed by similarly brief period of apnea.

Pharmacokinetics

- pH 6.9 (does not precipitate like thiopental); imidazole ring bestows water solubility in acidic solutions, and lipid solubility at physiologic pH. V_d large (relatively hypophilic and enters several compartments); protein binding 77% (mostly to albumin)
- Onset: one arm-brain circulation; rapid due to high lipid solubility and large nonionized fraction at physiological pH
- Offset: 3–8 minutes; terminated by redistribution from the brain to other compartments. Duration of action is linearly related to the dose, with each 0.1 mg/kg providing about 100 seconds of unconsciousness
- Elimination. Plasma clearance of 25 mL/kg/min results in a t-elimination ½ life of 5.5 hours. Metabolized in the plasma by ester hydrolysis (carboxylic acid) and in the liver (N-dealkylation) to inactive metabolites, which are then excreted in urine (78%) and bile (22%). Less than 3% is excreted unchanged in the urine. Clearance is 5 times > thiopental.

Preparations

- IV only
- 2 mg/kg, prepared in 35% propylene glycol solution

Adult Dose

- Induction: 0.2–0.6 mg/kg IV
- Maintenance: 10 mcg/kg/min IV with nitrous and opiate

Pediatric Dose

- Rectal 6.5 mg/kg onset of 4 minutes

Adverse Events

- Adrenocortical suppression. Dose-dependent inhibition of 11B-hydroxylase (enzyme that converts 11-deoxycortisol to cortisol); results in increased cortisol precursors (11-deoxycortisol, 17-hydroxyprogesterone). Effect lasts ~4–8 h after an induction dose. Should be considered during high-stress surgery or bedside/ICU intubations
- Pain with injection; thrombophlebits up to 72 h post injection (20% of cases where administered through small IV)
- Nausea and vomiting
- Fentanyl increases plasma levels and prolongs elimination half-life

Ketamine

Nina Singh-Radcliff, MD and Ellen Wang, MD

Clinical Uses/Relevance to Anesthesiology

- Induction agent with sympathetic effect on cardiopulmonary system; useful for hypovolemia, shock, trauma; asthma or reactive airway disease
- Maintenance adjunct; although capable of LOC, amnesia, and analgesia, typically administered in conjunction with propofol, nitrous, volatiles
- Sedation with unique ability to maintain SV; useful in prone procedures (eg, vertebroplasty), positioning and placement of regional/neuraxial blocks (eg, hip fractures), or awake FOB
- IM, oral, rectal sedation of pediatric or mental retardation where IV access unavailable and PO medication not possible
- Increases MEP/SSEP potentials
- Acute pain. Perioperative use can decrease overall opioid use and side effects (PONV) as well as improve analgesia.
- Chronic pain. Component of multimodal therapy (cancer, chronic peripheral and central neuropathic, phantom and ischemic limb, and visceral pain; fibromyalgia, complex regional pain syndrome, and migraines).
- Treatment of bronchospasm
- Not a malignant hyperthermia trigger

Pharmacology

- Phencyclidine derivative ($1/10$ the potency, maintains many of its psychomimetic effects)
- Inhibition of N-methyl-D-aspartate (NMDA), opioid, adrenergic, muscarinic, and voltage-sensitive ion channel receptors. Unlike several other sedatives/induction agents, does not interact with GABA
- CNS. Produces dissociative anesthetic: thalamic sensory impulses to the cerebral cortex and the limbic cortex, which function in awareness of sensation, are dissociated. Results in a "cataleptic" state where eyes remain open; cough, swallow, and corenal relexes may be maintained; and purposeless movements of the arms, legs, trunk, and head. Increases $CMRO_2$, which increases CBF and ICP; may be blunted by hypocapnia. EEG activity is increased; affects SSEPs by decreasing latencies and increasing amplitudes. Emergence delirium can occur in up to 30% of pts (out-of-body experience, hallucinations; benzodiazepines can be prophylactic as well as therapeutic)
- Cardiac. In vitro cardiac depressant. In vivo administration results in centrally mediated sympathetic stimulation as well as inhibits reuptake of norepinephrine with resultant increases in MAP, HR, CO, and SVR and myocardial O_2 consumption (coadministration of benzodiazepines, opioids, inhaled anesthetics may blunt). However, if catecholamine stores are depleted (critically ill), has a direct depressant effect on the myocardium.

- Pulmonary. Respiratory drive is maintained and respiratory response to hypercapnea is preserved. Only IV induction agent capable of bronchodilation. Transient hypoventilation, apnea (rare) can follow rapid administration or large IV doses. Despite presence of cough and swallow reflexes, airway protection is not necessarily maintained. In children, laryngospasm from increased salivation may occur (premedication with anticholinergics may reduce risk). Increases PAP; avoid in pts with pulmonary hypertension.

Pharmacokinetics

- pH 7.5; protein binding 12% (low). Highly lipid-soluble (5–10 times greater than thiopental) which results in a large volume of distribution; some water solubility.
- Onset: IV 30–60 seconds (one arm-brain circulation) due to high lipid solubility, low molecular weight, and pKa ~ pH. IM: 10–15 m.
- Offset: 5–15 m; effects of single bolus are terminated by redistribution to inactive tissue sites
- Elimination: plasma clearance 12–17 mL/kg/min results in short t-elimination ½ life (2–4 h). Metabolism is primarily hepatic (involves N-demethylation by the cytochrome P450 system). Norketamine, the primary active metabolite, is less potent ($^1/_3$ to $^1/_5$ the potency of ketamine) and is subsequently hydroxylated and conjugated into water soluble inactive metabolites that are excreted in the urine. The short context-sensitive ½ life makes attractive for sedation; full orientation to person, place, and time occurs within 15–30 m.
- Oral and intranasal routes have significant first-pass metabolism

Routes

- Oral, IV, oral, rectal, epidurally, intranasal spray

Adult Dose

- Induction: 1–2 mg/kg IV; 4–6 mg/kg IM
- Maintenance: 30–90 mcg/kg/minute; when given with adjunct (nitrous, propofol, dexmedetomidine, volatile) 15–45 mcg/kg/minute
- Subanalgesic: 3–5 mcg/kg/minute
- Epidurally 0.5–1 mg/kg (off-label use, needs to be preservative free)

Pediatric Dose

- <1 mg/kg IV for dressing changes

Adverse Events

- Hallucinations (benzodiazepines can prevent, or treat). Derivative of phencyclidine; disturbing, vivid, colorful dreams and out-of-body experiences; increased and distorted visual, tactile, and auditory sensitivity; can be associated with fear and confusion; may have euphoric state that is responsible for the addiction potential. Children usually with lower incidence, less severe emergence reactions. Larger doses, rapid administration predisposes to a higher incidence.

- Increased secretions may be reduced with anticholinergics given prophylactically

---

Clinical Case Scenario

A 36-year-old, 62-kg woman with PMH of HIV and chronic HCV infection is admitted to the ICU for respiratory failure and sepsis, likely due to pneumonia. She is intubated and mechanically ventilated, requiring increasing doses of propofol and midazolam infusions for sedation. On hospital day 7, the patient develops a rash on chest, shoulders, and neck, and multiple abnormal lab test values (elevated triglycerides, amylase, lipase, CK, abnormal liver function tests).

- **Background**: The patient is displaying early signs/symptoms of propofol infusion syndrome.

- **Pathophysiology**: A multifactorial syndrome that may occur in patients with genetic mitochondrial abnormalities. Propofol causes abnormalities consistent with disruption of fatty acid oxidation and failure of the mitochondrial respiratory chain. Risk factors include high dose propofol for prolonged periods and concomitant catecholamines or corticosteroids.

- **Treatment**: Taper and discontinue propofol, consider adding phenobarbital for sedation.

Chapter 2.2

Barbiturates

Katherine C. Normand, MD

Role in the Practice of Anesthesiology/Relevance to Anesthesiology

- IV induction agent. Has fallen out of favor since the introduction of propofol. However, due to its low cost, utilized in the developing world and possibly in rural areas.
- Rectal or IM administration can sedate or induce anesthesia in uncooperative or pediatric pts
- Intracranial hypertension treatment when other therapies (hyperventilation, diuresis) are unsuccessful
- Improves outcome of *focal* cerebral ischemia (not effective in *global* cerebral ischemia). Utilized preemptively when there is a potential for ischemia ("barbiturate coma") or when neuromonitoring indices suggest ischemia
- Potent anticonvulsants, especially in the face of continuous seizure activity.
- Electroconvulsive therapy; methohexital is capable of ↑ seizure duration

Pharmacodynamics

- Derivatives of barbituric acid. Drugs within this class have unique sedative-hypnotic properties and pharmacokinetics that result from substitutions at the number 2 and 5 carbon atoms of the acid.
- The Reticular Activating System (RAS) is located in the brain stem and is responsible for regulating state of consciousness; it functions as a "command center" and sends and receives input to and from neural structures above and below it. Inhibitory input to the RAS ↑ the rate of GABA neurotransmitter release, whereas excitatory impulses ↓ the rate of release. GABA, or gamma-aminobutyric acid, is the principle inhibitory neurotransmitter in the human CNS. When it binds to the GABA receptor (GABA$_A$) it results in chloride ion channel opening, chloride influx, membrane hyperpolarization, and ↓ neuron firing.
- Barbiturates bind to postsynaptic GABA receptors in the RAS and other areas of the CNS. Receptor binding *enhances* the effects of *inhibitory* GABA neurotransmitter, which results in ↑ frequency of chloride ion channel opening, ↑chloride influx, membrane hyperpolarization, and ↓ neuron depolarization.

- Barbiturates also *inhibit* presynaptic *excitatory* neurotransmitter release (gluta-mate and Ach) in the RAS and other areas of the CNS; thereby ↓ frequency of ion channel opening, ↓ ion flow, and ↓ neuron depolarization.
- CNS. ↓ CBF results from both potent vasoconstriction and ↓ $CMRO_2$; in turn, there is a ↓ in CBV and hence ↓ ICP. Additionally, because barbiturates vasoconstrict healthy cerebral vasculature, blood flow may be diverted to is-chemic or injured areas; Robin Hood phenomenon. Reductions in $CMRO_2$ (up to 50%) result from inhibition of neuron electrical activity only. Barbiturates do not affect basal cell metabolism and function, and therefore, there is a ceiling-effect on $CMRO_2$ reduction when electrical "silence" has occurred. The ↓ in $CMRO_2$ (O_2 demand) is harnessed to offset ↓ O_2 supply and ↓ the incidence of focal ischemia. Because EEG monitoring reflects cortical electrical activity, it can assist with optimal barbiturate titration when the goal is to max-imally ↓ $CMRO_2$ (electrical silence). CPP is generally maintained due to ↓ ICP and baroreceptor reflexes (blunt drops in BP). Not analgesic; antialgesic responses have been described.
- Cardiovascular. Affects preload and contractility. Barbiturates inhibit the medul-lary vasomotor response center, resulting in peripheral venodilation and pooling of blood (↓ preload). Cardiac contractility is directly depressed secondary to ↓ Ca^{++} availability (baroreceptor reflexes may offset). HR ↑ in response to the resul-tant hypotension, either due to baroreceptor reflexes or a central vagolytic effect (generally able to maintain CO). HD changes can be ↓ with slower injections and ↓ dosaging. Hypovolemic pts or those with high sympathetic tone can experience significant hypotension. QT interval prolongation has been described.
- Respiratory. Blunts the medullary ventilatory response center in a dose-dependent fashion and is enhanced in pts with chronic lung disease. A "double apnea" ventilatory pattern has been described where there is apnea for a few seconds followed by a few breaths with good TV, then a longer apneic period. Furthermore, also reduces hypoxic and hypercarbic respiratory responses. Are not capable of blunting airway reflexes (laryngospasm, cough-ing, bucking, bronchospasm) to the same extent as propofol during laryngos-copy and intubation.
- Hepatic. ↓ hepatic blood flow and induction of metabolic enzymes.
- Renal. ↓ RBF and GFR.

Pharmacokinetics

- Acidic drugs, prepared in highly alkaline salt solutions (acidemia results in a higher fraction of non-ionized drug that can cross the BBB)
- Onset is very rapid. Highly lipid soluble and nonionized (allows for enhanced crossing of the BBB). Maximum brain uptake occurs within 30 seconds or "one arm-brain circulation."
- Redistribution, primarily to the skeletal muscle, occurs over the next 5 mins, and is responsible for termination of effect (not metabolism). This is followed by accumulation into fat over the next 30 mins. Repeat administration results

in saturation of these compartments and hinders redistribution; clinical termination of action becomes dependent on metabolism.

- Highly protein bound to albumin. Hypoalbuminemia (renal and hepatic disease, neonates, malnourishment) results in more free drug available (active form) and ↑ sensitivity to boluses (consider ↓ accordingly). Additionally, co-administration of drugs with high albumin binding result in competition for the site, and more drug in its free, active form.
- Vd is large due to its ↑ lipid solubility (redistributes to muscle and fat stores). In cases where Vd is ↓ (shock, lean body mass, age), consider ↓ dosing
- Metabolism. All barbiturates, with the exception of Phenobarbital, are hepatically metabolized into inactive, water-soluble metabolites that are excreted in the urine. Renal excretion is the primary form of elimination for Phenobarbital, with 60%-90% of the drug excreted unchanged.
- Elderly experience delayed awakening due to ↑ CNS sensitivity, ↓ metabolism, and a ↓ central Vd (↓ redistribution)
- Children have a more rapid awakening with a faster total body clearance.

Phenobarbital

- Phenyl side group attachment at C_5 bestows anticonvulsant properties. Protein binding 20%-40% (low) results in shorter duration of action. Drug is excreted mostly in its unchanged/unmetabolized form (60%-90%) in the urine. As a result, urine alkalinization can hasten diuresis (acidic drug and will become charged in a basic environment, preventing reabsorption from the tubule to the bloodstream).

Thiopental

- The sulfur atom at C_2 increases lipid solubility, with a resultant increase in potency and onset of action. Protein binding ~80% results in increased duration of action. Can be administered IV and rectally (uncooperative pts). Cholinergic stimulation may be responsible for the increased incidence of bronchospasm. Avoidance in pts with sulfa allergy.

Table 2.2.1 Side Effects/Adverse Reactions

Hepatic enzymatic induction occurs can occur for 2–7 days after exposure. Other hepatically cleared drugs may have ↓ serum and effective concentrations

Precipitation can occur when mixed with acidic solutions within the same syringe or IV line (eg, succinylcholine, atropine).

Acute exacerbation of porphyria. Results from hepatic induction of microenzyme P-450 which can cause excessive production and excretion of aminolevulinic acid (ALA) and porphobilinogen (PBG).

Intra-arterial injection can cause intense pain with significant vasoconstriction of the artery (may lose pulses). Treatment includes injection of saline to dilute drug concentration and intentional vasodilation with lidocaine or sympathectomy via stellate ganglion block.

Coughing, hiccupping, tremors and twitches (excitatory responses), urticarial rash, and the feeling of experiencing a garlic or onion taste during administration.

Methohexital

- Methyl side group bestows "convulsant" properties; long hydrocarbon chain bestows lipid solubility. Utilized for electroconvulsive therapy to enhance therapeutic effects of shock therapy by increasing seizure duration. High hepatic metabolism results in speedier psychomotor function recovery. Can be administered IV and rectally (uncooperative pts)

Clinical Case Scenario #1

45-year-old female undergoing right MCA aneurysm clipping. While under general anesthesia with EEG monitoring, the surgeon requests burst suppression for temporary clip of MCA.

Usually dose for initial burst suppression with Thiopental is 4–5 mg/kg. After a quick bolus of thiopental, the blood pressure will expectantly drop with a subsequent rise in heart rate. Therefore, phenylephrine is the choice of vasopressor after thiopental bolus.

Within 30 seconds of administration, the EEG will show burst suppression. See Figure 2.2.1.

Burst suppression is a characteristic signal in the EEG described as a periodic pattern of low voltage less than 10 μV and a relatively shorter pattern of higher amplitude complexes. This pattern can only be recognized on with EEG monitoring. Burst suppression reflects a decrease in CMR02 of approximately 40%-50%. It is believed to be neurologically protective in face of focal ischemia, such as during temporary clipping of a cerebral vessel. Another alternative to causing burst suppression is bolusing propofol.

References

1. Stoelting, RK. *Pharmacology and Physiology in Anesthetic Practice.* Philadelphia: Lippencott Williams & Wilkins; 1995:82–93.

2. Pong, RP, Lam AM. In: JE Cottrell, WE Young, eds. *Cottrell and Young's Neuroanesthesia.* 5th ed. Philadelphia: Mosby/Elsevier; 2010:82.

3. Mori K, Shingu K, Nakao S. In: R. Miller, ed. *Miller's Anesthesia.* 7th ed. Philadelphia: Churchill, Livingstone/Elsevier; 2010:3008–3009.

4. Reves JG, Glass PSA, Lubarsky DA, McEvoy MD, Martinez-Ruiz R. In: R. Miller, ed. *Miller's Anesthesia.* 7th ed. Philadelphia: Churchill, Livingstone/Elsevier; 2010:730–733.

5. Dilger JP, Boguslavsky R, Barann M, Katz T, Vidal AM. Mechanisms of barbiturate inhibition of acetylcholine receptor channels. *J Gen Physiol.* 1997;109: 401–414.

6. Brunto L, Parker K, Blumnethal D, Buxton I. In LS Goodman, A Gilman, L Brunton, eds. *Goodman and Gillman's Manual of Pharmacology and Therapeutics.* 11th ed. New York: McGraw-Hill; 2008:272–274.

7. Hudson RJ, Stanski DR, Burch PG. Pharmacokinetics of methohexital and thiopental in surgical patients. *Anesthesiology.* 1983;59:215–219.

8. Nelson E, Powell JR, Conrad K, Likes K, Byers J, Baker S, Perrier D. Phenobarbital pharmacokinetics and bioavailability in adults. *J Clin Pharmacol.* 1982;22:141–148.

9. Methohexital package insert.

Chapter 3

Pain Medications

Chapter 3.1

Opioids

Thomas H. Scott MD and Jane C. Ballantyne MD

Clinical Uses and Indications

- First-line therapy for acute pain of all kinds, particularly for intraoperative and postoperative pain. They are also used in chronic cancer and nonmalignant pain. (Table 3.1.1)
- Opioids are also used alone and in combination with local anesthetics neuraxially to provide effective analgesia while minimizing sympathectomy and sensorimotor block.
- Morphine used for both vasodilatory and cardioprotective properties as well as analgesic properties in acute coronary syndrome
- Currently 3% of the US population is prescribed an opioid, and the incidence of overdose and death is also proportional to opioid dose

Clinical Case Scenario #1

You are consulted by a general surgery intern regarding conversion from intravenous hydromorphone to oral oxycodone. The patient is a healthy 27-year-old man who is postoperative day 3 from a hernia repair. Over the past 24 hours he has used a total of 3 mg of intravenous hydromorphone, which he states has controlled his pain effectively. With what dose of oxycodone would it be appropriate to send him home?

Answer: 3 mg of intravenous hydromorphone is equivalent to 20 mg of intravenous morphine (see Table 3.1.2). This converts to 60–120 mg of oral morphine as a 24-hour requirement. Erring on the conservative side, especially since we are changing opiates, let's reduce that amount by 50% and call his 24-hour morphine need is 40–60 mg or 20–40 mg of oxycodone. Thus, 40 mg of oxycodone divided into 4 daily doses is about 10 mg/dose. Thus a combination tablet of acetaminophen/oxycodone 325/10, 1 tablet every 4–6 hours should effectively and safely manage his pain in the outpatient setting

Table 3.1.1 Useful Opioid Pharmacokinetic and Pharmacodynamic Parameters

Opioid	pKa	V_D (L/Kg)	Octanol/water partition coefficient	Distribution Half-life(min)	Eliminaiton Half-life (h)	Time to Peak Effect (IV) (min)	Time to Peak Effect (PO) (h)	Duration of Effect
Morphine	7.9	4	0.7	1.7; 19.8	3	15–30	1.1	3 to 6
Meperidine	8.5	2.8–4.2	38.8	10	3 to 5	15–20	1 to 2	2 to 3
Hydromorphone	8.1	2.9	525	1.27; 14.7	2.3	10–20	0.5 to 1	2 to 3
Fentanyl	8.4	3.2–4.2	717	1.0; 19	3.6	3–6	N/A	0.5 to 1
Sufentanil	8	2.5–3.0	1778	1.4; 23	2.6[1]	1	N/A	0.5 to 1
Alfentanil	6.5	0.4–1.0	130	0.67; 20	1.5–2	1	N/A	0.2 to 0.3
Remifentanil	7.1	0.2–0.3	17.9	1; 9	10–20 min	1	N/A	0.1 to 0.2
Codeine	8.2	2.6–3.5	3.98	xxxx	2.5–3	N/A	1 to 2	4 to 6
Hydrocodone	8.9	xxxx	xxxx	xxxx	3.8	N/A	1.3	4 to 8
Oxycodone	8.5	2–3	0.7	3	3.5–5	30	1.3 to 2	4 to 6
Tramadol	9.41	2.6–2.9	xxxx	xxxx	5.6–6.7	<30	2 to 3	4 to 6
Methadone	8.3	3.6	xxxx	34–37 hours	13 to 50	15	2	4 to 8
Propoxyphene	6.3	16	xxxx	xxxx	6–12	N/A	2 to 2.5	3 to 5
Nalbuphine	8.7	3.8	xxxx	5	2.2	30	N/A	3 to 6
Naloxone	7.9	1.8–3.5	xxxx	4.7	0.5–1.2[2]	2–3	N/A	0.6

[1]Elimination half-life is 100 minutes in infants, and 499 minutes in neonates.
[2]Elimination half-life is much longer in neonates 2.5–3.5 hours.

Pharmacodynamics

- There are four accepted classes of opioid receptors: μ, κ, δ, and nociceptin-orphanin. All receptors mediate analgesia to varying degrees, however, κ receptors may be involved in dysphoria. In contrast, μ receptors seem to be primarily involved in analgesia. δ receptors bind endogenous opioids rather than opioid analgesics used in clinical practice. However, at high doses, in a tolerant patient, some δ receptor activity may be apparent. δ receptors meditate analgesia mainly in the spine.
- μ-opioid receptors mediate most of the effects normally attributed to opioids: analgesia, respiratory and cough suppression, sedation, and constipation.
- μ opioid receptors are found in the dorsal horn of the spinal cord, as well as in the periacqueductal grey matter, limbic system, and the thalamus, and may also be induced by injury or inflammation peripherally
- Sites of action: Systemic opioid analgesics mainly exert their analgesic effect in the periacqueductal grey matter by allowing inhibition of ascending pain signals via the rostral ventral medulla from the dorsal horn. Neuraxial opioids mainly act via μ-opioid receptors found in the substantia gelatinosa in the dorsal horn of the spinal cord
- All opioid receptors are G-protein mediated molecules. Opioid receptor agonists
  - Inhibit voltage gated calcium channels, preventing neurotransmitter release in presynaptic neurons
  - Activate inwardly rectifying potassium channels, hyperpolarizing postsynaptic neurons

Pharmacokinetics

- Lipophilic opioids, such as fentanyl and its derivatives, rapidly penetrate membranes resulting in a rapid onset of action.
  - Lipophilicity also results in relatively rapid redistribution into the fatty compartments of the body resulting in a short duration of action following an initial dose.
  - Once equilibrium is reached with a lipophilic opioid, however, repeated doses will have much longer duration of action as elimination, rather than redistribution, accounts for opioid concentration in plasma.
- Morphine, the least lipophilic opioid, has a slower onset of action than lipophilic opioids, but the least accumulation in fatty tissues.
- Plasma, elimination, and terminal half-life can be extremely misleading in predicting the duration of opioid effects.

Clinical Case Scenario #2

A 35-year-old male with a history of HIV and IVDU on methadone maintenance develops cough, fever, odynophagia, and mild nausea. His primary care physician believes this might be esophageal candidiasis and community acquired pneumonia. He initiates treatment with oral fluconazole for the thrush, ciprofloxacin for suspected pneumonia, and ondansetron for the nausea. Two days later, he is found dead at home. What was his likely cause of death?

HIV is extremely common in former IV drug users, many of whom are on methadone maintenance. Methadone prolongs the QT interval and is metabolized by the CYP3A4 pathway. Both fluconazole and ciprofloxacin are inhibitors of the CYP3A4 enzyme and can increase methadone levels. In addition, both ciprofloxacin and ondansetron prolong the QT interval.

Answer: Sudden cardiac death from Torsades de Points.

Side Effects/Adverse Reactions

- Central
  - Respiratory Depression
  - Euphoria
  - Dysphoria
  - Cough Suppression
  - Meiosis
  - Sedation
  - Seizures (mainly through meperidine metabolite normeperidine)
- Using Naloxone to treat meperidine associated seizures will worsen seizure activity
  - Hyperalgesia (generally with high doses)
  - Pruritis (μ receptor NOT histamine mediated)
  - Pruritis best treated with 5HT3 antagonists (ondansetron), μ-opioid receptor antagonists or mixed agonist/antagonists, propofol, and opioid sparing
- Cardiovascular
  - Hypotension
  - Bradycardia (reports of asystole when combined with beta-blockers)
  - High dose opioid anesthetics may decrease intraoperative hemodynamic variability.
  - Minimal to no effect on myocardial contractility
- Endocrine
  - Decreased LH, FSH, ACTH, norepinephrine, epinephrine
  - Increased ADH, and prolactin
  - Slightly lowered body temperature

- Renal
  - Urinary retention
  - Minimal to no effect on GFR
- GI
  - Decreased LES tone
  - Decreased GI motility
  - Decreased gastric emptying
  - Increased biliary sphincter tone
  - Increased GI secretions
  - Increased PONV
  - Patients on preoperative opioids, more likely to have "full stomach" regardless of last PO intake.
- OB
  - Decreased fetal heart rate variability
  - Fentanyl may be preferable to morphine for egg harvesting since morphine showed decreased rates of IVF in sea urchin eggs (no human data available)
  - Meperidine may increase uterine tone and contractions, and the effect is not reversible with naloxone
  - Fentanyl and morphine are concentrated 2–3x in breast milk, but clinical incidence of newborn narcosis is extremely rare.
  - For opioid tolerant or addicted parturients, methadone maintenance during pregnancy and delivery may result in improved outcomes relative to methadone assisted tapering during pregnancy.
- Immune
  - Decreased macrophage, NK cell, T cell activity 30–60 minutes after morphine

Clinical Case Scenario #3

A 26-year-old white woman was discharged from the hospital following cesarean section and given acetaminophen with codeine for pain control. Initially she felt no benefit so she was told to double her dose. This resulted in only minimal clinical benefit from the pills despite being narcotic naïve prior to her surgery. Why might her pain medicine not be working and what treatments are safe for nursing her child.

Codeine, a prodrug, is a particularly poor choice of opioid for nursing mothers. 10% of the population lacks the CYP2D6 gene to metabolize codeine into the biologically active morphine. Moreover, the FDA issued a warning that nursing mothers who are rapid metabolizers (a rare condition more common to those of East African descent) may pass on a lethal concentration of morphine passed to their newborn.

Answer: This patient is most likely in the 10% of the population that lacks the CYP2D6 polymorphism required to metabolize codeine to morphine. Switching her to morphine would give her excellent analgesia without serious risk to her child. Oxycodone and hydrocodone are suboptimal choices since both are metabolized by CYP2D6.

- Other Considerations
  - *Renal Impairment*: Metabolites morphine 6-gluconuride (M6G) and norme-peridine accumulate in renal insufficiency. Morphine and meperidine are therefore not ideal choices in this patient group.
  - *Hepatic Impairment*: There is a slightly longer elimination time in some opioids (especially meperidine and alfentanil). Metabolism and elimination of most opioids are not significantly affected by liver failure.
  - *Tolerance*: Tolerance means that with continued exposure to opioids, a higher dose of opioid is required to produce the same effect. At the beginning of treatment, dose may be increased until an effective analgesic level is reached. Tolerance to the centrally mediated side effects of opioids can be clinically beneficial since analgesic efficacy is often maintained despite full tolerance to side effects. Constipation (a peripheral opioid effect) is a notable exception. Constipation persists and requires prophylaxis or treatment throughout any prolonged course of opioid treatment.
  - *Opioid induced hyperalgesia* may arise in patients using opioids. This has been reported in the acute setting after intraoperative remifentanil. More commonly, it has been described in the chronic setting, especially with very high doses of opioids.

Neuraxial Opioids

- With the discovery of μ-opioid receptors in the dorsal horn of the spinal cord in the 1980s, neuraxial opioids have allowed anesthesiologists to provide excellent analgesia with lower doses of local anesthetics and thus avoiding dense sensory and motor blocks.
- Neuraxial opioids must be given in preservative free forms since these preservatives are neurotoxic.
  - The first opioid widely used in clinical practice was morphine. Despite excellent analgesia, sudden apnea was noted in a small fraction of patients as much as 18–24 hours after receiving neuraxial morphine. This was felt to be due to bulk flow of CSF migrating cephalad with the water soluble morphine. Thus, morphine is used less commonly in favor of more lipid soluble compounds such as fentanyl.
  - Common doses for neuraxial analgesia and anesthesia
    - Morphine:

- Adults: Epidural 3–5 mg max 10 mg in 24 hours; spinal 0.2–1 mg
- Children: Epidural 0.033–0.05 mg/kg; Spinal 0.01 mg/kg
- Patients should be monitored for 24 hours after neuraxial morphine due to risk of sudden apnea
- Hydromorphone: epidural 0.5–1.5 mg given in 5–15 mL normal saline; spinal 40–200 mcg.
- Fentanyl: epidural 50–100 mcg; spinal 10–25 mcg
  - Children: epidural 0.5–1 mcg/kg;
- Sufentanil: epidural 20–50 mcg; spinal 3–10 mcg
  - Spinal and epidural opioids have been reported to cause transient fetal bradycardia after administration.
- Treating Opioid Induced Respiratory Depression:
  - Naloxone is recommended for reversing opioid overdose, the standard dose being 0.4 mg IV naloxone. In the acute postsurgical setting this dose is likely to reverse virtually all μ-opioid receptor binding resulting in severe pain.
    - For postsurgical patients, we recommend diluting 0.4 mg of naloxone into 10 mL saline and then giving 1 mL aliquots of 40 mcg IV every 30–60 seconds until respiratory function recovers. Since the half-life of naloxone is significantly shorter than most opioids, repeated doses and infusions are often required.
- Opioid Conversion:
  - Approximate equianalgesic values are included in Table 3.1.2. In general when converting from one opioid to another: (1) determine the 24-hour opioid requirement, (2) convert that dose to an equianalgesic dose of morphine, (3) reduce that dose by 50%, (4) convert to the opioid you wish to use and divide the doses based on the dosing frequency of the opioid. Be very conservative when converting opioids. This is because individual variation in pharmacodynamics and incomplete cross-tolerance is unpredictable.
- Methadone has unique toxicities as well as slow and unpredictable elimination and should only be used by experienced clinicians. The precise conversion ratio is not well known, but appears dependent on the amount of morphine being taking prior to switching to methadone, with relatively less methadone being required at higher doses of morphine. For example, if one switches to methadone from another opioid and titrates to analgesic effect too rapidly (ie, changing doses more often than every 4–5 days) toxicity and overdose may result.

Individual Opioids

Morphine: Least lipophilic opioid. It has a longer analgesic duration (4–6 hours) than plasma half-life (3 hours), which limits accumulation. Most morphine is rapidly metabolized in liver, but morphine 6-gluconuride (M6G) is a renally cleared metabolite that has both analgesic and respiratory depressant

Table 3.1.2 Equianalgesic Doses and Common Starting Doses

Opioid	Equianalgesic Parenteral Dose (mg)	Equianalgesic PO Dose (mg)	Starting Dose Adults (>50kg)	Strating Dose Children (<50kg)
Morphine	10	30–60[1]	15 mg PO	0.05–0.1 mg/kg IV
Meperidine	75	300	12.5 mg[2] or 100 mg IV	1 mg/kg (max 100 mg/dose)
Hydromorphone	1.5	4–6	2–6 mg PO	0.015 mg/kg IV
Fentanyl	0.1	N/A	0.5–2 mcg/kg IV	1–10 mcg/kg
Sufentanil	0.01[3]	N/A	0.5–2 mcg/kg IV[c]	0.1–5 mcg/kg[c]
Alfentanil	1[3]	N/A	50–150 mcg/kg IV[c]	5–50 mcg/kg[3]
Remifentanil	0.1[3]	N/A	1–4 mcg/kg[c]	0.4–1 mcg/kg[a]; 0.25–1 mcg/kg[b]
Codeine	120	200	30–60 mg PO	0.5–1 mcg/kg (2–6 y/o)
Hydrocodone	N/A	20–30	5mg PO	0.125 mg/Kg
Oxycodone	N/A	20–40	5–20 mg PO	0.1 mg/kg
Tramadol	100[4]	300–600	25–50 mg PO	Not established in children
Methadone	2.0	6,7, 1[6]	2.5–5 mg PO	0.1 to 0.2 mg/kg q6 max 10 mg/dose
Propoxyphene	N/A	65–100mg	65–100 mg PO	Not established in children
Nalbuphine	N/A	N/A	10 mg IV	0.05–0.1 mg/kg
Naloxone	N/A	N/A	0.4 mg–2 mg IV[d]	0.1 mg/kg IV[d]

Because of incomplete cross-tolerance and significant variation in pharmacodynamics between individuals, extreme caution must be employed when converting from one opioid to another. The equianalgesic values presented here are approximate and intended to demonstrate relative potency and not necessarily clinically precise opioid conversion values (eg, the methadone value is only for converting from methadone to morphine, NOT vice versa).

[1] 30 mg for chronic dosing, 60 mg for acute dosing

[2] 12.5 mg dose is for treating postoperative or amphotericin associated shivering, 100 mg for mild to moderate pain.

[3] Relative potency based on amount required to reduce MAC isoflurane by 50%

[4] Intravenous form not available in the United States

[5] Average dose needed for sedation in infants and neonates about 20 mcg/kg

[6] Converting from methadone to another opioid is complicated and should only be attempted by clinicians familiar with its use. 6.7 mg should be used for acute dose conversion, 1 mg should be used from chronic dose conversion from methadone to morphine.

[a] Dose for infants birth to 1 y/o

[b] Dose for children 1–12 y/o

[c] Infusion rates and loading doses vary depending on whether the goal is sedation, analgesia, or anesthesia. Loading doses should be given gradually, over 2–5 minutes. Boluses are often associated with apnea and chest wall rigidity. Infusion rates depend on nature and duration of surgery for sufentanil, alfentanil, and remifentanil are 0.1–1mcg/kg/**hr**, 0.5–3 mcg/kg/min, and 0.1–0.4 mcg/kg/min. In children and infants, sufentanil may be used for sedation or anesthesia (usually cardiac). For ICU sedation in children, bolus of 0.1–0.5 mcg/kg followed by infusion of 0.005–0.01 mcg/kg/min, or for anesthesia (usually cardiac) with a bolus of 1–5 mcg/kg followed by 0.01–0.05 mcg/kg/min.

[d] Consider starting with 40 mcg (0.001–0.015 mcg/kg in children) in patients who are immediately postsurgical so as to avoid profound distress from hyperalgesia.

*Withdrawn from US market by FDA in November 2010 due to increased cardiac arrhythmia risk.

activities. Thus, morphine should be used with caution in patients with renal insufficiency due to risk of accumulation of M6G.

Hydromorphone: Slightly more potent (5–7x) than morphine with a shorter duration of action and available in both PO and IV formulations in the United States.

Meperidine: Slightly faster onset and offset of action compared to morphine. Normeperidine is a toxic metabolite causing seizures that accumulates in patients with renal insufficiency. Other unique properties include: local anesthetic, weak inhibitor of serotonin reuptake (fatal interactions with MAOIs), and highly effective at treating rigors associated with anesthesia and amphotericin.

Fentanyl: Fat soluble synthetic opioid with rapid onset of 3–5 minutes after intravenous bolus. Large volume of distribution results in rapid offset after initial dose due to redistribution. Repeated or large doses, however, accumulate and result in longer duration of effect.

Sufentanil: Most fat soluble and potent of the fentanyl derivatives. It has a shorter context sensitive half-life than fentanyl, allowing it be very useful for longer surgeries which require profound analgesia, but may facilitate extubation conditions more rapidly than fentanyl.

Alfentanil: The fastest onset (<2min) and offset (~15min) of all the fentanyl derivatives. Like fentanyl, however, repeated or large doses can accumulate with termination depending on elimination rather than redistribution.

Remifentanil: The only opioid with a rapid onset and offset and virtually no accumulation with prolonged infusion or large doses. This is due to its unique mechanism of elimination, via nonspecific esterases (NOT pseudocholinesterase) mostly in skeletal muscle.

Codeine: Prodrug of morphine and it MUST be converted to morphine in the liver in order for analgesia to result. About 10% of the population lacks the cytochrome p450 2D6 isoenzyme required to convert codeine to morphine, thus limiting its clinical usefulness. There are also reports of rapidly metabolizing nursing mothers passing lethal doses to their infants.

Hydrocodone: μ-opioid receptor prodrug of with similar activity to morphine. Commonly combined with acetaminophen. As with codeine and oxycodone, about 10% of the population is unable to metabolize hydrocodone to morphine metabolites.

Oxycodone: A μ-opioid receptor that is metabolized to oxymorphone (which has greater μ-opioid receptor affinity) with similar properties to morphine. It may also have some kappa receptor activity which may be more beneficial in patients with visceral or pancreatic pain. Oxycodone is metabolized to oxymorphone via CYP2D6 to exert its analgesic effect. Like codeine, and hydrocodone, 7% of Caucasians, 3% of African Americans, 1% of Asian Americans are poor metabolizers of CYP2D6 substrates and may lack analgesic benefit with oxycodone. The extended release tablet has been commonly abused by crushing the tablet in order to receive a large dose of opioid rapidly. A new gel coated capsule of the extended release oxycodone tablet, may make abuse more difficult and was approved by the FDA in 2010.

Tramadol: Weak μ-opioid receptor agonist. It also inhibits the reuptake of norepinephrine and serotonin, suppressing pain transmission from the spinal cord. It reduces the seizure threshold and can interact with other antidepressants causing serotonergic crisis.

Propoxyphene: Commonly combined with acetaminophen. Norpropoxyphene is a metabolite thought to be cardiotoxic with a long half-life of 30–60 hours. Propoxyphene was withdrawn from the US market in November 2010 due to concerns over cardiac arrhythmias.

Methadone: Two enantiomers R and S. The R isomer has an 8–50 times greater affinity for the μ-opioid receptor than the S isomer. The S isomer, however, is an NMDA antagonist and is thus thought to reduce opioid tolerance and withdrawal. Methadone prolongs the QT interval and must be used with great caution. Since the elimination half-life (~34 hours) greatly exceeds the analgesic duration (4–8 hours), toxic accumulation is possible if titrating rapidly to an analgesic end point. Thus, methadone should only be used by practitioners very familiar with its pharmacokinetics.

Chapter 3.2

Skeletal Muscle Relaxants

Chitra Ramasubbu, MD and Anita Gupta, DO, PharmD

Clinical Uses/Relevance to Anesthesiology

- Low back pain; 35% of pts visiting their PMD for low back pain are prescribed muscle relaxants (among the top 200 drugs dispensed in the United States in 2006). The American Pain Society and the American College of Physicians recommend acetaminophen and NSAIDs as first-line therapy, and skeletal muscle relaxants only as alternative therapy secondary to their side effects. Furthermore, the FDA approves use for 1–3 wks; however, they are commonly prescribed on a long-term basis.

- Other indications include fibromyalgia, myofascial pain syndrome, and tension headaches.
- Literature regarding skeletal muscle relaxants is limited. Most active comparator trials of patients with spasticity showed tizanidine, baclofen, dantrolene and diazepam to improve spasticity equally.
- Clinical data shows that skeletal muscle relaxants are more effective than placebo in the treatment of acute low back pain. No data shows one agent being more efficacious than another.
- Skeletal muscle relaxants should be considered as an alternative to NSAIDs, in patients in whom NSAID toxicity is a concern.
- Because of their CNS depressant effects, they should be used with caution in patients who are on opioids, anxiolytics, etc.
- There is evidence to support the use of tizanidine, carisoprodol and cyclobenzaprine in the treatment of acute low back pain. However evidence regarding long-term use is poor.
- Choosing the appropriate skeletal muscle relaxant depends on the side effect profiles, tolerability and cost.

Pharmacodynamics

- Skeletal muscle relaxants refer to a diverse range of medications that are not pharmacologically related. They produce their clinical effects through sedation as well as changes in the pain-spasm-pain cycle.

- Two categories. Antispasmodic agents: common musculoskeletal conditions (carisoprodol, cyclobenzaprine, metaxalone, methocarbamol). Antispastic agents: cerebral palsy and multiple sclerosis (baclofen, dantrolene).
- Spasticity is an upper motor neuron disorder characterized by muscle hypertonicity and involuntary jerks secondary to conduction interruption in the nerve pathways. Antispasticity drugs function by attempting to increase reflexes (diazepam and tizanidine have both antispastic as well as antispasmodic properties).

Antispasmodic Agents

Cyclobenzaprine
Clinical Uses/Relevance to Anesthesiology

- Acute pain musculoskeletal conditions; improves spasms, local tenderness, and range of motion
- Myofascial pain; however insufficient evidence supporting its use
- Fibromyalgia; shown to moderately improve sleep and pain (long-term benefits unknown)

Pharmocodynamics

- Pharmacologically related to TCAs. Acts centrally at the brain stem, rather than the spinal cord or muscle tissue
- Significant anticholinergic effects (avoid in elderly)

Pharmocokinetics

- Bioavailability of 33–55%
- Hepatic metabolism; 51% excreted unchanged by kidneys; elimination half-life 18 hrs.

Doses

- 5–10 mg PO TID (larger doses have more side effects)

Side Effects/Adverse events:

- Not associated with withdrawal symptoms after abrupt cessation with chronic administration (tapering is still recommended)
- Sedation (16–39% incidence)
- Anticholinergic effects: drowsiness, dry mouth, urinary retention.
- Serotonin toxicity: coadministration with SSRIs may precipitate
- Increases IOP, seizures with concomitant use of tramadol; rare incidences of arrhythmias, MI

Carisoprodol
Clinical Uses/Relevance to Anesthesiology

- Skeletal muscle relaxant; commonly prescribed, controlled in several states
- Abuse potential; among ER visits in the year 2000, ranked #14 of most abused mood-altering substances in United States (greater than oxycodone)

Pharmacodynamics

- Carisoprodol and its active metabolite, meprobamate, block interneuronal activity and depress transmission of polysynaptic neurons in the descending reticular formation and spinal cord. Functions via indirect agonism at the GABA A receptor and affects CNS chloride ion channel conductance.
- Weak anticholinergic, antipyretic and analgesic effects; cross-tolerance to barbiturates

Pharmacokinetics

- Rapid absorption from GI tract and distribution throughout the CNS; onset 30 mins
- Hepatic metabolism via cytochrome P450 to active metabolite meprobamate; elimination half-life ~100 mins (meprobamate is ~6–17 hrs; can result in accumulation with chronic therapy). Duration of action 4–6 hrs

Dosing

- 350 mg PO TID; 250 mg PO TID-QID if combined with codeine or aspirin.

Side Effects/Adverse Events

- Alcohol enhances impairment of physical abilities and increases sedation, agitation, euphoria, confusion, and weakness.
- Abuse potential for sedative and relaxant effects. Furthermore, studies have demonstrated increased concomittant utilization of opioids
- Withdrawal syndrome secondary to meprobamate: insomnia, vomiting, tremors, muscle twitching, anxiety, and ataxia. Hallucinations and delusions may occur.
- Acute intermittent porphyria contraindication

Antispastic Agents

Baclofen

Clinical Uses/Relevance to Anesthesiology

- Spasticity including multiple sclerosis; FDA-approved.
- Intractable hiccups, bladder spasms, tetanus, and trigeminal neuralgia; off-label use
- Acute baclofen withdrawal; intrathecal baclofen is a medical emergency and requires critical care.

Pharmacodynamics

- GABA derivative that disrupts polysynaptic and monosynaptic reflexes at the level of the spinal cord; may affect supraspinal sites as well

Pharmacokinetics

- Onset 3–4 days, peak effect 5–10 days
- Renal excretion of 70–85%; 15% hepatic metabolism. Elimination half-life for systemic baclofen 2–4 hrs, intrathecal baclofen is 1.5 hrs. Consider dosage adjustment in renal impairment

Dosages

- 5–25 mg PO TID
- Intrathecal test dose: initially 50 mcg, with upward titration 25 mcg q24 hrs until clinical response obtained

Side Effects/Adverse Events

- Withdrawal: high fever, acute exacerbations in muscle spasticity, BP lability, CNS complications (AMS, seizures, delirium). No definitive, effective approach; baclofen (PO), benzodiazepines, propofol, and dantrolene. Avoidance by slow taper.

Antispastic and Antispasmodic Agents

Tizanidine

Clinical Uses/Relevance to Anesthesiology

- Spasticity from CNS disorders such as multiple sclerosis and spinal cord injury; FDA-approved.
- Chronic headaches; off-label use
- Lower back pain, often in conjunction with NSAIDs
- Consider preoperative liver function assessment due to ability to cause hepatotoxicity

Pharmacodynamics

- Chemically related to clonidine; central action as an alpha 2 agonist. Causes presynaptic inhibition of motor neuron hyperactivity. Has 1/10th-1/50th effect of clonidine on BP

Pharmacokinetics

- Onset: 1–2 hrs; duration of action: 3–6 hrs (should be reserved for time-dependent activities)
- Hepatic metabolism to nonactive metabolites that are renally excreted (60%); elimination half-life ~2 hrs

Dosages

- 4 mg PO initially (may be increased by 2–4 mg q6–8 hrs until relief achieved; not to exceed 36 mg PO QD)

Adverse Effects

- Hepatotoxicity, hypotension, sedation, prolonged QT interval, hallucinations, and dry mouth.
- Withdrawal and rebound hypertension may be seen upon discontinuation (chronic therapy, high doses). Tapering is recommended.
- Decreased effectiveness with oral contraceptives

Clinical Case Scenario

A 19-year-old male with history of cerebral palsy underwent a posterior spinal fusion for scoliosis. History is significant for an intrathecal baclofen pump placed 5 years ago for spastic quadriplegia. On POD 2, he developed abrupt onset of delirium with worsening spasms. He was febrile with T-101.2, HR -135, BP 155/87. On POD 3 he had an episode of seizure.

- **Background:** Baclofen is a GABA derivative that disrupts polysynaptic and monosynaptic reflexes at the level of the spinal cord. Action at the supraspinal sites may also be involved.

- **Pathophysiology:** Probable cause for withdrawal syndrome was small nick in intrathecal pump catheter tubing during the dissection process. Chronic use of baclofen use results in down-regulation of GABA receptors. Withdrawal is associated with rebound excitations at all levels of the neuroaxis.

- **Differential Diagnosis:** Baclofen withdrawal, baclofen overdose, sepsis, neuroleptic malignant syndrome, autonomic dysreflexia, serotonin syndrome, malignant hyperthermia

- **Treatment**: Goal is to prevent and treat worsening muscle spasticity, blood pressure lability, and CNS conditions like seizures and delirium. Definitive treatment is restoration of drug administration by the same route. Oral therapy has a much slower onset. The common adjuvant therapies include benzodiazepines and propofol. Cyproheptadine may be helpful for symptoms involving serotonergic syndromes, while dantrolene may be helpful with excessive spasticity. Tizanidine may represent a viable option for patients with spasticity and blood pressure lability

References

1. Jackson KC, Argoff CE. In: HT Benzon, PP Raj, et al, eds. *Raj's Practical Management of Pain.* 4th ed. Philadelphia: Mosby-Elsevier; 2008.

2. Dillon C, Paulose-Ram R, Hirsch R, et al. Skeletal muscle relaxant use in the United States: Data from the Third National Health and Nutrition Examination Survey (NHANES III). *Spine.* 2004;29:892–896.

3. Drugtopics.com. *Top 200 generic drugs by units in 2006.* https://www.drugtopics.com/drugtopics/data/articlestandard//drugtopics/092007/407652/article.pdf. Accessed January 14, 2008.

4. See S, Ginzburg R. Skeletal muscle relaxants. *Pharmacotherapy.* 2008;28(2):207–213.

5. Tulder MW, Touray T, Furlan AD, Solway S, Bouter LM. Muscle relaxant for nonspecific low back pain: A systemic review within the framework of the Cochrane collaboration. *Spine.* 2003;28(17):1978–1992.

6. *Physicians' Desk Reference.* Montvale, NJ: Medical Economics Company, 2006.

7. Upsher-Smith Laboratories, Inc. Baclofen tablet product labeling. Minneapolis, MN; 2002. Available http://dailymed.nlm.nih.gov/dailymed/fdaDrug Accessed April 10, 2007.

8. Chou R, Peterson K, Helfand M. Comparative efficacy and safety of skeletal muscle relaxants for spasticity and musculoskeletal conditions: a systematic review. *J Pain Symptom Manage*. 2004;28(2):140–175.

9. Van Tulder MW, Touray T, Furlan AD, et al. Muscle relaxants for nonspecific low back pain. *Cochrane Database Syst Rev* 2003. CD004252.

Chapter 3.3

Non-Steroidal Anti-Inflammatory Drugs

Matthew Lesneski, MD and Peter Yi, MD

Role in the Practice of Anesthesiology/Relevance to Anesthesiology

- NSAIDs are among the most widely used analgesics worldwide.
- NSAIDs are first-line treatment for acute and chronic pain and are recommended as part of a multimodal approach to postoperative pain therapy.
- The use of NSAIDs to supplement systemic and neuraxial opioid therapy has demonstrated improved analgesia, opioid sparing, and a reduction in opioid-induced respiratory depression and nausea.
- According to the American Society of Regional Anesthesia consensus guidelines, NSAIDs (including aspirin) do not increase the risk of hematoma in patients receiving neuraxial anesthesia nor does the use of NSAIDs alone interfere with the performance of neuraxial blocks or the timing of neuraxial catheter removal.
- Despite ubiquitous use in the community these drugs carry significant risk.
- NSAIDs have a ceiling dose; once a maximum dose is achieved, the incidence of side effects increases but does not offer additional analgesia.
- Anesthesia professionals should know how these drugs affect the hematologic, gastrointestinal, cardiovascular, and renal systems to mitigate risk in the perioperative period.

Pharmacodynamics

- The primary effect of NSAIDs is cyclooxygenase inhibition, blocking the transformation of arachidonic acid to prostaglandins, prostacyclins, and thromboxanes.
- Prostaglandins, prostacyclins, and thromboxanes are lipid mediators that regulate body homeostasis and inflammation.
- Prostaglandin E2 (PGE2) is involved in the inflammatory process and mediates both peripheral and central pain sensitization.
- Prostacyclin regulates renal blood flow through vasodilatation of the kidney's afferent arteriole.
- Thromboxane A2 (TXA2) causes vasoconstriction and platelet aggregation.

- The cyclooxygenase enzyme exists in two forms: COX-1 and COX-2.
- COX-1 is constitutively expressed in most human tissues including platelets, the GI tract, and kidneys. COX-1 synthesized prostaglandins regulate platelet function, gastric mucosa integrity, and renal blood flow.
- COX-2 is found in the kidneys and central nervous system and induced at sites of tissue damage. COX-2 synthesized prostaglandins are involved in the inflammatory response and potentiate pain sensation on central and peripheral nociceptors.
- Prostaglandin mediated hyperalgesia regulates pain perception at sites of tissue damage as well as in the brain stem and spinal cord.
- NSAIDs inhibit COX-1 and COX-2 prostaglandin production decreasing both the inflammatory response and the sensitizing effects of prostaglandins on central and peripheral nociceptors.

Pharmacokinetics

- Weak acids with pKa values between 3–5.
- Good absorption from GI tract; food does not substantially change bioavailability.
- Peak concentration 1–4 hr, 95–99% protein bound—mostly to albumin.
- Hepatic biotransformation (cyctochrome P-450 oxidation, glucuronide conjugation) is the main elimination pathway, with less than 10% renal excretion of nonmetabolized drug.

Side Effects/Adverse Reactions

- Adverse effects of NSAIDs are attributed to disruption of prostaglandin-mediated homeostatic function and platelet inhibition.
- Aspirin covalently modifies COX-1 on platelets, irreversibly inhibiting thromboxane production for the life of the platelet (7–10 days).
- Non-aspirin NSAIDs cause transient reduction in platelet function that resolves after most of the drug is eliminated, usually after 5 half-lives.
- NSAIDs displace albumin-bound drugs and can potentiate the anticoagulant activity of warfarin.
- NSAIDs are contraindicated for perioperative pain control in the setting of coronary artery bypass surgery due to increased risk of myocardial infarction and stroke.
- Inhibition of COX-1 in gastric epithelial cells decreases production of cytoprotective prostaglandins leading to gastric ulcers and possible bleeding.
- NSAID treatment with proton pump inhibitors or misoprostol has been show to reduce ulcer risk.
- Gastric bleeding can occur at anytime during treatment, often without warning.
- Gastric bleeding is increased in the elderly, patients with prior bleeding episodes, and those taking anticoagulants.

- NSAIDs inhibit prostacyclin mediated vasodilation on the afferent arteriole and significantly decreases renal blood flow in patients with renal insufficiency and volume depletion.
- Hypersensitivity to NSAIDs can cause vasomotor rhinitis and asthma.
- Higher doses and longer durations of therapy can increase the adverse effects of NSAIDs.

Aspirin

Clinical Uses/Relevance to Anesthesiology

- The use of aspirin for chronic pain and inflammation is limited by a high incidence of severe gastropathy.
- Aspirin is used mostly for its antiplatelet effects; commonly used for the prevention of myocardial infarction, thrombotic stroke, and claudication.
- Used in conjunction with clopidogrel in patients with peripheral vascular disease and those with drug-eluting coronary stents.
- Perioperative use is common for patients undergoing cardiac stenting, coronary artery bypass grafting, and vascular surgical procedures.

Pharmacodynamics

- Covalently modifies COX-1 and COX-2, irreversibly inhibiting COX activity.
- The utility of aspirin in the treatment of vascular occlusive disease has been ascribed to its blockade of platelet thromboxane, a potent inhibitor of vascular smooth muscle contraction and platelet aggregation.
- After aspirin ingestion, COX-1 platelet thromboxane production is inhibited for the life of the platelet (7–10 days).

Pharmacokinetics

- Simple organic acid with pKa of 3.5
- Metabolized by the liver with minimal renal excretion of nonmetabolized drug.
- Rapidly absorbed from GI tract with peak plasma concentration within 1–2 hours
- Half-life 2–3 hours, onset 5–30 minutes, duration 3–6 hours.

Dose

- Pain/Fever: Adult: 325–650 mg PO q4–6 hr. Pediatric: 10–15 mg/kg q4–6 hr
- MI and stroke prophylaxis: 81–325 mg

Preparations

- Oral (regular, enteric coated, buffered): 81, 165, 325, 500, 650, and 800 tablets.
- Rectal: 120, 200, 300, and 600 mg suppositories.

Side Effects/Adverse Reactions

- Major side effects of aspirin in the perioperative period include risk of bleeding and risk of thrombosis secondary to aspirin withdrawal.
- The risk of bleeding must be balanced against the risk of predisposing the patient to a thromboembolic complication, such as a coronary event or stroke. Patients taking aspirin for coronary stents should continue perioperatively. Patients undergoing minor surgery do not need to stop aspirin.
- Risk of bleeding while taking aspirin is increased in transurethral prostatectomy, retinal, major orthopedic, and intracranial surgery. Patients should discontinue aspirin 7–10 days prior to these procedures.
- The American Society of Regional Anesthesia guidelines report aspirin use does not increase the risk of hematoma in patients having neuraxial anesthesia.
- Use in pediatric patients with varicella or influenza-like illness is associated with increased incidence of Reye's syndrome.

Ibuprofen

Clinical Uses/Relevance to Anesthesiology

- Treatment of mild to moderate pain, minor fever, and inflammatory conditions.
- Concomitant administration of ibuprofen with aspirin antagonizes the irreversible platelet inhibition induced by aspirin.
- Treatment with ibuprofen in patients with increased cardiovascular risk may limit the cardioprotective effects of aspirin.
- IV formulation for PDA closure in premature infants.

Doses

- Adult Dose: 200–400 mg q4–6 hr, not to exceed 3200 mg per day.
- Half-life 2–4 hours, onset 30 minutes, duration 4–6 hours.
- Pediatric Dose: 5–10 mg/kg q6 hr
- Minimal risk of severe gastropathy with daily dose < 2400 mg.

Preparations

- Liquid gel
- Topical cream
- Oral: 50, 100, 200, 300, 400, 600, and 800 mg tablets, suspension 100 mg/5 mL
- Intravenous: 10 mg/mL

Naproxen

Clinical Uses/Relevance to Anesthesiology

- Half-life of 13 hours provides for twice-daily administration

- Causes less GI bleeding than aspirin

Preparations
- 200, 220 mg OTC; 250, 275, 375, 500, 550 mg
- Oral suspension 25 mg/mL

Doses
- 500 mg every 12 hours

Pharmacokinetics
- Half-life 13 hours, duration 4–7 hours, onset 1 hour.

Diclofenac

Clinical Uses/Relevance to Anesthesiology
- Gastrointestinal ulceration may occur less frequently than with other NSAIDs.
- Topical preparations available for osteoarthritis, acute pain, and treatment of actinic keratoses.
- A 0.1% ophthalmic preparation is used for prevention of postoperative ophthalmic inflammation—used after intraocular lens implantation and strabismus surgery.

Preparations
- Oral: 50 mg tablets, 25, 50, 75, and 100 mg delayed release tablets.
- Ophthalmic: 0.1% solution
- Topical: 3% gel, 180 mg patch, 1.5% solution
- Combination diclofenac and misoprostal for patient at high risk for development of NSAID-induced ulcers.

Doses
- 50 mg PO every 8 hours

Pharmacokinetics:
- Oral: half-life 1–2 hours, topical: half-life 1–2 hours.

Ketorolac

Clinical Uses/Relevance to Anesthesiology
- Only parenteral NSAID for clinical analgesic use in the United States—useful for NPO patients and perioperative pain control.
- Ketorolac is used for the short-term management of moderately severe, acute pain. Ketorolac is not indicated for use in minor or chronic painful conditions.

- The total combined duration of parenteral and/or oral ketorolac therapy in adults is not to exceed 5 days because of an increased frequency and severity of adverse effects associated with more prolonged therapy.
- Ketorolac demonstrates analgesia beyond its anti-inflammatory properties.
- Analgesic efficacy similar to 6–12 mg of morphine.
- Opioid sparing with absence of ventilatory and cardiovascular depression.

Pharmacodynamics
- Onset IV / IM 10 minutes, PO 30 minutes.
- Half-life 2–4 hours, duration 6–8 hours.

Dose
- Adult: Parenteral Dose: 30mg IV initial, 15mg IV subsequent q6hr, limit treatment to 5 days. Oral Dose: Oral administration only indicated as continuation of IV or IM dosing. Total daily dose no more than 40 mg for no more than 5 days due to GI toxicity.
- Decrease the daily dose in patients > 65 years, < 50 kg, or moderately elevated serum creatinine level; the maximum daily dose in these patients should not exceed 60 mg.
- Pediatric Dose: 1mg/kg as single loading dose IV up to 60 mg, 0.5 mg/kg up to 30 mg for initial and subsequent doses.

Preparations
- Oral: 10 mg tablets; parenteral: IV and IM 15, 30 mg/mL; ophthalmic: 0.4, 0.5% solution; intranasal: 15.75 mg / per 100 mcq spray.

Side Effects/Adverse Reactions
- Bleeding and renal failure are the most feared adverse effects of ketorolac. Since made available for clinical use, there have been reports of death caused by GI and operative site bleeding.
- Contraindicated before major surgery or intraoperatively when hemostasis is critical.
- Ketorolac may precipitate renal failure in patients with preexisting renal insufficiency, hypovolemia, hypotension, and those with concomitant use of nephrotoxic drugs.
- Ketorolac should not be used in obstetric patients as a preoperative medication or for analgesia during labor since inhibitors of prostaglandin synthesis may affect uterine contractions and fetal circulation (PDA closure).

Selective COX 2 Inhibitors

Matthew Lesneski, MD, and Peter Yi, MD

Role in the Practice of Anesthesiology/Relevance to Anesthesiology

- COX-2 selective inhibitors (Coxibs) were developed to inhibit prostaglandin synthesis at sites of inflammation without disrupting the homeostatic function of the COX-1 enzyme on GI mucosa, the kidney, and platelets.
- COX-2 selective inhibitors have analgesic, antipyretic and anti-inflammatory effects equivalent to traditional NSAIDs with 50%-60% less GI adverse effects and no effect on platelet function.
- Coxib use in the immediate postoperative period has been shown to reduce opioid consumption. Perioperative use of COX-2 inhibitors has been shown to improve pain outcomes.
- The more favorable side effect profile of COX-2 inhibitors make them useful for the chronic treatment of pain from osteoarthritis, rheumatoid arthritis, and dysmenorrhea.

Pharmacodynamics

- COX-1 is constitutively expressed on GI mucosa, platelets, and kidneys where it is involved in prostaglandin-mediated homeostatic regulation.
- COX-2 is expressed constitutively in the kidneys and central nervous system and is induced by noxious stimuli that cause inflammation in peripheral tissues.
- Cell damage associated with inflammation causes release of arachidonic acid. The COX pathway of arachidonate metabolism produces prostaglandins that intensify the sensation of pain at sites of tissue damage or inflammation.
- Inhibition of COX-2 enzyme responsible for prostaglandin synthesis leads to analgesic and anti-inflammatory effects.

Pharmacokinetics

- Rapid and complete absorption from the GI tract; food does not substantially change bioavailability
- Peak concentration occurring within 1 to 4 hours
- Extensively protein bound (95%-99%).
- Metabolized by the liver with minimal renal excretion of nonmetabolized drug.
- COX-2 inhibitors are different from NSAIDS in that they are highly lipophilic, nonacidic, and neutral molecules

Side Effects/Adverse Reactions

- Risk of gastric ulceration and bleeding is reduced approximately 50% when compared with conventional NSAIDs however the risk of gastropathy and bleeding is still present.

- Chronic use of COX-2 inhibitors has demonstrated increased risk of myocardial infarction and stroke when compared to placebo.
- The prothrombotic effects of COX-2 inhibitors are attributed to an imbalance between vasodilatory prostacyclins and procoagulant thromboxanes on platelets.
- Coxibs inhibit COX-2 synthesized prostacyclin on endothelial cells, leading to vasoconstriction. The lack of COX-2 inhibition on platelets promotes thromboxane mediated vasoconstriction and platelet aggregation.
- The relative prothrombotic state caused by COX-2 inhibitors significantly increases the risk of myocardial infarction and stroke in patients with preexisting cardiac, hypertensive, renal, and vascular disease.

Celecoxib

- First COX-2 inhibitor approved by FDA.
- Effective for acute and perioperative pain.
- Chronic use for osteoarthritis, rheumatoid arthritis, acute pain, dysmenorrhea, and familial adenomatous polyposis.

Pharmacokinetics
- Half-life 11 hours.

Preparations
- 50, 100, 200, and 400 mg capsules.

Doses
- Acute pain: 400 mg once, followed by 200 mg qd or bid
- Chronic pain: 200 mg qd or 100 mg bid

Side Effects/Adverse Reactions
- FDA "black box" warning concerning cardiovascular risk.
- Contraindicated in patients with sulfonamide allergy.

Parecoxib

- IV prodrug of valecoxib available for use in Europe.
- Short-term treatment postoperative pain.

Doses
- Acute: 40 mg once
- Chronic: 20 to 40 mg every 6–12 hours

Clinical Case Scenario

65-year-old female with past medical history significant for osteoarthritis, coronary artery disease, and lumbar back pain presents for total hip arthroplasty. Her medications include low dose aspirin, naproxen, acetaminophen-oxycodone, and omeprazole. What are the perioperative considerations regarding NSAID use in this patient?

Practice guidelines for perioperative acute pain management recommend that all patients should receive NSAIDs, COX-2 inhibitors, or acetaminophen unless contraindicated.

Risk of Bleeding

Perioperative use of NSAIDs may predispose patients to bleeding. Patients undergoing elective surgical procedures with significant bleeding risk are instructed to discontinue aspirin 7–10 days prior to surgery. Use of COX-2 inhibitors preoperatively does not increase bleeding risk.

Bone Healing

NSAIDs prevent ectopic bone formation (heterotopic ossification) in humans. Alterations in bone healing may be of concern for procedure such as spinal fusion, where bone healing is crucial. However, short-term use of NSAIDs perioperatively may not compromise bone healing.

Cardiovascular

COX-2 inhibitors have been shown to increase the risk of MI and stroke compared to placebo. This risk is significant in patients who are already at high risk for cardiovascular complications. Celecoxib remains the only COX-2 inhibitor on the market in the United States and contains a black box warning for potential adverse cardiovascular events. Patients with coronary stents should continue aspirin unless contraindicated.

Regional Anesthesia

NSAIDs (including aspirin) do not significantly increase the risk of hematoma in patients receiving epidural or spinal anesthesia. The use of NSAIDs alone should not interfere with the performance of neuraxial blocks or the timing of neuraxial catheter removal.

References

1. Vane JR. (1971). Inhibition of prostaglandin synthesis as a mechanism of action for aspirin-like drugs. *Nature: New Biology*. 1971;231(25):232–235.

2. Malmberg A, Yaksh T. Hyperalgesia mediated by spinal glutamate or substance P receptor blocked by spinal cyclooxygenase inhibition. *Science*. 1992;257:1276–1279.

3. Morita I. Distinct functions of COX-1 and COX-2. *Prostaglandins Other Lipid Mediat.* 2002;68–69:165–175.

4. Graff J, Skarke C, Kinkhardt U, Watzer B, Harder S, Seyberth H, et al. Effects of selective COX-2 inhibition on prostanoids and platelet physiology in young healthy volunteers. *J Thromb Haemost.* 2007;5(12):2376–2385.

5. Rostom, A., Dube, C., Wells, G., Tugwell, P., Welch, V., Jolicoeur, E., et al. Prevention of NSAID-induced gastroduodenal ulcers. *Cochrane Database Syst Rev.* 2002;4:CD002296.

6. Kearney PM, Baigent C, Godwin J, Halls H, Emberson JR, Patrono C. Do selective cyclo-oxygenase-2 inhibitors and traditional non-steroidal anti-inflammatory drugs increase the risk of artherothrombosis? Meta-analysis of randomized trials. *BMJ.* 2006;332(7553),1302–1308.

7. FitzGerald GA. Coxibs and cardiovascular disease. *N Engl J Med.* 2004;351:1709–1711.

8. Bresalier RS, Sandler RS, Quan H, et al. Cardiovascular events associated with rofexocib in a colorectal adenoma chemoprevention trial. *N Engl J Med.* 2005;352:1081–1091.

9. Patrono C, Dunn MJ. The clinical significance of inhibition of renal prostaglandin synthesis. *Kidney Int.* 1987;32:1–12.

10. Klein M, Andersen LP, Harvald T, Rosenberg J, Gogenur I. Increased risk of anastomotic leakage with diclofenac treatment after laparoscopic colorectal surgery. *Dig Surg.* 2009;26(1): 27–30.

11. Deguchi M, Rapoff AJ, Zdeblick TA. Posterolateral fusion for isthmic spondylothesis in adults: analysis of fusion rate and clinical results. *J Spinal Disorders.* 1998;11:459–464.

12. Glassman SD, Rose SM, Dimar JR, Puno RM, Campbell MJ, Johnson JR. The effect of postoperative nonsteroidal anti-inflammatory drug administration on spinal fusion. *Spine.* 1998;23:834–838.

13. Reuben SS, Ekman EF. The effect of cyclooxygenase-2 inhibition on analgesia and spinal fusion. *J Bone Join Surg Am.* 2005;87:536–542.

14. Rahman MH, Beattie J. Peri-operative medication in patients with cardiovascular disease. *Pharm J.* 2004;272(7291):352–354

15. Burger, et al. Low-dose aspirin for secondary cardiovascular prevention: cardiovascular risks after its perioperative withdrawal versus bleeding risks with its continuation: review and meta-analysis. *J Intern Med.* 2005;257:399–414.

16. Horlocker, TT, Wedel DJ, Schroeder DR. Preoperative blood platelet therapy does not increase the risk of spinal hematoma associated with regional anesthesia. *Anesth Analg.* 1995;80:303–309.

17. Moote C. Efficacy of nonsteroidal anti-inflammatory drugs in the management of postoperative pain. *Drugs.* 1992;44(supp 5):14–29, discussion 29–30.

Chapter 3.4

Acetaminophen

Chitra Ramasubbu, MD and Anita Gupta, DO, PharmD

Clinical Uses /Relevance to Anesthesiology

- Acute and chronic pain management. FDA-labeled indications also include fever, headache, and dysmenorrhea.
- Doses within recommended range have minimal effect on cardiovascular, respiratory, and coagulation systems.
- IV form OFIRMEV recently FDA-approved, which may expand perioperative and intraoperative role.
- Hepatotoxicity may be seen at high doses. It can be used in patients with alcoholic liver disease as long as the recommended 4 g over 24 hours is not exceeded.

Pharmacodynamics

- Mechanism of action of acetaminophen remains unknown after more than 100 years of its synthesis. Potential actions include inhibition of cyclooxygenase isoenzymes, interaction with the endogenous opioid pathway, activation of the serotoninergic-bulbospinal pathway, involvement of the NO pathway, and an $\uparrow$ in the cannabinoid tone.
- The two cyclooxygenase isozymes (COX-1 and COX-2) catalyze the conversion of arachidonic acid to prostaglandins, thromboxanes, and prostacyclins. Prostaglandins are mediators of fever, pain, and inflammation. Acetaminophen reduces the enzyme to its inactive form (centrally > peripherally is likely reason for the lack of gastric side effects and platelet activity inhibition).
- The analgesic effect may involve interaction between the spinal and supraspinal sites with recruitment of endogenous opioid pathways. This property has been dubbed "self-synergy."
- There is substantial evidence that the descending serotonergical pathway originating from the raphe nuclei in the brain stem exerts an inhibitory (analgesic) effect on the pain signal.
- Does not bind to cannabinoid receptors itself. However its metabolites display cannabinoid-like activity. Therefore it could activate the endocannabinoid system by acting as a prodrug.

Pharmacokinetics

- Onset: PO single dose 0.5 hrs; peak: 2–3 hrs; bioavailability 60%-80% with rapid absorption; half-life of 4.5 min; able to cross the BBB. PO absorption in spinal cord injury is ↓ secondary to ↓ GI motility/gastric emptying. Rectal: benefit of rectal administration is restricted by slow onset time and unpredictable bioavailability

- Duration: PO single dose 4 hrs; extended-release formulation releases for up to 8 hrs (however, 95% has been released by the 5th hr)

- Metabolism: first-pass metabolism up to 25%. Hepatic metabolism results in up to 90% to glucuronides and sulfates (nontoxic). Less than 5% is conjugated by cytochrome P450 CYP2E1 to a toxic metabolite, N-acetyl-p-benzo-quinone imine (NAPQI).

- NAPQI is irreversibly conjugated by glutathione; however in an overdose, this pathway is overwhelmed and binds to macromolecules in the hepatocyte causing cell death and hepatic necrosis.

Side Effects/Adverse Reactions

- Acetaminophen overdose results in more calls to the poison control centers in the United States than overdose of other pharmacological substance. Furthermore, toxicity is the most common cause of acute liver failure in the United States; 307 cases were reported to the US FDA from January 1998 to July 2001 (40% mortality). Patients present with coagulopathy, hepatic encephalopathy, and renal failure; massive overdose can produce coma, hyperglycemia, and lactic acidosis. The Rumack-Matthew nomogram is utilized to predict potential hepatoxicity and indication for acetylcysteine therapy (↓ morbidity). After 4 hrs of ingestion, a serum concentration of acetaminophen is drawn and plotted. The nomogram does not apply to cases of chronic ingestion or multiple doses.

- Coagulation. Unlike NSAIDS, does not influence platelet function. However, pts on chronic warfarin therapy who receive 4 grams for 14 days can have an ↑ in INR and a ↓ in vitamin K dependent clotting factors. Thus, consider monitoring PT/INR values in these pts when acetaminophen is initiated, or during sustained therapy with large doses.

- Sensitivity. Dermatologic reactions include pruritic maculopapular rash and urticaria; laryngeal edema, angioedema, and anaphylactoid reactions may occur rarely. Some formulations may contain sulfite, which can cause allergic-type reactions including asthma and anaphylaxis.

- Blood dyscrasias. p-aminophenol derivatives may cause thrombocytopenia, leukopenia, and pancytopenia (especially with prolonged use, large doses). Acetaminophen may cause neutropenia, agranulocytosis, and thrombocytopenic purpura.

- Anticonvulsants (including pheyntoin, barbiturates, carbamazepines) that induce hepatic microsomal enzymes ↑ acetaminophen conversion to hepatotoxic metabolites. Use and dosage should be limited.

- FDA pregnancy risk factor: B. Adequate, well-controlled studies in pregnant women have not shown increased risk of fetal abnormalities despite adverse findings in animals, or, in the absence of adequate human studies, animal studies showed no fetal risk. The chance of fetal harm is remote but remains a possibility.
- The benefit of rectal administration is restricted by slow onset time and unpredictable bioavailability.

Dosages/Preparation

- Adult dosing: PO 650–1000mg q4 hrs prn; max 4000 g/24 hrs. Rectal: 650–1000 mg q4–6 hrs; max 6 suppositories/ 24 hrs. Chronic renal disease: no dosage adjustments, however, consider ↑ intervals to 6 hrs in moderate renal failure, and 8 hrs with severe renal failure. Chronic hepatic disease: therapeutic doses may be safely administered
- Pediatric dosing: 10–15 mg/kg/dose orally every 4–6 hours; max 5 doses/day. Age 1 to 3 years: 80 mg rectally q4 hrs. Age 3 to 6 years: 120–125 mg rectally q4–6 hrs; max 720 mg/24 hours. Age 6 to 12 years: 325 mg PO q4–6 hrs; max 2.6 g/24 hrs

Clinical Case Scenario

A 57-year-old male underwent an emergent right inguinal hernia repair for strangulation. His history is significant for alcohol abuse. He drinks 12 cans of beer a day. He was sent home on POD 5 on percocet (5/325mg) two tablets every 4–6 hours as needed for pain. One week later, he was in the emergency room with malaise, nonspecific abdominal pain, nausea, and vomiting. He admitted to have taken additional doses due to inadequate pain control. Physical exam showed hepatomegaly and icteric sclerae with diffuse abdominal tenderness. Labs showed total bilirubin -3.5 mg/dl ALP -300 IU/ml, AST-3750 IU/ml and ALT 3960 IU/ml.

Background: The patient presents with acute liver injury secondary to acetaminophen overdose in the setting of underlying chronic alcohol abuse.

Pathophysiology: This patient likely had depleted glutathione stores due to underlying malnutrition. He also probably had cytochrome enzyme induction from chronic alcohol use leading to rapid accumulation of toxic intermediate metabolites.

Alternative: Consider therapeutic misadventure as a possible complication even at therapeutic doses of acetaminophen in patients with underlying malnutrition and liver disease. Use opiate analgesics alone instead.

Treatment: Treat with N-acetyl cysteine (NAC) to replete glutathione stores. Recognize and treat complications of acute liver injury such as acidosis, renal failure. Monitor for acute liver failure and hepatic encephalopathy for early referral to a liver transplant center.

References

1. Toussaint K, Yang XC, Zielinski MA, Reigle KL, Sacavage SD, Nagar S, Raffa RB. What do we (not) know about how paracetamol (acetaminophen) works? *J Clin Pharm Ther.* 2010;35(6):617–638.

2. Pickering G, Loriot MA, Libert F, Eschalier A, Beaune P, Dubray C. Analgesic effect of acetaminophen in humans: first evidence of a central serotonergic mechanism. *Clin Pharmacol Ther.* 2006;79:371–378.

3. Pickering G, Esteve V, Loriot MA, Eschalier A, Dubray C. Acetaminophen reinforces descending inhibitory pain pathways. *Clin Pharmacol Ther.* 2008;84:47–51.

4. Douglas D, Sholar J, Smikstein M. A pharmacokinetic comparison of acetaminophen products (Tylenol extended relief vs regular Tylenol). *Acad Emerg Med.* 1996;3:740–744.

5. Larson AM, Polson J, Fontana RJ, et al. Acetaminophen-induced acute liver failure: results of a United States multicenter, prospective study. *Hepatology.* 2005;42(6):1364–1372.

6. *Physicians Desk Reference.* 61st ed. Montvale, NJL Thomson PDR; 2007, p. 1871.

7. McEvoy GK, ed. *American Hospital Formulary Service. AHFS Drug Information.* American Society of Health-System Pharmacists, Bethesda, MD. 2007; p. 2181.

8. Oscier CD, Milner QJ. Peri-operative use of paracetamol. *Anaesthesia.* 2009;64(1):65–72.

9. Mattia A, Coluzzi F. What anesthesiologists should know about paracetamol (acetaminophen). *Minerva Anestesiol.* 2009;75(11):644–653.

Chapter 3.5

Benzodiazepines

Ellen Wang, MD

Clinical Uses

- Anxiolysis and amnesia; often used as a premedication, in IV, IM, or PO form
- Sedation for procedures or ventilated patients; may be administered as an infusion
- Emergence delirium; prophylaxis and treatment
- Withdrawal of abuse drugs
- Induction of anesthesia (high doses); however longer onset and duration than other available induction agents
- Anticonvulsant
- Nausea and vomiting
- Antipruritic effects
- Chronic refractory headache
- Insomnia
- Does not trigger malignant hyperthermia

Pharmacodynamics

- Benzene ring (5 carbon atoms) fused to a seven-member diazepine ring (2 nitrogen atoms, 5 carbon atoms); side groups are responsible for the property variations between drugs of this class
- The GABA neurotransmitter binds to the GABA receptor ($GABA_A$) and results in chloride ion channel opening. When chloride ions flow into the cell, the membrane becomes hyperpolarized and neuron firing is inhibited. Benzodiazepines bind to the alpha subunit at $GABA_A$ and enhance the effects of GABA neurotransmitter; results in increased frequency of chloride channel opening, hyperpolarization, and inhibition of neuron firing.
- A "ceiling effect" exists with respect to CNS depression. Additionally, differential properties are the result of different receptor subtypes and/or concentration-dependent receptor occupancy (20% receptor occupancy = anxiolysis; 30–50% occupancy = sedation; > 60% occupancy = hypnosis). The reduced electrical activity results in a proportional reduction in $CMRO_2$ and CBF, decreasing ICP; does not affect cerebrovascular autoregulation.

Additionally, decreases IOP (does not protect against transient increases during laryngoscopy, intubation); reduces the MAC of volatile anesthetics (up to 30%); anterograde amnesia (from there-on and forward); anticonvulsant effects (burst-suppression pattern at high doses); spinally mediated muscle relaxant properties; minimal effect on SSEPs (less than volatiles); no neuro-protective activity or intrinsic analgesic properties.

- Cardiac. Minimal cardiovascular effects, though decreases SVR and BP with large doses; decreased preload/afterload; depresses compensatory barore-ceptor reflex mechanisms
- Pulmonary. Dose-dependent respiratory depression (pronounced when coad-ministered with other respiratory depressants); decreased TV and MV; tran-sient rightward shift in the CO_2 response curve; blunts upper airway reflexes/swallowing reflex

Pharmacokinetics

- Onset. Rapid distribution to vessel-rich groups; lipid solubility increases onset.
- Elimination. Hepatic p450 metabolism (oxidation and glucuronide conjuga-tion); metabolites are excreted in the urine. Metabolism is decreased with severe liver disease, advanced age, and drugs that bind cytochrome P-450 (cimetidine).

Side Effects/Adverse Reactions

- Burning with injection
- Cytochrome P450 interactions. Inhibitors (erythromycin, clarithromycin, cimetidine) will decrease clearance and enhance sedative effects, inducers (rifamycin, phenytoin) will decrease effects.
- Paradoxical reactions; caution in depressed patients (can result in hypomania/mania, and worsening of suicidal ideation)
- Nausea, vomiting, diarrhea
- Pregnancy-Risk Category D (positive evidence of risk to human fetus; poten-tial benefits may still justify its use during pregnancy); increased risk of birth defects if taken during pregnancy; some drug is excreted in breast milk—recommend discontinue drug or bottle feed
- Schedule IV drug. Risk of dependence or tolerance in long-term use, risk of death if overdose; abrupt withdrawal can lead to seizures; recommend taper of drug, sometimes over months

Diazepam

- Potent; high lipid solubility allows rapid crossing of the BBB. Large Vd, how-ever, results in drug accumulating in fat, particularly with chronic dosing, or elderly or obese pts. This, combined with active metabolites (desmethyldiaz-epam, 3-hydroxydiazepam) leads to prolonged effects; secondary conjugation converts to inactive compounds.

- Heparin can increase free drug concentration by 200% (displaces it from protein-binding sites).
- Prepared in propylene glycol (causes pain on injection), available as a lipid emulsion that is not painful, but has less bioavailability. Good PO absorption from GI tract, however IM injection can be slow, erratic, and painful.

Lorazepam

- Strong GABA receptor binding prolongs effect despite its small Vd (does not redistribute into fat and accumulate). Its poor lipid solubility is responsible for its small Vd and also slows its onset (does not cross BBB easily).
- Directly conjugated to glucuronic acid, forming an inactive compound
- Prepared in propylene glycol solution; well absorbed with PO and IM administration

Midazolam

- Potent due to high lipid solubility and high affinity to $GABA_A$
- Imidazole ring can open and close. Opens in acidic solutions and bestows hydrophilicity (allows preparation in acidic salt solution; pH 3.5). The ring closes in physiologic pH, bestowing lipophilicity and speeding onset (can easily cross cell lipid membranes).
- Decreases vagal tone (BP and HR) to a greater extent than other drugs in its class.
- Oxidation to alpha-hydroxymidazolam (metabolite with minimal activity) and high hepatic clearance (despite high Vd) result in short duration of action. Nonetheless, renal failure may prolong sedation due to metabolite build-up; erythromycin inhibits metabolism, leading to 2- to 3-fold prolongation of effects.
- Good IM absorption

Chapter 4

Muscle Relaxants

Chapter 4.1

Nondepolarizing Neuromuscular Blockers

Jared Feinman, MD and Nina Singh-Radcliff, MD

Clinical Uses/Indications

- Optimize intubating conditions (midline vocal cords and facilitate mouth opening; reduce coughing, gagging)
- Prevent fasciculations and other complications from succinylcholine when a small amount is administered prior (defasciculating dose)
- Optimize surgical conditions
- Optimize conditions for mechanical ventilation (reduce bucking, coughing, breath stacking)

Pharmacodynamics

- Competitive antagonist that blocks neurotransmission at postsynaptic acetylcholine receptors (AchR)
- The action potential (AP) results from cell depolarization (resting potential $\sim-90mV$). When both alpha subunits of the AchR are bound by Ach, it undergoes a conformational change that allows $Na+$, $Ca++$ to flow intracellularly (increases voltage, makes positive). When a membrane threshold of -30 mV is attained (~10–20% of AchR channels opened), voltage gated ion channels open and fully depolarize the membrane, producing the AP.
- Nondepolarizing neuromuscular blockers (NDNMB) compete with Ach at the alpha subunit binding sites; thus, the relative concentrations of the NDNMB and Ach determine whether neurotransmission is blocked.
- In addition to redistribution of NDNMB out of the NMJ, neuromuscular blockade can be reduced by administering an acetylcholinesterase inhibitor (ie, neostigmine). Acetylcholinesterase inhibitors reduce the breakdown of Ach in the NMJ and increases Ach concentration. The increased ratio of Ach to NDNMB increases the incidence that two Ach molecules bind to 2 alpha subunits on the AchR. The result is increased ion channel opening, cell depolarization, and muscle contraction. Reversal, however, is not possible if the concentration of NDNMB at the NMJ is very high (after administration of a large dose); the increase in Ach concentration may not be enough to overcome the neuromuscular blockade.

- Recurarization occurs if the acetylcholinesterase administered (neostigmine) has a shorter half-life than the remaining NDNMB. Despite a period of successful reversal of neuromuscular blockade, the ratio of Ach to NDNMB changes (reduced); results in reduced postsynaptic depolarization and muscle contraction ("weakness").
- Two main chemical classes of NDNMBs: steroidal (-curonium) and benzylisoquinolinium (-acurium). Benzylisoquinoliniums tend to be more potent, slower in onset, are eliminated by the kidneys or Hofmann elimination, and can promote histamine release. Steroidal compounds are less potent with faster onset, are eliminated by the liver, and are not associated with histamine release.
- Divided into short-acting (15–20 min), intermediate acting (20–50 min), and long-acting (>50 min).

Pharmacokinetics

- Recovery from blockade occurs initially through redistribution, but later via metabolism and elimination of the drug (may be prolonged in renal failure).
- Highly ionized molecules with small volume of distribution (hydrophilic, remains in vasculature)
- Potency is inversely related to speed of onset (lower ED_{95} = faster onset of blockade). Less potent medications must be given in larger doses, making more drug molecules available to diffuse into the NMJ, resulting in a faster speed of onset.
- Intubating dose is usually twice the ED_{95}, while dose for muscle relaxation alone is slightly less than the ED_{95}. A rough rule of thumb for intubating dose: administer 1 mL of drug for every 10 kg of pt body weight.
- Monitoring of neuromuscular blockade is performed with a nerve monitor. Two electrodes are applied to the ulnar, facial, or posterior tibial nerves. Recovery of blockade consists of 4 phases that can be followed with the nerve monitor:
- Intense blockade: occurs within 3–6 minutes after administration of drug. No response to TOF or posttetanic count (PTC).
- Deep blockade: no TOF but PTC ≥1 present. The number of PTC twitches elicited is proportional to the depth of the block.
- Moderate blockade: TOF count 1–3. Degree of blockade (depression of single twitch height) is 90–95% with TOF 1.
- Recovery: Return of fourth TOF twitch. Degree of blockade may still be as high as 60%-85%.

Side Effects/Adverse Effects

- Significant. One retrospective analysis demonstrated that NDNMBs were responsible for 7.3% of deaths; another study showed that they were responsible for 50%-70% of anaphylactic reactions.
- Potential for histamine release (particularly the benzylisoquinolinium compounds; also seen with the steroidal compounds). Can result in erythema, a brief drop in blood pressure, moderate HR increase, and very rarely bronchospasm. Usually seen with the initial dose and can be reduced by injecting slowly.

- The following can potentiate the effects of NDNMBs: inhaled anesthetics (desflurane > sevoflurane > isoflurane > halothane), antibiotics (especially aminoglycosides), hypothermia, magnesium sulfate, lithium, local anesthetics, dantrolene, and tamoxifen.
- The following can antagonize the effects of NDNMBs: calcium, antiepileptic drugs, azathioprine, and steroids.

Pancuronium

- 1 mg/mL in 10 mL vial, or 2 mg/mL in 2 mL or 5 mL vials.
- pH 3.8–4.2. Prepared with sodium acetate and benzyl alcohol as a preservative.
- Adults: Intubating dose 0.1 mg/kg IV. Supplemental dose for relaxation 0.01–0.03 mg/kg IV.
- Pediatrics: Dosage is same as adults, except in neonates, who are very sensitive to NDNMBs. Test dose of 0.02 mg/kg IV should be given in neonates.
- Pancuronium is associated with moderate tachycardia due to decrease in vagal tone, likely due to inhibition of cardiac muscarinic AchRs.

Vecuronium

- Supplied as sterile, buffered cake of crystalline particles in 10 mg or 20 mg vials. May be reconstituted in any common IV fluid. Reconstituted solution is acidic and should not be mixed with alkaline solutions.
- pH 3.5–4.5. Contains citric acid anhydrous, sodium phosphate dibasic anhydrous, mannitol, sodium hydroxide, and/or phosphoric acid.
- Adults: Intubating dose 1 mg/kg IV. Maintenance dose is 0.01–0.015 mg/kg IV. A maintenance infusion can also be started at 1 mcg/kg/min and titrated to 90% twitch suppression. Average infusion rates are 0.8–1.2 mcg/kg/min.
- Pediatrics: Age > 10 dosage is same as adults. Children < 10 years may require higher doses.

Atracurium

- Utilized in renal or hepatic disease
- 10 mg/mL.
- pH 3.25–3.65. Benzenesulfonic acid added for pH adjustment and benzyl alcohol added as preservative. Should be refrigerated.
- Adults: Intubating dose 0.5 mg/kg IV. Maintenance dose 0.08–0.1 mg/kg IV or an infusion of 5–9 mcg/kg/min IV can be run.
- Pediatrics: Dose is the same in children > 2 years of age. In children < 2 years the intubating dose is 0.3–0.4 mg/kg IV.

Cisatracurium

- Utilized in renal or hepatic disease
- 2 mg/mL in 5 mL and 10 mL vials, and 10 mg/mL in 20 mL vials.
- pH 3.25–3.65, adjusted with benzenesulfonic acid. The 10 mL vial contains benzyl alcohol as a preservative. Should be refrigerated.
- Adults: Intubating dose 0.2 mg/kg IV. Maintenance dose 0.03 mg/kg IV or infusion at 1–2 mcg/kg/min IV.
- Pediatrics: Children aged 2–12 years, intubating dose 0.1–0.15 mg/kg IV. Children < 2 years of age, intubating dose 0.15 mg/kg IV.

Rocuronium

- Alternative for succinylcholine when rapid onset is desired, but succinylcholine contraindicated
- 10 mg/mL.
- pH 4, adjusted by addition of acetic acid.
- Adults: Intubating dose is 0.6 mg/kg IV, or 1.2 mg/kg IV for rapid-sequence intubation. Maintenance dose 0.1–0.2 mg/kg IV. A maintenance infusion can be started at 10–12 mcg/kg/min IV and titrated to twitch response.
- Pediatrics: Intubating dose 0.45–0.6 mg/kg IV.

Mivacurium

- 2 mg/mL. Available in most of the world but not sold in the United States.
- pH 3.5–5, adjusted with HCl. Benzyl alcohol added as a preservative.
- Adults: Intubating dose 0.15–0.25 mg/kg IV. 0.25 mg/kg dose often given as divided dose to minimize hypotension from histamine release. Maintenance dose 0.1 mg/kg IV. Infusion can be started at 5–7 mcg/kg/min and titrated to twitch response.
- Pediatrics: Intubating dose 0.2 mg/kg IV for children 2–12 years old. Mivacurium has not been studied in children under 2 years.
- Acetylcholinesterase-inhibitor administration was suspected to possibly prolong block due to inhibition of plasma cholinesterase and reduced drug breakdown, but this effect is dwarfed by the increase in Ach at the NMJ and has no real clinical significance.

Clinical Case Scenario

A 45-year-old woman is undergoing a laparoscopic cholecystectomy. She has received several doses of vecuronium during the case, and is now 1/4 on TOF at the facial nerve at the end of the case. After reversal she is 4/4 on TOF and is extubated. She quickly develops respiratory distress and has to be reintubated.

Significant neuromuscular blockade (about 70%) may still be present with 4/4 twitches on TOF. As a result, TOF is less reliable than other methods like 5-second head lift or hand grip to evaluate suitability for extubation. The location of TOF measurement must also be considered, as distal nerve monitoring (ie, ulnar nerve) is more representative of the ability to maintain upper airway protection than proximal placement (ie, facial nerve).

References

1. Anaesthetists and the reporting of adverse drug reactions. *BMJ (Clin Res Ed)*. 1986;292:949.

2. Mertes PM, Lambert M, Gueant-Rodriguez RM, et al. Perioperative anaphylaxis. *Immunol Allergy Clin N Am*. 2009;29:429–451.

Chapter 4.2

Succinylcholine

Jared Feinman, MD and Nina Singh-Radcliff, MD

Clinical Uses/Indications

- Rapid sequence intubation
- Optimize intubating conditions when rapid onset or short duration is desired
- Short surgical procedures
- Electroconvulsive therapy
- Infusion for surgical procedures requiring profound relaxation (laryngoscopies)
- Provide muscle relaxation at end of case when only short duration is needed
- Optimize insertion and placement of laryngeal mask airway

Pharmacodynamics

- Diacetylcholine; 2 acetylcholine (Ach) molecules linked through acetate methyl group.
- Only clinically approved depolarizing neuromuscular blocker today. Succinylcholine is an acetylcholine receptor (AchR) agonist; provides sustained, but reversible muscle cell depolarization that prevents subsequent depolarization and muscle activity.
- Normal neuromuscular junction (NMJ) physiology: Site where nerve action potential (AP) is transmitted/transformed into a muscle AP by Ach neurotransmitter. When the nerve AP reaches the NMJ, Ach storage vesicles in the prejunction are released into the NMJ and bind to AchR on the postjunctional muscle cell. AchR is made up of 5 subunits (two α, and one each of β, δ, and ε) that surround an ion channel. At rest, the channel pore is closed. When Ach binds to both α subunits, the channel opens, Ca^{2+}, Na^+ flow into the cell, K^+ flows out, the membrane depolarizes, Ca++ is released from the sarcoplasmic reticulum (SR) intracellularly, Ca++ binds with troponin/myosin, and the muscle contracts. The AP is terminated by Ach hydrolysis by acetylcholinesterase within the NMJ and reuptake by the prejunctional membrane; the AchR ion channel closes, the membrane potential returns to -90 mV via Na/K ATPase, Ca++ is reuptaken into the SR, and the muscle relaxes.

- Succinylcholine mimics the action of Ach at the NMJ. One succinylcholine molecule binds the two α subunits, which opens the ion channel (Na^+, Ca^{2+} influx ; K^+ efflux) and depolarizes the muscle cell, causing contraction. Unlike Ach, however, succinylcholine cannot be broken down by NMJ acetylcholinesterases and must diffuse out of the NMJ to be broken down by plasma cholinesterases.
- After the muscle contraction induced by succinylcholine, a time-dependent lower gate closes within the AchR, preventing further ion movement. A voltage-dependent upper gate, however, remains open due to the presence of succinylcholine, preventing the muscle end plate from repolarizing. As long as the AchR is in this conformational state it cannot be depolarized again by additional acetylcholine activity. This is the method by which succinylcholine induces neuromuscular blockade.
- Phase I block. Seen with succinylcholine depolarization. Train of four (TOF) = no fade; Posttetanic facilitation (PTF): none, since the effect on the AchR is noncompetitive.
- Phase II block. Seen with repeated boluses, or prolonged infusions that exceed 6 mg/kg; or with genetically abnormal plasma cholinesterase. TOF = fade; PTF = fade (similar to nondepolarizing muscle relaxants). In normal patients, can be antagonized by a cholinesterase inhibitor (may prolong the block in pts with abnormal plasma cholinesterase, use cautiously).

Pharmacokinetics

- ED_{95} = 0.51–0.63 mg/kg (recent studies estimated an ED_{95} < 0.3 mg/kg, indicating greater potency than previously thought).
- Intubating dose = 1 mg/kg IV (2 mg/kg IV for infants and small children); complete suppression of response to neuromuscular stimulation within 60 seconds. May be given IM (dose to 3–4 mg/kg, onset 2–3 m).
- 90% recovery of muscle strength at 9–13 minutes for 1 mg/kg IV dose.
- Hydrolyzed by plasma cholinesterase (pseudocholinesterase) to succinylmonocholine (very weak neuromuscular blocker) and choline. Plasma cholinesterase is extremely efficient (only ~10% of IV dose reaches the NMJ, reducing onset); elimination ½-life ~47 seconds.
- Plasma cholinesterase is only present in plasma (not NMJ). Termination of action requires diffusion back into plasma.
- Plasma cholinesterase activity is reduced in liver disease, advanced age, pregnancy, and with multiple drugs including OCPs, MAOIs, and esmolol (usually clinically insignificant). Maybe significantly prolonged in pts with genetically abnormal plasma cholinesterase, however.
- Dibucaine number. Measures the inhibition of plasma cholinesterase activity; atypical variant is inhibited to a lesser extent than the normal enzyme.
- Avoid administering after neostigmine or other anticholinesterase; these drugs prolongs succinylcholine blockade by inhibiting plasma cholinesterase

- A small dose (5%-10% of ED_{95}) of nondepolarizing NMB given 2 min prior to succinylcholine prevents muscle fasciculation. However, increases muscle resistance to succinylcholine, and dosing by ~50%; may prolong the onset of neuromuscular block.

Side Effects/Adverse Effects

- Cardiovascular. Dysrhythmias; sinus bradycardia (SB) from binding of muscarinic AchRs at SA node. Prominent in young children (can avoid with atropine premedication). Sinus tachycardia may also occur from binding of nicotinic AchRs at the ganglia of sympathetic nerves innervating the heart. Junctional rhythms and ventricular dysrhythmias are also seen.
- Malignant Hyperthermia trigger. Autosomal disorder of SR ryanodine receptor; triggers cause uncontrolled skeletal muscle hypermetabolism (increased CO_2, temperature, O_2 consumption). Masseter spasm, a premonitory sign of MH, may be seen in normal patients after succinylcholine.
- Hyperkalemia. Opening of AchR ion channels allow K^+ efflux from the cell into the circulation. Normally raises plasma K^+ by ~ 0.5mEq/dL. In hyperkalemia, or abnormal proliferation of extrajunctional AchRs (disuse or damage to muscle tissue: hemi- or paraplegia, burn or crush injuries, muscular dystrophy, Guillain-Barre, etc), may cause cardiac dysrhythmias. May use safely in burn or crush injury, within the first 24–48 hrs (length of time for proliferation of AchRs to occur).
- Elevated ICP. Unclear mechanism. Transient; pretreatment with nondepolarizing NMB can attenuate
- Increased intraocular pressure. Mechanism likely due to tonic contraction of myofibrils and/or dilation of choroidal blood vessels, lasts 5–6 min. Cautious use with open globe injuries.
- Increased intragastric pressure. Mechanism likely due to fasciculations of abdominal skeletal muscles. Variable; pretreatment with nondepolarizing NMB may prevent
- Myalgias. May be due to unsynchronized muscle contraction. Neck, back, abdomen. Variable occurrence, increased in minor procedures, ambulatory surgery, and women. May be reduced with defasciculating dose; Mg reduces fasciculation, not myalgias. NSAIDS to treat.
- Pediatrics: routine use in young children is strongly discouraged. Undiagnosed neuromuscular disease (Duchenne's Muscular Dystrophy) can lead to cardiac arrest. If succinylcholine is going to be used, premedication with atropine should occur to prevent severe bradycardia.

Preparation and Dose

- 20 mg/mL
- pH adjusted to 3.5 mL with addition of HCl. Becomes unstable in alkaline solutions.

- 0.1% methylparaben is added as a preservative. Should be refrigerated to prolong potency.
- Adults: Intubating dose 0.5–1.5 mg/kg IV. An infusion can also be used with an initial rate of 0.5–10 mg/min and a maintenance rate of 0.04–0.07 mg/kg (neuromuscular monitoring should be used to prevent overdose [Phase II blockade]).
- Children: Intubating dose 2 mg/kg in infants and small children, 1 mg/kg in older kids. IM dose is 3–4 mg/kg (not to exceed 150 mg).

Clinical Case Scenario #1

A 24-year old man presents to the OR for emergency lower extremity fasciotomy after an MVC. Anesthesia is induced with propofol and succinylcholine and the case proceeds uneventfully. 48 hours later he returns to the OR for closure of his fasciotomy wounds and is again induced with propofol and succinylcholine. As the surgeon is closing, he develops VT and progresses to V fib.

When succinylcholine binds to AchRs, K^+ effluxes into the circulation. This leads to an increase of plasma K^+ level of 0.5 mEq in normal patients, but can cause dangerous hyperkalemia in patients with preexisting neuromuscular disease, burns, or trauma. After an injury it takes 24–48 hrs for AchR upregulation to occur, so succinylcholine can often be used safely in the immediate posttrauma setting. On EKG, hyperkalemia will present with peaked T waves, widened QRS, and finally VT and V fib.

Clinical Case Scenario #2

An 18-month-old boy presents to the OR for tonsillectomy. An inhalational induction with sevoflurane is done, and he is given succinylcholine to facilitate intubation. He becomes profoundly bradycardic to the 50s, but responds to atropine. As the case progresses he becomes increasingly hyperthermic, and hypercarbic, eventually developing severe hemodynamic instability. The boy as treated with dantrolene and transferred to the ICU.

MH can be triggered by succinylcholine. Its use is often avoided in young children, especially boys, who may have undiagnosed muscular dystrophy and associated MH. If succinylcholine is used in children, it should be administered with atropine or glycopyrrolate to counteract bradycardia.

Reference

1. Kopman AF, Klewicka MM, Neuman GG. An alternate method for estimating the dose-response relationships of neuromuscular blocking drugs. *Anesth Analg.* 2000;90:1191–1197.

Anticholinergics and Anticholinesterases

Chapter 5.1

Anticholinesterases

Devin Tang, MD and Anita Gupta, DO, PharmD

Clinical Uses/Relevance to Anesthesiology

- "Reversal" of neuromuscular blockade; increases acetylcholine (Ach) at neuromuscular junction (NMJ). Given in conjunction with antimuscarinic drugs
- Myasthenia gravis (MG) diagnosis and treatment.
- Alzheimer's Disease symptomatic treatment
- Anticholinergic syndrome treatment
- Chronic primary open-angle glaucoma; topical treatment
- Postoperative delirium in the elderly

Pharmacodynamics

- Acetylcholinesterase enzyme (AChE) is found in the NMJ, sympathetic and parasympathetic nervous system, and brain. It is responsible for breaking the Ach neurotransmitter down into choline and acetate. Ach functions as a neurotransmitter at both muscarinic and nicotinic receptors. However, Ach receptor antagonists, NMBD and antimuscarinics, are specific to nicotinic and muscarinic Ach receptors, respectively.
- Anticholinesterase drugs reversibly bind to the enzyme and prevent the breakdown of Ach; indirectly increasing Ach.
- NMJ. Neuromuscular blocking drugs (NMBD) compete with Ach at the nicotinic Ach receptors and prevent neurotransmission/muscle contraction. Their action is terminated by diffusion away from the NMJ and metabolism by the liver, kidneys, bile, or pseudocholinesterase. When faster recovery is desired, anticholinesterases can be administered to block Ach breakdown. By increasing levels of Ach neurotransmitter available to compete with NMBD at nicotinic Ach receptors, neurotransmission/muscle contraction can be reestablished. Additionally, edrophonium may have prejunctional effects that enhance release of Ach; and neostigmine has a direct agonist effect on nicotinic receptors in the NMJ
- Myasthenia Gravis. Autoimmune disease where abnormal production of antibodies results in blocking and destroying nicotinic Ach receptors; prevents normal Ach neurotransmitter binding and muscle contraction.

Anticholinesterases are utilized for symptomatic treatment by increasing Ach levels to compete with the antibodies and compensate for the reduction in available Ach receptors. Pyridostigmine is commonly utilized due to its greater duration of action (requires reduced frequency).

- Sympathetic nervous system (SNS) and parasympathetic nervous systems (PNS). The PNS releases Ach neurotransmitter at both the preganglionic (muscarinic and nicotinic receptors) and postganglionic junctions (muscarinic receptors). Ach binding results in nerve transmission to the heart (bradycardia), lungs (increased respiratory secretions and bronchoconstriction), and GI tract (peristaltic activity and glandular secretions). The SNS release Ach at the preganglionic junction (nicotinic and muscarinic) only; the postganglionic junction releases noradrenaline. Anticholinesterases increase Ach throughout the SNS and PNS

- Alzheimer's disease may be due to abnormal destruction of cholinergic neurons; results in reductions of Ach levels. PO anticholinesterases capable of crossing the BBB are utilized for symptomatic treatment [donepezil (*Aricept*), galantamine (*Razadyne*), and rivastigmine (*Exelon*)]. They are not curative.

- Anticholinergic syndrome. Results from the competitive antagonism with Ach at muscarinic Ach receptors. Signs and symptoms include "dry as a bone, red as a beet, hot as a hare, blind as a bat, mad as a hatter, stuffed as a pipe" ; and refers to the inhibition of sweating, flushing, mydriasis, delirium, and ileus that can result. Can result from antihistamines, antiparkinson drugs, antipsychotics, antispasmodics, plants, TCAs, and opthalmics. Physostigmine is often used as an antidote since it can cross the BBB; however, if the diagnosis is incorrect, can result in cholinergic toxicity

- Chronic primary open-angle glaucoma. Degenerative process in the trabecular meshwork, including deposition of extracellular material within the meshwork and beneath the endothelial lining of Schlemm's canal. Echothiophate irreversibly inhibits acetylcholinesterase, causing miosis, thereby facilitating the outflow of aqueous humor, and reducing intraocular pressure

- Postoperative delirium. Elevated serum anticholinergic activity in pts with delirium suggests that cholinergic medications (or anticholinesterases) may be useful in treatment. IM neostigmine has been shown to improve symptoms within 10–15 minutes, lasting up to 1 hour. PO neostigmine and pyridostigmine can provide clinical improvement up to 6 hrs.

Pharmacokinetics

- Hepatic metabolism (25%-50%) and renal excretion (50%-75%)

Side Effects/Adverse Reactions

- Prolongation of succinylcholine. Anticholinesterases have variable inhibitory effects on pseudocholinesterase (plasma enzyme that metabolizes succinylcholine) as well as increases motor end plate potential by increasing Ach in the NMJ

- Cholinergic crisis can occur with overdosage or incorrect administration of anticholinesterases. An abnormal increase in Ach can result in increased salivation, bradycardia, miosis, diarrhea, and weakness.

- Unwanted muscarinic effects. Although anticholinesterases are most commonly administered to reverse NMBD at nicotinic Ach receptors, the increased Ach neurotransmitter can combine with nicotinic and muscarinic Ach receptors. The muscarinic receptor response includes bradycardia, bronchoconstriction, mydriasis, flushing, and increased GI motility. Coadministration with an antimuscarinic to match onset and duration can prevent this.

Neostigmine

- The carbamate moiety covalently binds to AChE
- Lipid insoluble due to quaternary ammonium group; does not cross the BBB. Therefore, not useful for delirium or Alzheimer's therapy.
- Available in 10 mL vial of 1mg/mL, 0.5 mg/mL, or .25 mg/mL
- *Dosing:* 0.04–0.08 mg/kg (up to 5 mg in adults)
- Recommended anticholinergic: glycopyrrolate 0.2 mg per mg of neostigmine
- May cross placenta, high doses can result in Ach receptor blockade; Side effects: nausea, vomiting, fecal incontinence, delayed recovery room discharge, bradycardia

Pyridostigmine

- The carbamate moiety covalently binds to AChE
- Lipid insoluble due to quaternary ammonium group; does not cross the BBB. Therefore, not useful for delirium or Alzheimer's therapy
- Available in 5 mg/mL solution
- *Dosing:* 0.1 0.4 mg/kg (up to 20 mg in adults)
- Recommended anticholinergic: glycopyrrolate 0.05 mg per mg of pyridostigmine

Edrophonium

- May be more effective than neostigmine for reversal of mivacurium blockade; may have less muscarinic effects than neostigmine or pyridostigmine; useful to differentiate cholinergic crisis from MG weakness (quick onset and offset)
- Noncovalently binds to AChE.
- Lipid insoluble due to quarternery ammonium group; does not cross the BBB. Therefore, not useful for delirium or Alzheimer's therapy
- Available in 10 mg/mL solution. Also available with atropine as combination drug (10 mg edrophonium & 0.14 mg atropine / mL)
- *Dosing:* 0.5–1 mg/kg
- Recommended anticholinergic: atropine 0.014 mg per mg of edrophonium

Physostigmine

- Utilized for delirium, anticholinergic overdose, and prevention of postoperative shivering due to its ability to cross the BBB (lacks quaternary ammonium group and is lipid soluble); not useful for NMBD reversal
- The carbamate moiety covalently binds to AChE
- Metabolized by plasma esterases
- Available in 1 mg/mL solution.
- *Dosing:* 0.01–0.03 mg/kg
- Clinical dosages rarely cause bradycardia (though anticholinergic should be immediately available when using this drug)

Clinical Case Scenario

A 68-year-old female was admitted to the hospital 1 week ago for SBO. Conservative therapy was initially implemented with NG tube and IV fluids. Earlier this AM, however, the patient developed localized abdominal tenderness with rebound. The surgeon decides to take her to the OR for an exploratory laparotomy. Her past medical history includes a TAH/BSO 4 years ago. She has no known allergies. Her height is 4'10" and she weighs 90 pounds. Her labs show a WBC count of 15 000, a progressively worsening metabolic acidosis, normal electrolytes. Although the patient has been NPO, she still continues to drain from her NG tube. She has been induced with RSI using propofol, succinylcholine, fentanyl. She is maintained with isoflurane, vecuronium, and 1.5 mg hydromorphone. Intraoperatively, small bowel perforation was found and the area of small bowel was resected. At the end of the case, pt had 3/4 twitches at the end of the case, and the patient was reversed with 5 mg of neostigmine with 0.6 mg glycopyrrolate. Just prior to extubation, there was no end-tidal isoflurane detected, pt had been breathing 450 mL tidal volume with PS 8 cm H2O just prior to reversal. She followed commands and was subsequently extubated. During transport, the patient appeared somnolent, and in the PACU, the pt was apneic and unresponsive. She was reintubated and transferred to the SICU for further management. Several hours later, the patient was breathing spontaneously again and successfully extubated.

Discussion

The patient received a large dose of neostigmine (>5 mg/kg) for her weight. This resulted in an excess of Ach in the synapse and a desensitization of the postsynaptic receptor. Clinically, flaccid paralysis and respiratory failure was observed.

References

1. Morgan GE, Mikhail MS, Murray MJ. *Clinical Anesthesiology.* 4th ed. New York: Lange Medical Books/McGraw-Hill Medical Publishing Division; 2006.

2. Geula C, Mesulam MM. Cholinesterases and the pathology of Alzheimer disease. *Alzheimer Dis Assoc Disord.* 1995;9(Suppl 2):23–28.

3. Stahl SM. The new cholinesterase inhibitors for Alzheimer's disease, Part 2: illustrating their mechanisms of action. *J Clin Psychiatry.* 2000;61(11):813–814.

4. Birks J. (2006). Cholinesterase inhibitors for Alzheimer's disease. *Cochrane Database Syst Rev.* 2006;(1):CD005593.

5. Cole MG. Delirium in elderly patients. *Am J Geriatr Psychiatry.* 2004;12(1):7–21.

6. Cohen JA, Oosterbaan RA, Berends F. Organophosphorus compounds. *Meth Enzymol.* 1967;11:686.

7. Wax PM. Anticholinergic toxicity. In: Tintinalli JE, ed. *Emergency Medicine: A Comprehensive Study Guide.* Chapter 183. New York: McGraw-Hill, Medical Pub. Division; 2004.

8. Ropper AH, Samuels MA. Myasthenia gravis and related disorders of the neuromuscular junction. In: Victor M, Ropper AH, Adams RD, Samuels MA, eds. *Adams and Victor's Principles of Neurology.* Chapter 53. New York: McGraw-Hill Medical; 2009.

9. Hill GE, Stanley TH, Sentker CR. Physostigmine reversal of postoperative somnolence. *Can Anaesth Soc J.* 1977;24(6):707–711.

10. Pestronk A. *Autonomic pharmacology & physiology.* Neuromuscular Disease Center. 18 Feb 2002. http://neuromuscular.wustl.edu/nother/autonomic/autonfcn.htm.

11. Acetylcholinesterase inhibitor. *Wikipedia.* 28 June 2010. http://en.wikipedia.org/wiki/Acetylcholinesterase_inhibitor.

12. Neostigmine methylsulfate injection. Drugs.com. http://www.drugs.com/pro/neostigmine-methylsulfate-injection.html.

13. Edrophonium. Drugs.com. http://www.drugs.com/mtm/edrophonium.html.

14. Physostigmine salicylate. Drugs.com. http://www.drugs.com/ppa/physostigmine-salicylate.html.

15. Pyridostigmine. Drugs.com. http://www.drugs.com/cdi/pyridostigmine.html.

16. Echothiophate iodide. Drugs.com. http://www.drugs.com/ppa/echothiophate-iodide.html.

Chapter 5.2

Anticholinergics

Anita Gupta, DO, PharmD and Amna Mehdi, BS

Clinical Uses/Indications

- Anticholinergic drugs are used for treating neurologic as well as nonneurologic disorders.
- Anticholinergic drugs are used in treating a variety of conditions, such as disorders of gastrointestinal (including nausea and vomiting), genitourinary, and respiratory systems.
- Atropine, an anticholinergic agent, is used as premedication in anesthesia to reduce upper respiratory secretions.

Pharmacodynamics

- Anticholinergics are substances that block the neurotransmitter acetylcholine in the central and peripheral nervous systems and are administered to reduce the effects mediated by acetylcholine on acetylcholine receptors in neurons through competitive inhibition.
- Anticholinergic agents are classified into 2 categories according to the receptors that they act on:

  1. Antimuscarinic agents constitute the majority of anticholinergic drugs; they act on the muscarinic acetylcholine receptors.
  2. Antinicotinic agents act on the nicotinic acetylcholine receptors. The majority of these are nondepolarizing skeletal muscle relaxants for anesthetic use.

- A classical example of antimuscarinic agents is atropine, which blocks acetylcholine receptor sites, opposes the actions of the vagus nerve, increases firing of the sinoatrial node and conduction through the atrioventricular node of the heart, and decreases bronchiole secretions.
- Atropine is used to lower the parasympathetic activity of PNS-mediated muscles and glands regulated by the parasympathetic nervous system because acetylcholine is the main neurotransmitter used by the parasympathetic

nervous system. Therefore, it may cause swallowing difficulties and reduced secretions.

Pharmacokinetics

- Anticholinergic compounds compete with ACh and other muscarinic agonist for a common binding site on the muscarinic receptor. Since antagonism by atropine is competitive, it can be overcome if the concentration of ACh at muscarinic receptor of the effectors organ is increased sufficiently.

Side Effects/Adverse Effects

- Anticholinergic syndrome
- Anhidrosis: Sweat glands are innervated by muscarinic receptors, so anticholinergic medications produce dry skin.
- Anhydrotic hyperthermia: Interference with normal heat dissipation mechanisms (ie, sweating) frequently leads to hyperthermia.
- Cutaneous vasodilation: occurs as a means to dissipate heat by shunting blood to the skin, in order to compensate for the loss of sweat production
- Nonreactive mydriasis: muscarinic input contributes to both pupillary constriction and effective accommodation. Anticholinergic medications generally produce pupillary dilation and ineffective accommodation that frequently manifests as blurry vision.
- Delirium, hallucinations: blockade of muscarinic receptors in the central nervous system (CNS) accounts for these findings. Manifestations may include: anxiety, agitation, dysarthria, confusion, disorientation, visual hallucinations, bizarre behavior, delirium, psychosis, coma, and seizures.
- Urinary retention: the detrusor muscle of the bladder and the urethral sphincter are both under muscarinic control; anticholinergic substances reduce detrusor contraction thereby reducing or eliminating the desire to urinate and prevent normal opening of the urethral sphincter
- Tachycardia

Atropine

- Adult Dosage: Inhibit salivation and secretions (preanesthesia): IM, IV, SubQ: 0.4–0.6 mg 30–60 minutes preop and repeat every 4–6 hours as needed. Oral: 0.4 mg; may repeat in 4 hours if necessary; 0.4 mg initial dose may be exceeded in certain cases and may repeat in 4 hours if necessary
- Adult Dosage: Bradycardia: IV: 0.5 mg every 3–5 minutes, not to exceed a total of 3 mg or 0.04 mg/kg
- Adult Dosage: In adjunct to neuromuscular blockade reversal: IV: 25–30 mcg/kg 30–60 seconds before neostigmine or 7–10 mcg/kg 30–60 seconds before edrophonium

- Pediatric Dosage: Inhibit salivation and secretions (preanesthesia): Oral, IM, IV, SubQ: Children <5 kg: 0.02 mg/kg/dose 30–60 minutes preop then every 4–6 hours as needed. Use of a minimum dosage of 0.1 mg in neonates <5 kg will result in dosages >0.02 mg/kg. There is no documented minimum dosage in this age group. Children >5 kg: 0.01–0.02 mg/kg/dose to a maximum 0.4 mg/dose 30–60 minutes preop; minimum dose: 0.1 mg
- Pediatric Dosage: Bradycardia: IV, IO: 0.02 mg/kg, minimum dose 0.1 mg, maximum single dose: 0.5 mg; may repeat once in 3–5 minutes to a maximum total dose of 0.04 mg/kg or 1 mg

Glycopyrolate

- Adult Dosage: Reduction of secretions: Preoperative: IM: 4 mcg/kg 30–60 minutes before procedure, Intraoperative: IV: 0.1 mg repeated as needed at 2- to 3-minute intervals
- Adult Dosage: Reversal of neuromuscular blockade: IV: 0.2 mg for each 1 mg of neostigmine or 5 mg of pyridostigmine administered or 5–15 mcg/kg glycopyrolate with 25–70 mcg/kg of neostigmine or 0.1–0.3 mg/kg of pyridostigmine
- Pediatric Dosage: Reduction of secretions: Preoperative: IM: <2 years: 4–9 mcg/kg 30–60 minutes before procedure, >2 years: 4 mcg/kg 30–60 minutes before procedure, Intraoperative: IV: 4 mcg/kg not to exceed 0.1 mg; repeat at 2- to 3-minute intervals as needed

Scopolamine

- Adult Dosage: Antiemetic: SubQ: 0.6–1 mg, Preoperative: IM, IV, SubQ: 0.3–0.65 mg
- Pediatric Dosage: Antiemetic: SubQ: 0.006 mg/kg, Preoperative: IM, IV, SubQ: Children 6 months to 3 years: 0.1–0.15 mg, Children 3–6 years: 0.2–0.3 mg

Clinical Case Scenario

A 55-year-old man is undergoing thoracic surgery. Patient is given atropine to block responses to vagal reflexes like increase in bronchospasm and secretions, which are induced by surgical visceral traction of the chest wall. Atropine or glycopyrolate is used with neostigmine to block parasympathomimetic effects when neostigmine is used to reverse skeletal muscle relaxation after surgery.

Reference

1. Su M, Goldman, M . Anticholinergic poisoning. *UpToDate*. Jan. 2011. Web. 03 Nov. 2011. <http://www.uptodate.com.ezproxy.lmunet.edu/contents/anticholinergic-poisoning?source=search_result>.

Chapter 6

Vasopressors and Inotropes

Priscilla Nelson, MD, Jonas A. Nelson, MD, and
Nina Singh-Radcliff, MD

Clinical Uses/Relevance to Anesthesiology

- Treatment for hypoperfusion and shock; improves and preserves perfusion to organs and tissues
- Vasopressors constrict veins and arteries; ↑ preload (↑ SV directly, ↑ SBP indirectly) and ↑ afterload (↑ DBP and MAP)
- Inotropes ↑ myocardial chronotropy (↑ HR), ↑ contractility (↑ SV, ↑ CO, ↑ SBP, and ↑ MAP), and lusiotropy
- Drug selection should be based on the underlying etiology of hypotension or shock. Dose should be titrated to effect and requires careful assessment of vital signs, invasive monitor measurements, clinical signs of perfusion, and labs. If increasing doses are not yielding the desired effects or are producing side-effects, a second agent may be chosen or coadministered to augment perfusion via a different mechanism.

Pharmacology

- Adrenergic receptors are ubiquitous in the CNS and periphery; receptor activation can result in myocardial, vascular and nonvascular smooth muscle, and metabolic effects. Furthermore, vasopressors and inotropes often have affinities to more than one receptor (often dose-dependent). Thus, a clear understanding of receptor location and physiologic response is necessary when choosing and utilizing these potent medications.
- α-1 Receptor. Gq coupled receptor located mostly on postsynaptic sympathetic nerve terminals on vascular as well as nonvascular smooth muscle (veins and arteries in the heart, brain, skin, GI tract, and kidneys; ureters, uterus, GI tract, and sphincters). Receptor binding results in activation of phospholipase C, which in turn ↑ IP_3 and Ca^{++}, resulting in contraction. In vascular smooth muscles, this results in ↑ preload (↑ SV with resultant ↑ SBP, ↑ MAP) and ↑ afterload (↑ DBP, ↑ SVR, and ↑ MAP). In the myocardium, receptor activation ↑ the duration of myocardial contraction *without* ↑ chronotropy (↑ SV and ↑ CO). In the liver and fat cells, glycogenolysis and gluconeogenesis take place (metabolic effects). Sphincter receptor activation causes contraction.

- α-2 Receptor. Gi coupled receptor that is located on presynaptic and post-synaptic central and peripheral nerves. Possesses a *mixed* effect. *Pre*synaptic receptor binding inhibits adenyl cyclase, which ↓ cAMP and hence protein ki-nase A activation. This results in ↓ noradrenaline release and blunting of sym-pathetic activity (limits α-1 receptor agonist effects). *Post*synaptic receptors are found on blood vessels and cause contraction. Additionally, receptor binding in the GI tract ↓ motility and ↑ sphincter tone; in the pancreas insulin release is ↓ while glucagon is ↑; fat cell lipolysis is ↓; and platelet aggregation may ↑

- β-1 Receptor. Gs coupled receptor located mainly in the heart. Agonist binding converts ATP to cAMP, which results in ↑ inotropy, chronotropy (↑ SA nodal firing), and impulse conduction in the heart. Minimal vasodilation.

- β-2 Receptor. Gs coupled receptor located mostly in vascular and bronchial smooth muscles as well as the uterus and sphincters. Agonist binding converts ATP to cAMP, which ↓ intracellular Ca^{++} and causes vasodilation, broncho-dilation, and uterine and sphincter relaxation. In the liver glycogenolysis and gluconeogenesis occurs; in fat cells lipolysis.

- Dopamine-1 Receptor (D-1). Gs coupled receptor located mostly in the CNS (eg, substantia nigra), but also in mesenteric, cerebral, coronary, and renal vas-cular beds. Agonist binding *activates* adenylyl cyclase, which converts ATP to cAMP with consequent vasodilation (↓ BP) as well as diuresis and natriuresis.

- Dopamine-2 Receptor (D-2). Gi coupled receptor located mostly in the CNS (eg, substantia nigra), but also in the adrenal medulla, heart, sympathetic nerve termi-nals, and kidney (locations and effects overlap with D1 receptors; however quan-titative ratios and signaling cascades differ). Agonist binding *inhibits* adenyl cyclase and ↓ cAMP, resulting in ↓ noradrenaline release (vasodilation) and ↑ GFR

- Vasopressin Receptors (V1,V2,V3). V1 receptors are G-protein coupled receptors located in systemic, brain, splanchnic and coronary arteries; activa-tion stimulates phospholipase C, resulting in vasoconstriction. V2, V3 recep-tors are located in the kidneys and liver; activation stimulates adenylyl cyclase and ↑ cAMP, resulting in an antidiuretic effect and concentration of urine as well as the release of clotting factors.

Norepinephrine

Clinical Uses/Relevance to Anesthesiology

- Potent vasoconstrictor (greater than phenylephrine)
- Vasodilatory, cardiogenic, anaphylactic, and septic shock
- Useful when heart rate stimulation is undesirable

Pharmacodynamics

- Endogenous catecholamine that functions as a neurotransmitter in the CNS and periphery as well as a hormone. In the CNS, it plays a role in alertness and arousal; in the periphery, norepinephrine is released by the postsynaptic terminal of the SNS. It is also secreted into the blood by the adrenal medulla, and functions as a hormone. Negative feedback mechanism exists to down-regulate norepinephrine's effects via α-2 presynaptic receptors.

- Exogenously administered norepinephrine has strong α-1 receptor agonism at higher doses. Binding results in smooth muscle contraction of veins, arteries, and sphincters; the cardiac receptors $\uparrow$ inotropy. Results in $\uparrow$ preload ($\uparrow$ SV, $\uparrow$ SBP/MAP), $\uparrow$ afterload ($\uparrow$ DBP/MAP), and $\uparrow$ contractility ($\uparrow$ SBP, and $\uparrow$ but less pronounced CO). Coronary blood flow $\uparrow$ due to $\uparrow$ DBP and indirect stimulation of cardiomyocytes (release local vasodilators). Metabolic effects include glycogenolysis and gluconeogenesis. Weaker B1-receptor agonism is seen at lower doses and $\uparrow$ chronotropy and inotropy.

Pharmacokinetics

- Rapid onset, duration 1–2 min; half-life 2.5 mins (continuous infusions often utilized)
- Rapid inactivation by catechol-O-methyltransferase (COMT) and monoamine oxidase (MAO) located in the liver, tissues, and nerve synapses; metabolites are renally excreted. Also reuptake by the presynaptic cell.
- β-1 receptor effects at lower dosages, α-1 receptor effects at higher dosages

Side Effects/Adverse Reactions

- Reflex bradycardia from $\uparrow$ BP
- $\uparrow$ myocardial O_2 consumption ($\uparrow$ pressure and volume work; $\uparrow$ contractility)
- Pulmonary vascular resistance $\uparrow$ (caution in pulmonary hypertension)
- Mesenteric ischemia, renal failure, and peripheral hypoperfusion (digit necrosis). Consider simultaneous infusion of low dose dopamine to prevent nephrogenic pathology
- Hepatic blood flow $\downarrow$ may impair clearance of hepatically metabolized drugs
- Tissue necrosis from extravasation into surrounding tissues; treat with phentolamine.
- Hypertension (especially in nonselective β-blockade).
- Cardiac myocyte toxicity from prolonged use; apoptosis through protein kinase A activation and $\uparrow$ cytosolic calcium influx.

Dosages

- IV: 0.01–3 mcg/kg/min; 0.5–1mcg/min with titration to effect

Phenylephrine

Clinical Uses/Relevance to Anesthesiology

- Hypotension postinduction or with spinal anesthesia as well as for aortic stenosis, nitrate or sildenafil usage; peripheral vasoconstriction
- $\uparrow$ coronary perfusion without chronotropic effects; useful in vascular, cardiac patients

- Low SVR (<700 dynes x sec/cm5); not recommended if SVR >1200 dynes x sec/cm^5
- Obstructive hypertrophic cardiomyopathy; ↓ outflow gradient
- Mydriasis
- Paroxysmal supraventricular tachycardia (reflex bradycardia)
- Nasal decongestant and prior to nasotracheal intubation, NG tube placement; vasoconstriction reduces "stuffiness" and reduces bleeding
- Adjunct to local anesthetics (SQ, epidurally, regional blocks); vasoconstriction of surrounding vessels ↓ vasculature uptake (↑ duration and onset, ↓ toxicity)

Pharmacodynamics

- Synthetic, selective and pure α-1 agonist (no beta effect like norepinephrine).
- α-1 receptor binding (coupled to Gq protein and phospholipase C system) ↑ release of Ca^{++} from the sarcoplasmic reticulum, causing vasoconstriction. Results in ↑ preload (↑ SV/SBP) and ↑ afterload (↑ DBP, MAP, and SVR).

Pharmacokinetics

- IV: Rapid onset, duration 15–30 mins; half-life of 5–10 mins
- SQ/IM: onset 10–15 mins; IM duration 30–120 mins (SQ 60 mins)
- Intranasal/mydriatic have longer duration of action
- Termination of action by presynaptic reuptake as well as metabolism in the liver, synapses, and tissues by MAO

Side Effects/Adverse Reactions

- Reflex bradycardia from ↑ BP
- ↑ myocardial O$_2$ consumption; ↑ volume and pressure work
- Pulmonary vascular resistance ↑ (caution in pulmonary hypertension)
- ↓ hepatic blood flow results in impaired clearance of hepatically metabolized drugs
- Tissue necrosis from extravasation into surrounding tissues; treat with phentolamine
- Hypertension (especially in nonselective β-blockade)

Dosages

- Bolus: 50–100 mcg IV; titrate to effect
- Infusion: 0.4–9.1ug/kg/min
- Can be administered IM, SC, IV push, continuous infusion, and nasally
- SVT 50–100 mcg IV bolus, repeat q20–30 seconds; avoid exceeding 500 mcg, SBP >160

Epinephrine

Clinical Uses/Relevance to Anesthesiology

- Cardiac arrest (asystole, pulseless electrical activity, ventricular fibrillation), shock states

- Test dose in epidurals and peripheral nerve blocks to rule out vascular placement
- Coadministration with local anesthetics ↓ toxicity, ↑ duration and hastens onset
- Mast cell stabilization and bronchodilation for reactive airway disease
- Anaphylaxis; mast cell stabilization, blood pressure support, and bronchodilation

Pharmacology

- Endogenous catecholamine that is synthesized by the adrenal medulla in response to ACTH and stress triggers. Functions as a hormone neurotransmitter at α-1, α-2, β-1, and β-2 adrenergic receptors to elicit a coordinated "fight-or-flight" response. ↑ blood flow to vital organs (↑ contractility, HR, SV, CO combined with vasodilation and vasoconstriction to divert blood appropriately) plus ↑ energy substrates to provide the fuel (glucose and fatty acids are ↑ via glycogenolysis, glycolysis, glucagon secretion, and lipolysis). Additionally, ACTH also triggers the cortisol system to simultaneously coordinate the "fight-or-flight" response in a parallel manner. Does not have a negative feedback mechanism.
- Exogenously administered epinephrine binds to α-1, α-2, β-1, and β-2 adrenergic receptors; receptor predilection is determined by dose and location where it is administered. β-1 receptor activation ↑ inotropy, chronotropy, lusiotropy, cardiac conduction (↑ SV, HR, CO, SBP, O_2 consumption). β-2 receptor activation relaxes smooth muscles in the vasculature and bronchial trees (↓ DBP, PIP). α-1 receptor activation results in vasoconstriction; ↑ SVR, SBP, DBP, MAP and hence vital organ perfusion (myocardium, cerebrum) while decreasing nonvital organ perfusion to the splanchnic, intestinal, renal and integumentary systems.

Pharmacokinetics

- Rapid metabolism by COMT and MAO (synaptic cleft, liver, tissues) and uptake (synaptic cleft)
- Metabolites are renally excreted or recycled

Dosages

- Cardiogenic arrest, shock: 1mg IV bolus, q3–5 mins
- Anaphylaxis. 0.5mg IM, repeat q5 mins. 0.3 mg IV (0.3 mL of a 1:1000 solution), repeat q10–15 mins. Continuous IV dose 1–4 mcg/min
- Endotracheal administration 2–2.5 x IV dose (dilute to 10 mL with NS or distilled water prior to administration)
- Asthma. Inhalational form: 1 inhalation, may repeat in 1 min (do not use again for at least 3 hrs). SQ 0.2–0.5 mg (0.2–0.5 mL of a 1:1000 solution), q2 hrs however in severe attacks, may be repeated q20 mins for a maximum of 3 doses

Side Effects/Adverse Reactions

- Ventricular arrhythmias, severe hypertension resulting in cerebrovascular hemorrhage, cardiac ischemia, and sudden cardiac death

- Mesenteric ischemia from vasoconstriction; may be greater than equivalent doses of NE or dopamine in severe shock.
- Cardiac toxicity to arterial walls (high doses) leading to myocardial contraction band necrosis as well as through direct stimulation of myocyte apoptosis.

Ephedrine

Clinical Uses/Relevance to Anesthesiology

- Hypotension (inotropy and vasopressor)
- Prophylactically to prevent hypotension for labor epidural placement (IM)
- Pressor of choice during labor and cesarean section (animal studies demonstrate reduced fetal hypoxia, acidosis, and bradycardia; possibly from increased uterine blood flow)
- Bronchial dilation (IV and oral)
- Increased muscle strength in myasthenia gravis
- Hiccups
- Nasal decongestant

Pharmacodynamics

- Synthetic drug with binding at α-1, β-1, and β-2 receptors, but with less potency (mini epinephrine); direct effect. Indirect sympathomimetic effects via release of endogenous NE stores. Depletion of NE stores, as seen with trauma, multiorgan failure, repeated doses may have $\downarrow$ effects or tachyphylaxis.
- β-1 receptor activation $\uparrow$ inotropy, $\uparrow$ chronotropy, $\uparrow$ coronary blood flow, and $\uparrow$ myocardial O_2 consumption. β-2 receptor activation results in vasodilation, bronchodilation (oral administration results in slower onset, less potent, and longer duration than SQ ephedrine or inhaled epinephrine), and sphincter relaxation. $\uparrow$ glycogenolysis in the liver (less than epinephrine). α-1 receptor activation results in vasoconstriction.
- Conditions for α-1, β-1, and β-2 receptor binding are not dose dependent like epinephrine; factors for predilection are still unclear. Thus, peripheral, cerebral, and pulmonary vessels may either constrict or dilate.
- Central nervous system excitation and treatment of hiccups have unclear mechanism

Pharmacokinetics

- Immediate onset with IV administration; duration up to 1 hr; elimination half-life 3–6 hrs (urine pH dependent)
- Rapid onset (slightly slower and with a longer duration of action compared to epinephrine)
- Excreted renally in unchanged form; small amounts are hepatically metabolized

Dosages

- IV bolus: 2.5–25 mg IV q5–10 min
- IM bolus: 25–50 mg IM, not to exceed 150 mg in 24 hrs

Side Effects/Adverse Effects

- Increased myocardial O_2 consumption
- Arrhythmias (PACs, PVC, VT, and VF); increased occurrence if myocardium is sensitized by other drugs (halothane, digitalis) or ischemic/hypoxic states
- Tachyphylaxis with repeated use; ↓ effect with depleted NE storage states (trauma, multiorgan failure)
- CNS stimulation similar to amphetamines (less pronounced)

Dobutamine

Clinical Uses/Relevance to Anesthesiology

- CHF or cardiogenic shock in the presence of low cardiac output
- Refractory CHF or hypotension where catecholamine vasodilatory effects would be detrimental (eg, phosphodiesterase inhibitors, epinephrine)
- Inotropy (lacks vasodilation) when coming off of CPB

Pharmacodynamics

- Synthetic agent, acts primarily at the β-1 receptor (weak β-2 and α-1 receptor activity with minimal clinical effect).
- β-1 receptor activation ↑ contractility (↑ SV, ↑ SBP) and ↑ HR and hence CO (SV x HR = CO). By ↑ SV/EF, ↓ LVEDP (more complete emptying of the left ventricle) and hence ↑ coronary artery perfusion pressures.
- Lacks vasopressor activity (dilation may occur from β-2 receptor agonism; despite ↓ DBP, MAPs are maintained from ↑ SBP). No endogenous release of norepinephrine (unlike dopamine)

Pharmacokinetics

- Rapid onset 1–10 mins; peak 10–20 mins. Plasma half-life 2 mins.
- Metabolized by MAO and the COMT protein in the liver; metabolites excreted in urine

Side Effects/Adverse Reactions

- Tachycardia can result in severe CHF, RVR in patients with AF, cardiac ischemia, and hypotension; less pronounced than with dopamine
- Hypertension in β-blocked patients.

Dosages

- IV: 0.5–20 mcg/kg/min

Isoproterenol

Clinical Uses/Relevance to Anesthesiology

- Heart transplant recipients for chronotropy (nerve terminals have been severed and require direct action at SA node)
- Induction of arrhythmias during electrophysiology mapping
- Stokes-Adams disease
- Shock with high SVR/vasoconstriction
- Profound beta-blockade or overdose
- AV node heart block
- Carotid sinus hypersensitivity
- Pulmonary embolism ($\uparrow$ CO, $\downarrow$ PAP)
- Diagnosis of coronary artery disease ($\uparrow$ myocardial O_2 demand and unmasks $\downarrow$ supply from atherosclerosis or stenosis)

Pharmacodynamics

- Structurally similar to epinephrine; nonselective beta agonism
- β-1 receptor agonism, $\uparrow$ inotropy, and $\uparrow$ chronotropy results in $\uparrow$ SV $*$ $\uparrow$ HR = $\uparrow$ CO; $\uparrow$ SBP. $\downarrow$ conduction time and refractory period in the AV node.
- β-2 receptor agonism results in vasodilation and bronchodilation; $\downarrow$ DBP, $\downarrow$ preload, $\downarrow$ PIP, $\downarrow$ residual volume; $\uparrow$ glycogenolysis in the liver, $\uparrow$ insulin secretion from the pancreas, $\uparrow$ lipolysis in fat cells

Pharmacokinetics

- Immediate onset, duration 10–15 mins, half-life 2–5 mins
- Oral, sublingual, and rectal administrations have longer onset and duration of action.

Dosage

- Bolus 0.02–0.06 mg (in 1–3 mL of diluted solution)
- IV infusion 5 mcg/min
- IM/SQ 0.2 mg (in 1 mL)

Side Effects/Adverse Reactions

- Tachycardia, which can result in severe CHF, RVR in patients with AF, cardiac ischemia, and hypotension
- Vasodilation resulting in hypotension
- $\uparrow$ myocardial O_2 consumption
- No reduction in mortality with use

Dopamine

Clinical Uses/Relevance to Anesthesiology

- Shock with the goal of ↑ CO, ↑ BP, ↑ UOP
- Post CPB for ↓ CO
- May improve blood flow to renal and mesenteric beds during hypotension
- Hypotension associated with bradycardia

Pharmacodynamics

- Endogenous catecholamine neurotransmitter that binds to dopamine receptors in the brain (substantia nigra, CTZ) and SNS postsynaptic terminals that travel to the kidneys, carotid bodies, cerebral and myocardial arteries, GI, GU, and endocrine systems. Dopamine receptor agonism in the CNS plays a role in cognition, voluntary movement, motivation, mood, sleep, and several other functions. In the periphery, dopamine receptor agonism results in vasodilation, ↑ contractility, and ↑ natriuresis. Negative feedback mechanism exists to down-regulate effects at dopamine receptors in the presynaptic nerve terminal.
- Exogenous dopamine interacts at dopamine, β-1, and α-1 receptors. Receptor predilection depends on dose.
- D-1 receptor agonism (up to 3 mcg/kg/min). Vasodilation in renal, mesenteric, cerebral, and coronary beds. Some evidence that ↑ UOP is due to ↑ RBF and inhibition of aldosterone (↓ renal tubular Na^+ reabsorption, however, renal dose dopamine has not been shown to reduce renal morbidity.
- β-1 receptor agonism (3–10 mcg/kg/min). ↑ SV, ↑ HR, and hence CO; rates >5 mcg/kg/min stimulate the release of NE. Less myocardial O_2 consumption and tachyarrhythmias than isoproterenol.
- α-1 receptor agonism (>10 mcg/kg/min). Vasoconstricting effects predominate; initially in skeletal muscle vascular beds. Higher doses may compromise circulation of the limbs and override the beneficial effects of dopamine (reverse renal dilation and natriuresis). Infusion should be reduced or discontinued if drop in UOP at this rate.
- Indirect effects from NE release from storage sites

Pharmacokinetics

- Onset within 5 min, duration of 10 minutes
- Metabolized by the liver, kidney, and plasma by MOA and COMT. Metabolites are excreted via the kidneys.

Dosages

- D1 receptors: 2–3 mcg/kg/min
- β-1 receptors: 3–10 mcg/kg/min
- α-1 receptors: >10 mcg/kg/min

Side Effects/Adverse Reactions

- Severe hypertension, particularly in patients taking nonselective β blockers.
- Ventricular arrhythmias and cardiac ischemia
- Tissue ischemia or gangrene at high doses (due to α-1 effects).
- Improved mortality in shock has not been demonstrated; improved renal function or renoprotection at renal doses has not been demonstrated

Fenoldopam

Clinical Uses/Relevance to Anesthesiology

- Antihypertensive crisis (alternative to sodium nitroprusside)
- Hypertension postoperatively
- Renal protection in cardiac surgery; potentially ↓ in acute kidney injury and mortality

Pharmacodynamics

- Synthetic, selective D-1 receptor agonist; 6–9 times more potent than dopamine.
- Vasodilation of renal afferent and efferent arterioles results in natriuresis, diuresis, and ↑ RBF

Pharmacokinetics

- Onset 5–15 mins, peak activity 20–120 mins, duration 1 hr, half-life ~ 1 hr
- Metabolized in the liver, metabolites excreted in the kidneys; small percentage excreted in the feces.

Dosages

- Hypertension: IV 0.1–0.8 mcg/kg/min, with incremental titrations of 0.1
- Renoprotective dose: IV 0.1 mcg/kg/min (may vary depending on clinical scenario)

Side Effects/Adverse Effects

- ↑ norepinephrine
- Tachycardia
- Hypotension
- Hypokalemia
- Expensive, and outcome studies are underway

Milrinone

Clinical Uses/Relevance to Anesthesiology

- Acute and refractory CHF, usually NYHA Class III or IV; short-term treatment

- Cardiac surgery for ↓ cardiac output states
- Cor pulmonale (↑ right heart function, dilates pulmonary vasculature)

Pharmacodynamics

- Phosphodiesterase (PDE) inhibitor that blocks phosphodiesterase enzyme from breaking down cAMP to cGMP; thus, ↑ cAMP results in ↑ intracellular Ca^{++} and ↑ myocardial contraction. ↑ SV/EF reduces LVEDP and ↑ coronary perfusion pressure and also ↑ CO (↑ SBP). Additionally, milrinone ↑ myocardial cytoplasmic Ca^{++} uptake by ↑ Ca^{++}-ATPase activity on the sarcoplasmic reticulum; improving lusiotropy. Because it functions via a nonadrenergic receptor mechanism, PDE inhibitors are effective even in the setting of adrenergic receptor down-regulation (eg, heart failure). Lacks chronotropic function.
- Vasodilation results from ↑ cAMP in vascular smooth muscle. In hypotensive pts, consider coadministration of a vasoconstrictor (phenylephrine or norepinephrine) to blunt further ↓ BP
- Lacks tachyphylaxis
- Figure 6.1

Pharmacokinetics

- Onset 5–15 mins, half-life 2.5 hrs (greater than other inotropes)
- Primarily excreted unchanged in the urine

Dosages

- IV Bolus 50 mcg/kg over 10–30 mins; maintenance 0.375–0.75 mcg/kg/min with titration to effect
- Post CPB: Begin 15 mins prior to separation from CPB, followed by 50 mcg/kg IV over 20 mins, and then continuous infusion of 0.5 mcg/kg/min IV for 4 hours.

Side Effects/Adverse Reactions

- Arrhythmias
- Hypotension, cardiac ischemia
- Torsades de Pointes

Vasopressin

Clinical Uses/Relevance to Anesthesiology

- Diabetes insipidus treatment
- Cardiac arrest; has a role in ACLS algorithm
- Refractory shock with adequate fluid resuscitation
- Esophageal variceal bleed
- Refractory hypotension form angiotensin-converting enzyme inhibitors

Pharmacodynamics

- Endogenous peptide hormone primarily responsible for fluid and osmolarity homeostasis. Synthesized in the hypothalamus, stored in the posterior pituitary, and released in response to hyperosmolarity and/or dehydration. It binds to vasopressin receptors in the collecting tubules and increases water permeability in order to reabsorb and conserve water (concentrates urine, reduces urine volume). Additionally, vasopressin receptors are located in several vascular beds and receptor agonism results in vasoconstriction ($\uparrow$ BP).
- Exogenous vasopressin binds to V1, V2, and V3 receptors. V1 receptor agonism activates phospholipase C, which $\uparrow$ SR release of Ca^{++} and results in vascular smooth muscle constriction. Occurs primarily in capillaries and small arterioles, shifting blood flow to vital organs (brain, heart) from splanchnic, muscle, fat, and skin tissues (incorporated into ACLS algorithm).
- V2 receptor binding activates adenylyl cyclase, which $\uparrow$ cAMP and $\uparrow$ water permeability in the luminal surface of the distal convoluted tubule and collecting duct ($\uparrow$ urine osmolarity and $\downarrow$ urine volume)
- Esophageal variceal bleeds are treated by direct arterial injection into celiac or superior mesentery arteries, resulting in constriction of gastroduodenal, superior mesenteric, and splenic arteries (requires angiographic placement of the catheter; may also be given with low dose IV continuous infusion)

Pharmacokinetics

- Immediate onset, half--life 10–20 mins

Dosages

- Pulseless VT/VF 40 units IV single dose. May be administered endotracheally (40 units diluted into 10 mL of NS.
- Shock: 0.01–0.1 units/min
- GI hemorrhage. Continuous IV infusion: 0.5 milliunits/kg/hr. Dose can be doubled q30 minutes to a max of 10 milliunits/kg/hr. Taper off over 24–48 hrs.
- Diabetes insipidus. 5–10 units IM/SQ BID-QID, titrate to serum and urine osmolarity as well as fluid balance and UOP

Side Effects/Adverse Reactions

- Arrhythmias
- Hypertension, $\downarrow$ CO, cardiac ischemia, severe peripheral vasoconstriction (limb ischemia, splanchnic vasoconstriction)
- Overhydration
- Hypersensitivity reactions

Clinical Case Scenario #1

A 65-year-old male with a complicated PMH presents with chest pain radiating to his R shoulder and SOB. He deteriorates clinically in the ED. His pulse is elevated and his blood pressure is 75/40. EKG shows elevated ST segments, and labs reveal an elevated CKMB and Troponin I.

Treatment: The patient received O_2 therapy, nitroglycerin, morphine, and aspirin. With SBP of 75/40, he was initiated on dobutamine at the 0.375 mcg/kg/min (lowest suggested dose) and was titrated upward until his MAP was >65.

Background: The American college of cardiology and the American heart association guidelines for treating hypotension complicating acute myocardial infarction suggest dobutamine as a first-line agent if systolic pressure is between 70 and 100 without signs of shock. If signs of shock exist, therapy with dopamine is suggested. The data supporting use of either agent in these settings is lacking, however. It has been shown, however, that the combination of these agents at low to moderate doses may improve hemodynamics without the side effects seen at higher levels. If systolic pressure is lower than 70, NE may be beneficial. Finally, in cases where vasodilatory shock causing hypotension is refractory to NE treatment vasopressin can be added. Vasopressin has been shown to increase MAP without adversely affecting pulmonary wedge pressure.

Clinical Case Scenario #2

A 23-year-old male was admitted for acute pancreatitis secondary to alcohol abuse. This progressed to hemorrhagic pancreatitis, and after debridement he became febrile to 103, with persistent hypotension with MAPs in the 40s.

Treatment: He underwent fluid resuscitation and was then initiated on a norepinephrine infusion.

Background: The patient described above is likely in septic shock. Vasopressors are indicated to maintain an MAP > 65. The agents of choice are norepinephrine or dopamine. A recent randomized trial, however, showed norepinephrine to be slightly superior to dopamine in this situation as the initial vasopressor. Dobutamine may be utilized if CO remains low on inotropic and vasopressor therapy. Vasopressin may be utilized for salvage therapy, but not as first-line.

Clinical Case Scenario #3

A 57-year-old female with a history of R sided heart failure underwent three vessel, off pump, CABG without complication, but her cardiac index remained slightly low at the end of the procedure.

Treatment: She was initiated on prophylactic milrinone therapy.

Background: No single agent has been found to be superior in this setting, but dobutamine has the best profile of the β agonists, while milrinone increases flow through the graft, reduces MAP, and improves right sided heart performance in pulmonary hypertension. Additionally, both agents were found to improve hemodynamic parameters when used in randomized trial settings. Given the history of right heart failure, milrinone may be a drug of choice.

References

1. Overgaard CB, Dzavik V. Inotropes and vasopressors: review of physiology and clinical use in cardiovascular disease. *Circulation.* 2008;118(10):1047–1056.

2. De Backer D, Biston P, Devriendt J, Madl C, Chochrad D, Aldecoa C, et al. Comparison of dopamine and norepinephrine in the treatment of shock. *N Engl J Med.* 2010;362(9):779–789.

3. Mullner M, Urbanek B, Havel C, Losert H, Waechter F, Gamper G. Vasopressors for shock. *Cochrane Database Syst Rev.* 2004(3):CD003709.

4. Dunser MW, Mayr AJ, Ulmer H, Knotzer H, Sumann G, Pajk W, et al. Arginine vaso-pressin in advanced vasodilatory shock: a prospective, randomized, controlled study. *Circulation.* 2003;107(18):2313–2319.

5. Beale RJ, Hollenberg SM, Vincent JL, Parrillo JE. Vasopressor and inotropic support in septic shock: an evidence-based review. *Crit Care Med.* 2004;32(11 Suppl):S455-S465.

6. Gooneratne N, Manaker S. Uptodate: Use of vasopressors and inotropes. 2010 [updated June 3, 2010; cited 2010 September 1, 2010].

7. Glick DB. Chapter 12 – The autonomic nervous system. In: Miller RD, ed., *Miller's* Anesthesia. Philadelphia: Elsevier Saunders; 2009.

8. Lexicomp, Inc. Uptodate: Drug Information. 1978–2010 [cited October 15, 2010].

9. De Backer D, Creteur J, Silva E, Vincent JL. Effects of dopamine, norepinephrine, and epinephrine on the splanchnic circulation in septic shock: which is best? *Crit Care Med.* 2003;31(6):1659–1667.

10. Jones D, Bellomo R. Renal-dose dopamine: from hypothesis to paradigm to dogma to myth and, finally, superstition? *J Intensive Care Med.* 2005 Jul-Aug;20(4):199–211.

11. Landoni G, Biondi-Zoccai GG, Marino G, Bove T, Fochi O, Maj G, et al. Fenoldopam reduces the need for renal replacement therapy and in-hospital death in cardiovascu-lar surgery: a meta-analysis. *J Cardiothorac Vasc Anesth.* 2008;22(1):27–33.

12. Goldberg LI. Dopamine—clinical uses of an endogenous catecholamine. *N Engl J Med.* 1974;291(14):707–710.

13. Kusano E, Tian S, Umino T, Tetsuka T, Ando Y, Asano Y. Arginine vasopressin inhibits interleukin-1 beta-stimulated nitric oxide and cyclic guanosine monophosphate pro-duction via the V1 receptor in cultured rat vascular smooth muscle cells. *J Hypertens.* 1997;15(6):627–623.

Chapter 7

Antihypertensives

Chapter 7.1

Beta-Blockers

Anita Gupta, DO, PharmD and Amna Mehdi, BS

Clinical Uses/Indications

- Clinically have been effective in the treatment of hypertension, ischemia heart disease, congestive heart failure, and arrhythmias
- Also used as a treatment for akathisia, essential tremor, hypertrophic subaortic stenosis, pheochromocytoma, stable angina, tachydysrhythmias, thyrotoxicosis, congenital heart conditions, and for migraine headache prophylaxis and variceal hemorrhage prophylaxis
- Some beta-blockers have local anesthetic or membrane-stabilizing activity similar to lidocaine that is independent of B blockade. Such drugs include propranolol, acebutolol, carvedilol
- Beta-blockers lower blood pressure in patients with hypertension by blocking B_1 receptors and therefore blocking release of renin from juxtaglomerular apparatus
- Beta-blockers slow the heart rate and decrease myocardial contractility. Beta-blockers can be used to manage patients with acute myocardial infarction. This drug class decreases oxygen demand by reducing heart rate, blood pressure, and contractility, resulting in relief of ischemic chest pain. Bradycardia prolongs diastole and therefore improves coronary diastolic perfusion.
- Beta-blockers are beneficial in patients undergoing PCI, and should be administered intravenously before PCI as well as orally after the procedure
- Beta-blockers are effective in patients treated with antiarrhythmic drugs. The relative risks for all-cause mortality, cardiac death, arrhythmic deaths, and resuscitated cardiac arrest were lower for patients receiving beta-blockers along with amiodarone
- Nonselective B receptor antagonists such as propranolol block B_2 receptors in bronchial smooth muscle causing bronchoconstriction, which can be life threatening in patients with bronchospastic disease. Therefore drugs like celiprolol, which have B_1 receptor selectivity and B_2 receptor partial agonism, can be beneficial.

Pharmacodynamics/Pharmacokinetics

- Inhibition/competitive blockade of beta-adrenergic receptors
- Beta-blockers are distinguished clinically based on their selectivity for beta receptors. The nonselective beta-blockers antagonize both B_1 and B_2 adrenergic receptor. The selective beta-blockers are indicated for patients in whom B_2 receptor antagonism can increase risks like asthma.

Side Effects/Adverse Effects

- Cardiovascular: hypotension, bradycardia, first-degree heart block
- CNS: dizziness, fatigue, depression, sleep disturbances, sexual dysfunction
- Pulmonary: dyspnea, bronchospasm
- Nonselective beta-blockers can delay recovering from insulin induced hypoglycemia

Propranolol

- Can be administered intravenously for management of life threatening arrhythmias or patients under anesthesia. Dose: 1–3 mg administered slowly <1 mg/min
- Akathisia: Oral: 30–120 mg/day in 2–3 divided doses
- Essential tremor: Oral: 40 mg twice daily initially; maintenance doses: 120–320 mg/day
- Hypertension: Oral: 40 mg twice daily; increase dosage every 3–7 days; usual dose: 120–240 mg divided in 2–3 doses/day; maximum daily dose: 640 mg; usual dosage range 40–160 mg/day in 2 divided doses
- Hypertrophic subaortic stenosis: Oral: 20–40 mg 3–4 times/day
- Migraine headache prophylaxis: Oral: 80 mg/day divided every 6–8 hours; increase by 20–40 mg/dose every 3–4 weeks to a maximum of 160–240 mg/day given in divided doses every 6–8 hours
- Pheochromocytoma: Oral: 30–60 mg/day in divided doses
- Post-MI mortality reduction: Oral: 180–240 mg/day in 3–4 divided doses
- Stable angina: Oral: 80–320 mg/day in doses divided 2–4 times/day
- Tachyarrhythmias: Oral: 10–30 mg/dose every 6–8 hours, IV: 1–3 mg/dose slow IVP; repeat every 2–5 minutes up to a total of 5 mg; titrate initial or 0.5–1 mg over 1 minute; may repeat, if necessary, up to a total maximum dose of 0.1mg/kg
- Thyrotoxicosis: Oral: 10–40 mg/dose every 6 hours, IV: 1–3 mg/dose slow IVP as a single dose
- Variceal hemorrhage prophylaxis: Primary prophylaxis: Initial: 20 mg twice daily, Secondary prophylaxis: Initial: 20 mg twice daily

Timolol

- Hypertension: Oral: 10 mg twice daily, increase gradually every 7 days, usual dosage: 20–40 mg/day in 2 divided doses; maximum: 60 mg/day

- Prevention of myocardial infarction: Oral: 10 mg twice daily initiated within 1–4 weeks after infarction
- Migraine prophylaxis: Oral: 10 mg twice daily, increase to maximum of 30 mg/day
- Glaucoma: Ophthalmic: *Solution:* Initial: 0.25% solution, instill 1 drop twice daily into affected eye, increase to 0.5% solution if response not adequate; decrease to 1 drop/day if controlled; do not exceed 1 drop twice daily of 0.5% solution

Carvedilol

- Hypertension: Immediate release: 6.25 mg twice daily, Extended release: 20 mg once daily, maximum dose 80 mg once daily
- Heart failure: Immediate release: 3.125 mg twice daily for 2 weeks, Extended release: 10 mg once daily for 2 weeks
- Left ventricular dysfunction following MI: Immediate release: 3.125–6.25 mg twice daily, Extended release: 10–20 mg once daily

Metoprolol

- Angina: Immediate release: 50 mg twice daily maximum: 400 mg/day, Extended release: 100 mg/day maximum: 400 mg/day
- Atrial fibrillation/flutter, supraventricular tachycardia: IV: 2.5–5 mg every 2–5 minutes maintenance: 25–100 mg twice daily
- Heart failure: Extended release: 25 mg once daily
- Hypertension: Immediate release: 50 mg twice daily; effective dosage range: 100–450 mg/day in 2–3 divided doses, Extended release: 25–100 mg once daily, maximum: 400 mg/day
- Hypertension/ventricular rate control: IV: 1.25–5 mg every 6–12 hours
- Myocardial infarction: Acute: IV: 5 mg every 2 minutes for 3 doses in early treatment of myocardial infarction

Atenolol

- Hypertension: Oral: 25–50 mg once daily, may increase to 100 mg/day
- Angina pectoris: Oral: 50 mg once daily; may increase to 100 mg/day
- Postmyocardial infarction: Oral: 100 mg/day or 50 mg twice daily for 6–9 days

Esmolol

- Intraoperative tachycardia and/or hypertension: (immediate control) IV: Initial bolus: 80 mg (1 mg/kg) over 30 seconds, followed by a 150 mcg/kg/minute

infusion, adjust infusion rate as needed to maintain desired heart rate and/or blood pressure up to 300 mcg/kg/minute
- Supraventricular tachycardia or control of postoperative tachycardia/hypertension: IV: Loading dose: 500 mcg/kg over 1 minute; follow with a 50 mcg/kg/minute infusion for 4 minutes

Acebutolol

- Angina, ventricular arrhythmia: Oral: 400 mg/day, maintenance: 600–1200 mg/day, maximum: 1200 mg/day
- Hypertension: Oral: 400–800 mg/day, maximum: 1200 mg/day
- Chronic stable angina: 400 mg/day in divided doses, maintenance: 600–1200 mg/day, maximum: 1200 mg/day

Labetalol

- Hypertension: Oral: 100 mg twice daily, may increase to usual dose: 200–400 mg twice daily
- Acute hypertension (hypertensive emergency/urgency): IV bolus: 20 mg IV push over 2 minutes, may administer 40–80 mg at 10-minute intervals, up to 300 mg total cumulative dose, IV infusion: 2 mg/minute; titrate to response up to 300 mg total cumulative dose

Clinical Case Scenario

A 68-year-old woman is undergoing vascular surgery. Her past medical history is positive for coronary artery disease, hypertension, diabetes, and cigarette smoking. The surgeon identifies the patient as high cardiac risk and starts beta-blockers. If the patient is not identified until the morning of surgery, intravenous atenolol or metoprolol should be used. If the drug is started prior to the day of surgery, atenolol 25 mg PO QD is an appropriate starting dose. On the day of surgery the anesthesiologist may increase the dose or treat with intravenous beta-blockers. Intravenous metoprolol in 5 mg boluses is used. Standard dose is 10 mg IV to achieve heart rate less than 50 or systolic blood pressure less than 100 mm Hg. Also, it is recommended to continue patient on beta-blockers for 30 day postoperative cardiac care.

References

1. Goodman LS, Brunton LL, Chabner B, Knollmann, BC . *Goodman & Gilman's The Pharmacological Basis of Therapeutics.* New York: McGraw-Hill Medical; 2011.
2. Rosenson, RS, Reeder GS, Kennedy HL. Beta blockers in the management of acute coronary syndrome. *UpToDate.* June 2010.

Chapter 7.2

Other Antihypertensives

Onyi Onuoha, MD and Nina Singh-Radcliff, MD

Vasodilating Drugs

Hydralazine

Clinical Uses/Relevance to Anesthesiology

- Essential HTN refractory to first-line therapy. Often combined with a diuretic (↓ Na^+ retention, ↓ plasma volume) and/or beta-blocker (↓ reflex tachycardia) to prevent undesired side effects
- CHF to ↓ afterload and as a component of multimodal therapy. May ↓ mortality in black pts in combination with isosorbide dinitrate
- Acute treatment for severe, refractory, or malignant HTN or CHF exacerbation due to ↑ afterload.
- Pregnancy-induced hypertension, preeclampsia, eclampsia
- Idiopathic pulmonary hypertension; lacks consistent therapeutic efficacy
- Diagnosis of renovascular HTN

Pharmacodynamics

- HR: ↑ (reflexive); contractility: ↑ (reflexive), cardiac output: ↑ (indirect); BP: ↓; SVR/PVR: ↓ (direct), preload: mild ↓. Overall effect is a maintenance of, or ↑, coronary, cerebral, renal blood flow
- Alpha-1 receptors are located at postsynaptic vascular smooth muscles. Agonism results in a cascade of events that ultimately ↑ Ca^{++} from the endoplasmic reticulum and result in peripheral arterial/arteriolar constriction.
- Hydralazine selectively antagonizes catecholamine and sympathomimetic binding at alpha-1 receptors and inhibits ↑ in intracellular Ca^{++} resulting in vasodilation. This corresponds to ↓ SVR/afterload, ↓ BP (diastolic > systolic), and ↑ HR (reflex sympathetic response/baroreceptor reflex).
- ↓ afterload can result in ↑ SV, which when combined with ↑ HR will ↑ CO (↑ SV x ↑ HR = ↑ CO) and potentially offset some of hydralazine's hypotensive effects by ↑ SBP. Furthermore, ↑ SV will ↓ LVEDP and improve coronary artery perfusion (coronary perfusion = MAP − LVEDP) and O_2 delivery. ↓ afterload will also the ↓ tension and energy that the LV has to expend during contraction (↓ myocardial O_2 consumption)

- Venodilation results in ↓ CVP, ↓ preload, and ↓ RAP; however, because arterial vasodilation is greater than venodilation (and venous pooling), postural hypotension is less likely

Pharmacokinetics

- Onset: IV 10–15 mins; IM delayed
- first-pass hepatic metabolism via acetylation and metabolites are renally excreted (slow acetylators can have prolonged effect; present in up to 50% of population); elimination half-life 2–8 hrs

Dose

- PO: 12.5–50 mg BID (Oral dosing is $^1/_3$ – ¼ that of IV dosing)
- IV: 2.5–20 mg q15–20 mins for HTN (duration 2–4 h); 5–10 mg q 20–30 mins for preeclampsia (infusion of 0.5–10 mg/hr)
- IM: 10–50 mg q6 hrs

Side Effects

- Unpredictable ↓ in BP; more difficult to titrate than SNP or NTG due to its slower onset and longer duration
- Tachycardia ↑ myocardial O_2 consumption (consider beta blockade)
- Compensatory renin stimulation results in aldosterone secretion (↑ Na+ and ↑ fluid retention). Tolerance to antihypertensive effects can develop; consider diuretics to off-set.
- Cerebral autoregulation is affected; vasodilation ↑ blood flow which in turn ↑ ICP
- Perinatal outcomes have not been demonstrated, and may ↓ uteroplacental blood flow
- Diarrhea, nausea and vomiting, headache, palpitations, flushing, depression, drug-induced lupus, blood dyscrasias, peripheral neuritis

Minoxidil

Clinical Uses/Relevance to Anesthesiology

- Malignant or refractory HTN in pts who have failed first-line therapy. Often combined with a diuretic (↓ Na+ retention, ↓ plasma volume), beta-blocker (↓ reflex tachycardia), or methyldopa to minimize adverse effects. Has lost popularity with the advent of newer and safer drugs
- Central balding to promote hair growth

Pharmacodynamics

- HR: ↑ (reflexive); contractility: ↑ (reflexive); cardiac output: ↑ (indirect); BP: ↓; SVR/PVR: ↓ (direct); preload: mild ↓
- Vasodilator via selective alpha-1 receptor antagonism of catecholamines and sympathomimetics at postsynaptic vascular smooth muscles
- ↓ Ca^{++} release from the endoplasmic reticulum resulting in peripheral arterial/arteriolar vasodilation; results in ↓ SVR, ↓ BP (diastolic > systolic), and ↑ HR (reflex sympathetic response/baroreceptor reflex).

Pharmacokinetics

- Absorption: 90% absorbed from the GI tract. Peak levels within 1 hr; elimination half-life 4.2 h
- Metabolism: 90% of drug hepatically metabolized by conjugation with glucuronic acid
- Excretion: mostly renal (renal clearance corresponds to GFR); can be removed by dialysis.

Dose

- Adult: 2.5–10 mg PO QD or BID. Titrate to effect (max 100mg QD)
- Pediatrics: 0.2 mg/kg with titration in 50%-100% increments until optimal BP control; limited data
- Nursing: excreted in breast milk. Avoid in nursing mothers.

Side Effects

- Burning or irritation of the eyes; redness and irritation at the treated area
- Cardiovascular: Tachycardia, palpitations, angina and pericarditis, pericardial effusion, cardiac tamponade, and exacerbation of angina pectoris. Dose-dependent cardiac lesions (focal necrosis of papillary muscles and subendocardium in the left ventricle) have been demonstrated in animal studies.
- Dermatologic: Hypertrichosis (nonvirilizing); unwanted hair growth, enhanced pigmentation; rare reports of bullous eruptions including Stevens-Johnson syndrome
- Gastrointestinal: Nausea and/or vomiting
- ↑ renin secretion in response to ↓ BP; results in Na^+ and water retention, which may be offset by a diuretic

Angiotensin Converting Enzyme Inhibitors (ACEIs)

Clinical Uses/Relevance to Anesthesiology

- Chronic, acute, or malignant HTN
- CHF particularly with systolic dysfunction. Improves cardiac function indexes, symptoms, and functional capacity and can ↓ cardiac cachexia, malignant arrhythmias, and sudden cardiac death
- Post myocardial infarction; can ↓ ventricular remodeling, LV dilation and dysfunction
- DM; ↓ microvascular disease, particularly the progression of nephropathy and renal failure as well as stroke, heart failure, and death
- Chronic kidney disease from HTN or other nephropathies; ↓ progression
- Frail cachexic elderly patients without heart failure.

Pharmacodynamics

- HR: minimal; contractility: ↑ (reflexive); cardiac output: ↑ (indirect); BP: ↓; SVR/PVR: ↓ (direct); preload: ↓; renovascular resistance: ↓; natriuresis: ↑

- The renin-angiotensin-aldosterone system (RAAS) is normally triggered by hypotension, hypovolemia, or $\downarrow$ [Na^+] in the distal tubule. Renin (released by the renal juxtaglomerular apparatus) converts angiotensinogen to angiotensin-I. Angiotensin-I is converted to angiotensin-II by ACE (located in the pulmonary circulation and endothelium of blood vessels). Angiotensin-II stimulates aldosterone release from the adrenal cortex. Aldosterone $\uparrow$ BP by Na^+ reabsorption and subsequent H_2O retention.

- ACEIs block conversion of angiotensin-I to angiotensin-II. Angiotensin II has several maladaptive functions in disease processes. It is a potent vasoconstrictor of renal efferent arterioles ($\uparrow$ BP, $\uparrow$ GFR); $\uparrow$ release of aldosterone from the adrenal cortex; $\uparrow$ release of vasopressin (acts on kidneys to $\uparrow$ H_2O retention) from the posterior pituitary gland; and promotes ventricular remodeling of the heart in LVH, post MI, CHF.

- Classes are based on molecular structure (sulfhydryl-containing, dicarboxylate-containing, phosphate-containing)

Side Effects

- Refractory Hypotension with GA. The body has 3 systems to maintain BP: RAAS (inhibited by ACEI), sympathetic (inhibited by GA, opioids), and vasopressin. Treatment therefore may require vasopressin administration.

- Persistent dry cough and angioedema ($\uparrow$ kinins), headache, dizziness, fatigue, nausea

- Hyperkalemia from $\downarrow$ aldosterone

- Exacerbation of renal failure in renal artery stenosis; vasoconstricts the efferent arterioles of the glomeruli resulting in $\uparrow$ GFR

- Angiotensin "escape." Not all angiotensin arises from the RAAS system. ACE is contained in the heart and blood vessels where its local effects are harmful

- Avoid in pregnancy (congenital malformations and fetal abnormalities)

Captopril (Capoten); sulfhydryl-containing:

- First ACEI to be developed. May also have mood elevating properties. PO only. Minimal tachyphylaxis. Short duration of action; requires frequent dosing which may affect pt compliance. Taste disturbances (metallic or loss of taste, attributed to sulfhydryl moiety).

Enalapril (Vasotec, Renitec); dicarboxylate containing:

- Second ACEI to be developed. IV formulation (enalaprilat): useful in HTN emergency. A prodrug; metabolized in vivo to enalaprilat by esterases. Onset: PO 1 hr (duration 12–24 hrs); IV 5–15 mins (duration 6 hrs); IV 0.625–5 mg q6h. Biphasic elimination consists of an initial phase of renal filtration and excretion (elimination half-life of 2–6 hrs). The subsequent prolonged phase is due to equilibration from tissue distribution sites (elimination half-life 36 hrs). Accumulation and toxicity may be seen with renal dysfunction (CrCl < 20 ml/min).

Ramipril (Altace, Tritace, Ramace, Ramiwin); dicarboxylate containing:

- A prodrug; metabolized in vivo to active metabolite ramiprilat by liver esterase enzymes. Variable elimination half-life of 3–16 hrs. PO availability in 1.25–10 mg BID tablets (started at lowest dose with upward titration q 3–4 weeks prn).

Quinapril (Accupril):

- Prodrug; converted to active metabolite quinaprilat in the liver.

Lisinopril (Lisodur, Lopril, Novatec, Prinivil, Zestril):

- Hydrophilic; not a prodrug. Elimination half-life 12 hrs (allows for daily dosing and ↑ compliance). Dose PO 2.5–20 mg QD. Consider ↓ dose in elderly

Benazepril:

- Prodrug metabolized in vivo to active metabolite benazeprilat by liver esterase enzymes. Used as a single agent or in combination with hydrochlorothiazide (Lotensin) or amlodipine (Lotrel). Prepared as 5–40 mg PO tablet.

Fosinopril (Monopril); phosphonate-containing:

- Only currently marketed phosphate containing ACEI. Prodrug with the active metabolite fosinoprilat. Biliary excretion primarily; does not need to be adjusted with renal insufficiency. Poor bioavailability.
- See Table 7.2.1

Angiotensin II Receptor Blockers/Antagonists (ARBs)

Clinical Uses/Relevance to Anesthesiology

- Chronic HTN. ↓ incidence of stroke (particularly when combined with aspirin). Combination therapy with ACE I may have improved efficacy.
- CHF as second-line therapy; ↓ ventricular remodeling
- DM (↓ progression of nephropathy, renal failure)
- Renal disease due to HTN, IgA nephropathy, etc, to slow progression
- AF; ↓ recurrence
- Intolerance to ACEI

Pharmacodynamics

- HR: minimal; contractility: ↑ (reflexive); cardiac output: ↑ (indirect), BP: ↓; SVR/PVR: ↓ (direct), preload: ↓; renovascular resistance:↓; natriuresis: ↑
- The renin-angiotensin-aldosterone system (RAAS) is normally triggered by hypotension, hypovolemia, or ↓ [Na^+] in the distal tubule. Renin (is released by the renal juxtaglomerular apparatus) and converts angiotensinogen to angiotensin-I. Angiotensin-I is converted to angiotensin-II by ACE (located in the pulmonary circulation and endothelium of blood vessels). Angiotensin-II stimulates aldosterone release from the adrenal cortex and ↑ BP by Na^+ reabsorption and subsequent H_2O retention.

- Angiotensin II Receptor Blockers (ARBs) competitively antagonize angiotensin II binding at receptors located on blood vessels. ↓ arterial vasoconstriction and hence ↓ DBP > SBP
- ACEI cannot completely block angiotensin II formation due to alternate conversion pathways (angiotensin "escape"). Therefore, coadministration with ACEI results in more complete ↓ of angiotensin II effects.
- ARBs ↓ other maladaptive effects of angiotensin II: renal efferent arteriole vasoconstriction, aldosterone and vasopressin stimulation, ventricular remodeling in LVH, post MI, CHF
- No tachyphylaxis, or reflex tachycardia

Side Effects

- Cough (less than ACEI), hypotension, headache, dizziness, lightheadedness, drowsiness, rash, abnormal taste sensation, diarrhea, associated with sexual dysfunction.
- Kidney failure, liver failure, angioedema (rare, but serious effects)
- Avoid in pregnancy due to a predisposition to birth defects;
- Hyperkalemia from aldosterone reduction. Avoid K+ supplements, drugs that increase K+

Candesartan (Atacand):

- Specifically approved for chronic therapy in CHF (↓ mortality). Prodrug. PO 4–32 mg tablets QD. ↓ efficacy in black pts. Possibly secreted in breast milk (avoid in nursing mothers). Dizziness

Eprosartan (Teveten):

- PO 600 mg QD. No dosage adjustment in renal, hepatic disease.

Irbesartan (Avapro):

- PO: 75, 150, 300 mg tablets QD. Diarrhea and abdominal pain/heartburn.

Telmisartan (Micardis):

- No dosage adjustment needed for renal disease. PO 20, 40, 80 mg tablets QD. Caution in hepatic disease

Valsartan (Diovan):

- ↓ mortality in post MI. PO 40 mg BID in CHF, PO 40 mg QD HTN; (max 320 mg a day); clinical effect in 4 weeks. ↓ absorption when coadministered with food. May ↑ serum creatinine.

Losartan (Cozaar):

- first metabolite antagonizes angiotensin II as well. PO 25, 50, 100 mg tablets (max 100 mg daily). May be used in pediatric patients (>6 y.o.; 0.7 mg/kg; max 50 mg a day). Fluconazole/nizoral and NSAIDS (indomethacin, aspirin, ibuprofen, naproxen) have been shown to ↓ efficacy.

Olmesartan (Benicar):

- Available as single agent, or combined with hydrochlorthiazide. A prodrug. Dose adjustments not necessary in renal/hepatic dysfunction or advanced age.

Nitrovasodilators

Drug class comprised of nitrates, nitrites, and compounds that are converted in vivo to yield nitric oxide. Developed after the antianginal effects of amyl nitrate, first observed in 1857.

Nitroglycerin (NTG)

Clinical Uses/Relevance to Anesthesiology

- Angina pectoris (CAD)
- Coronary artery spasm
- CHF, acute and chronic
- HTN
- Prostate cancer
- Anal fissure (off-label use at reduced concentration in ointment form)
- Facilitate removal of retained placenta and treatment of uterine tetany
- Volume loading during aortic cross clamping or residual pump blood after CPB

Pharmacodynamics

- HR: ↑ (reflexive); contractility: ↑ (reflexive); cardiac output: variable (↓ SV and/or ↑ HR); BP: ↓; preload: ↓; SVR/PVR: ↓ (direct)
- Endogenous nitric oxide (NO) is a gas neurotransmitter that activates guanylyl cyclase in vascular smooth muscle to produce cGMP. cGMP begins a cascade of protein phosphorylation which eventually results in Ca^{++} sequestration into endoplasmic reticulum, vascular smooth muscle relaxation, and vasodilation.
- Nitroglycerin is converted by aldehyde dehydrogenase in mitochondria to yield NO. Low doses mainly affect venous and coronary arteries; higher doses ↑ arterial dilation. Vasodilatory function requires an intact endothelium.
- Venodilation ↑ venous capacitance, ↓ venous return and hence ↓ preload. By ↓ LV diameter, it ↓ myocardial wall tension and ↓ myocardial O_2 consumption. Vasodilation ↓ SVR and afterload which also ↓ wall tension (↓ resistance that LV has to pump against and thus ↓ cardiac work) and ↓ myocardial O_2 consumption.
- Additionally, ↓ LVEDP results in ↑ coronary perfusion pressure (CPP = MAP − LVEDP). Coronary perfusion may also be enhanced by coronary artery vasodilation (as long as MAP is not dropped drastically). ↑ blood flow leads to ↑ myocardial O_2 supply
- During ischemia, NTG may optimize the myocardial O_2 supply/demand balance and relieve symptoms

- Inhibits platelet aggregation ($\uparrow$ cGMP)
- Less rebound HTN after discontinuation
- Uterine relaxant via $\downarrow$ cytoplasmic Ca^{++}; utilized for breech extraction or uterine tetany

Pharmacokinetics

- Metabolized by glutathione-organic nitrate reductase found in liver and blood
- Elimination half-life: 1–3 mins
- Yields nitrite, which may react with hemoglobin to form methemoglobin (therapeutic rationale of nitrite in cyanide poisoning)

Doses/Formulations

- Translingual, transdermal, IV, topical/ointment, tablets, spray
- IV continuous: 0.5–10 mcg/kg/min; IV bolus 5–100 mcg. SL 0.15–0.6 mg; topical 2% ointment 0.5–2 inches q 4–8 hrs. Controlled release 5–10 mg q 24 hrs.

Side Effects

- Tolerance. Due to depletion of reactants needed for NO formation and from reflexive renin release (results in vasoconstriction)
- Reflexive tachycardia (consider beta blockade)
- Withdrawal symptoms; headaches, angina. Seen in workers in NTG manufacturing facilities.
- Headache, weakness, lightheadedness, dizziness, flushing of the head and neck, palpitations, nausea, painful urination, lack of sexual desire, $\uparrow$ bowel movements.
- Severe hypotension when combined with some antidepressants, antipsychotics, antiarrhythmics (quinidine, procainamide, diazepam), opiates, or erectile dysfunction medications (sildenafil [Viagra[R]], tadalafil [Cialis], vardenafil [Levitra]).
- Cerebral autoregulation is affected by vasodilation, $\uparrow$ CBF with resultant $\uparrow$ ICP.
- Hypoxic pulmonary vasoconstriction is hindered. Under normal circumstances, alveolar arterioles constrict when exposed to low alveolar PaO_2 in order to $\downarrow$ perfusion to poorly oxygenated alveoli, thereby $\downarrow$ shunting. NTG dilation prevents alveolar arterioles from constricting and results in V/Q mismatch and shunting. Not clinically significant.
- Not adequately studied in pregnant women
- Absorbed by polyvinyl chloride tubing

Sodium Nitroprusside (SNP)

Clinical Uses/Relevance to Anesthesiology

- Hypertensive emergency
- Severe CHF, AR, MR ($\downarrow$ afterload; $\uparrow$ cardiac output)
- AAA dissection (coadministered with beta-blocker to $\downarrow$ reflex tachycardia)

- Tight intraoperative BP control (eg, CEA, intracranial aneurysm clipping, paroxysmal HTN for pheochromocytoma)
- Afterload reduction with aortic cross-clamping ($\downarrow$ tension, afterload, myocardial work and O_2 consumption)
- Controlled hypotension to $\downarrow$ surgical blood loss
- Peripheral vasospasm (caused by ergot alkaloid poisoning); antidote

Pharmacodynamics

- HR: $\uparrow$ (reflexive); contractility: $\uparrow$ (reflexive); CO: variable ($\downarrow$ SV, $\uparrow$ HR); BP: $\downarrow$; SVR/PVR: $\downarrow$
- In the circulation, SNP binds to the Fe^+ moiety in oxyhemoglobin to yield methemoglobin and SNP- (reduced, unstable form). SNP- breaks down into nitric oxide (NO) and cyanide (CN). NO activates guanylyl cyclase in vascular smooth muscle, which $\uparrow$ cGMP (phosphorylation cascade of proteins) and Ca^{++} sequestration into the endoplasmic reticulum. Vascular smooth muscle relaxation occurs with dilatation of blood vessels.
- Venodilation will $\uparrow$ venous capacitance and $\downarrow$ venous return/preload and tension ($\downarrow$ diameter of LV). Arterial dilation $\downarrow$ afterload and tension ($\downarrow$ resistance that LV has to pump against) leading to $\downarrow$ myocardial O_2 consumption
- Coronary vasodilation and $\downarrow$ LVEDP (due to improved SV) will $\uparrow$ coronary perfusion pressure (CPP = MAP – LVEDP) and hence $\uparrow$ myocardial O_2 supply. However, if MAP is excessively $\downarrow$, then CPP may be hindered.
- Afterload $\downarrow$ in CHF, MR, and AR may be useful to $\uparrow$ cardiac output

Pharmacokinetics

- Onset of action: 1–2 mins.
- Elimination half-life: 1–2 mins; thiosulfate elimination half-life: 20 mins, thiocyanate elimination half-life: 3–4 days. Thiosulfate and thiocyanate are renally eliminated; therefore, in renal failure, elimination half-may be doubled or tripled.

Dose

- Bolus: 1–2 mcg/kg; Infusion: 0.5–10 mcg/kg/min

Side Effects

- Broken down into 1 NO (rapidly released) and 5 cyanide (more gradual release) molecules. CN- inhibits cytochrome oxidase and prevents mitochondrial oxidative phosphorylation (effective and efficient ATP production). The body resorts to anaerobic ATP production (inefficient ATP production that produces lactic acid) despite normal arterial oxygenation. The slow release of CN- typically allows the body time to detoxify before it interferes with cellular respiration.

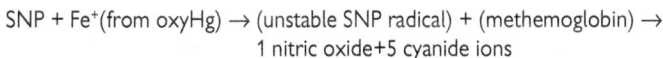

SNP + Fe^+(from oxyHg) $\rightarrow$ (unstable SNP radical) + (methemoglobin) $\rightarrow$
1 nitric oxide+5 cyanide ions

- Detoxification:

  Cyanide + thiosulfate = thiocyanate, via rhodanese enzyme in liver, kidney

  Cyanide + methemoglobin (2% of all Hgb) = cyanomethemoglobin
  (nontoxic, non–O2 carrying Hg).

- Thiosulfate becomes the "rate-limiting step" for cyanide toxicity; levels can be exhausted with high dose SNP or with low thiosulfate levels (eg, malnutrition, postoperative states). Tachyphylaxis or unresponsiveness to ↑ doses may indicate ensuing cyanide toxicity
- ↓ coronary blood flow to ischemic areas; "steal" mechanism (ischemic areas are already maximally dilated, with SNP dilating normal vessels and diverting blood away; stealing from the poor to give to the rich)
- Reflex tachycardia (consider beta blockade)
- Interferes with cerebral autoregulation; ↑ CBF with subsequent ↑ ICP. Consider hyperventilation as CO_2 responsiveness remains intact
- Hypoxic pulmonary vasoconstriction is affected. Under normal circumstances alveolar arterioles constrict when exposed to low alveolar PaO_2 and ↓ perfusion to poorly oxygenated alveoli, thereby ↓ shunting. SNP dilatation prevents alveolar arterioles from constricting and results in V/Q mismatch and shunting. Not clinically significant
- Renin is reflexively released in response to ↓ BP, with effects persisting after SNP is discontinued (rebound HTN).
- Unstable in light

Calcium Channel Blockers (CCB)

Clinical Uses/Relevance to Anesthesiology
- HTN; may be effective first-line drug combined with diuretic in black pts
- Isolated systolic HTN in the elderly
- Cerebral vasospasm
- Angina pectoris
- AF and atrial flutter rate control
- Migraines
- Raynaud's disease

Pharmacodynamics
- Normally, Ca^{++} enters the cytoplasm from extracellular compartments or the SR intracellularly. External entry of Ca^{++} will trigger Ca^{++} release from voltage-gated calcium channels on the SR membrane ("calcium-induced calcium release"). ↑ cytoplasmic Ca^{++} results in ↑ myocardial contractility, vascular smooth muscle contraction, or cardiac conductance.

- CCB block the voltage-gated calcium channels in the SR membrane, resulting in ↓ intracellular calcium. Based on the drug's affinity, they can ↓ cardiac contractility, vasomotor tone, or cardiac conductance
- Myocardium: ↓ cardiac contractility results in ↓ CO and ↓ BP with consequent ↓ myocardial O_2 consumption. Vascular smooth muscle: arterial vasodilation results in ↓ SVR, ↓ afterload, and ↓ LV wall tension with consequent ↓ myocardial O_2 consumption. Cardiac conduction system: ↓ conductance and ↓ HR with consequent ↓ myocardial O_2 consumption (heart beats fewer times) and ↑ myocardial O_2 supply (↓ HR allows for more time for diastolic perfusion of the LV).
- The dihydropyridines predominantly affect vascular tone and *treat BP* (↓ SVR, ↓ arterial BP but with reflexive tachycardia). The phenylalkylamines predominantly affect the myocardium and ↓ inotropy (↓ myocardial O_2 demand, with minimal vasodilation and minimal reflex tachycardia); also ↓ coronary vasospasm and can *treat angina*. The benzothiazepines possess both cardiac depressant and vasodilatory actions but can ↓ BP without producing the same degree of reflex tachycardia as seen with the dihydropyridines.

Side Effects

- Potentiation of NMBD
- Potentiation of volatile anesthetics (further depress contractility, AV node conduction, vasodilation)
- Magnesium supplements may potentiate effects
- Dihydropyridines: dizziness, headache, fluid retention in lower extremities, tachycardia, bradycardia, facial redness, gingival hyperplasia; peripheral edema, fatigue, depression, insomnia, impotence, GI discomfort, gynecomastia, palpitations.
- Nondihydropyridines: headaches, dizziness, lightheadedness, fluid retention, facial flushing, ecchymosis, gingival growth. Potential for profound toxicity with the slow release agents.

Amilodipine (Norvasc); dihydropyridine:

- HTN, exertional and vasospastic angina (predominant effect on vascular smooth muscle cells). PO 2.5–10 mg tablets QD. Metabolized mostly to inactive metabolites that are excreted in the urine. Avoid in cardiogenic shock, unstable angina, and severe aortic stenosis; nursing mothers.

Felodipine (Plendil); dihydropyridine:

- HTN. Effects on cardiac conductance (avoid in sick sinus syndrome, 2nd or 3rd degree heart block)

Nicardipine (Cardene, Carden SR); dihydropyridine:

- HTN, angina pectoris (chronic stable angina), PCI, controlled hypotension, Raynaud's phenomenon, CHF. Predominantly vascular smooth muscle effects. Selective for cerebral and coronary blood vessels. PO and IV formulations.

Nifedipine (Procardia, Adalat); dihydropyridine:

- Angina (particularly Prinzmetal's), HTN, and hypertensive emergencies, Raynaud's, premature labor (tocolysis), esophageal spasms, anal fissures, and rarely in pulmonary hypertension or high-altitude pulmonary edema (vascular smooth muscle dilator). High doses may ↑ mortality in patients with CAD

Nimodipine (Nimotop); dihydropyridine:

- Mainly utilized in prevention of cerebral vasospasm (common complication of SAH). For prophylaxis, current recommendations suggest initiating therapy 4 days after bleed and up to 3 weeks for prophylaxis; routine use is controversial. PO and IV formulations. Peak plasma concentration 1.5 hrs after PO. Metabolized by cytochrome P-4503A (first-pass metabolism), which can be inhibited by keto-conazole, valproic acid, or troleandomycin (↑ CaChB levels). Enzyme-inducing anticonvulsants ↓ drug concentrations. Metabolites are excreted renally.

Verapamil (Calan, Isoptin); phenylalkylamine:

- HTN, angina pectoris, cardiac arrhythmias (class IV antiarrhythmic agent), cluster headaches, migraines, mania and hypomania in pregnancy (nonterato-genic); intra-arterially for cerebral vasospasm. PO and IV formulations. Onset 1–2 hrs; highly protein bound, large Vd. first-pass metabolism (10%-35% bio-availability) to numerous inactive metabolites, one of which retains 20% of the vasodilatory properties of the parent drug. Excreted primarily in the urine (70%) and minimally in feces (16%). Elimination half-life 5–12 hrs.

Diltiazem (Cardizem); benzothiazepine:

- HTN, angina pectoris, certain cardiac arrhythmias (SVT such as reentrant, atrial flutter, AF; class IV antiarrhythmic agent), migraine prophylaxis, and management of cluster headaches (off-label), short-term treatment of anal fissures (oral or topical application; off-label). Potent coronary and peripheral vasodilator, ↓ HR (depression of AV and SA node conduction), and chro-notropy. May have a reflex sympathetic response to the negative inotropic, dromotropic, and chronotropic effects. Avoid in SA or AV nodal conduc-tion abnormalities (including WPW), sick sinus syndrome, CHF (with poor LV function), peripheral artery disease, COPD, Prinzmetal's angina. Cautious use with beta-blockers (↑ propensity for AV-nodal block and dysrhythmias).

Alpha-1-Adrenergic Blockers

Clinical Uses/Relevance to Anesthesiology

- HTN. May be effective first-line therapy when combined with a diuretic in black or young pts
- HTN with concurrent benign prostatic hypertrophy (by ↓ gland size it can serve a dual purpose)
- CHF to ↓ afterload
- Raynaud's syndrome to reverse vasospasm

- Pheochromocytoma, preoperative preparation; blunts effects of catecholamine excess particularly during surgical manipulation

Pharmacodynamics

- HR: minimal; contractility: minimal; BP: $\downarrow$; SVR/PVR: $\downarrow$; preload: $\downarrow$ (venous > arterial)
- α-1 Receptor agonism sets off a cascade of events that ultimately $\uparrow$ Ca^{++} and cause contraction at postsynaptic nerve terminals on vascular and nonvascular smooth muscle
- Selective alpha-1 receptor antagonism of catecholamine and sympathomimetic binding will therefore result in vasodilation by preventing release of Ca^{++} from the SR. Clinically, a $\downarrow$ SVR/afterload and $\downarrow$ venous return/preload are observed, with a resultant $\downarrow$ in myocardial O_2 consumption.
- Because there is no competitive binding to presynaptic alpha-2 receptors, inhibition of norepinephrine release goes unopposed. As a result, it lacks reflexive $\uparrow$ in CO, HR, or renin release seen with other drugs such as SNP or hydralazine.

Side Effects

- Orthostatic/postural hypotension. The greater effect on the venous compared to the arterial system results in venous pooling. This is further enhanced by unopposed alpha-2 receptor effects that inhibit norepinephrine release and reflexive responses.
- Fluid retention. Coadministration with a diuretic improves efficacy
- Concurrent use of NSAIDS may impair efficacy; mechanism unclear
- Urinary frequency and sexual dysfunction

Prazosin (Minipres):

- first-pass metabolism results in $\downarrow$ bioavailability. Elimination half-life ~3 hrs. PO 0.5–40 mg PO BID.

Terazosin (Hytrin):

- Elimination half-life 8–12 hrs. 1–20 mg PO QD.

Doxazosin (Cardura):

- Elimination half-life 9–13 hrs. 1–16 mg PO QD.

Tamsulosin (Flomax):

- Specifically for BPH; no effect on BP. 0.4–0.8 mg PO QD.

Alpha-2 Agonists/Centrally Acting Sympathomimetics

Clonidine (Catapres)

Clinical Uses/Relevance to Anesthesiology

- HTN particularly in moderate to severe, or renin-induced disease

- ↓ anesthetic requirements; contributes to MAC via ↓ in sympathetic activity and arousal
- Premedication for sedation (useful in pediatrics), ↓ HD lability, and potential cardioprotection (studies have suggested greater effect than perioperative beta-blockers).
- Regional and neuraxial anesthesia adjunct to local anesthetics. Additive analgesic effect and duration without some of the side effects seen with opioids
- Detoxification aid to suppress unpleasant sympathetic responses during withdrawal from narcotics, alcohol, nicotine
- Neuropathic pain (eg, postherpetic neuralgia); off-label use
- Migraine headaches
- Diagnosis of pheochromocytoma; failure of the "clonidine suppression test" to ↓ catecholamine release suggests diagnosis
- ADHD, Tourette's syndrome and tics, hyperarousal due to PTSD, insomnia, sleep disorders, anxiety, and ulcerative colitis are among a growing list of off-label uses

Pharmacodynamics

- HR: ↓ (indirect via vagal input to pacemakers and impairment of cardioaccelerator fibers); contractility: ↑ ; SVR/PVR: ↓; cardiac output: ↓; BP: ↓
- Alpha-2 receptors uniquely possess a "mixed effect:" ↓ of central and peripheral SNS output but with direct peripheral vasoconstriction. Alpha-2a receptors are primarily located presynaptically and normal physiologic agonism occurs when there is an "excess" of catecholamines (norepinephrine) and sympathomimetics that bind to alpha-1 receptors. Agonsim ↓ norepinephrine release and results in a "negative feedback" that is akin to "putting on the breaks" to SNS output; responsible for the antihypertensive, sedative, and analgesic properties that are observed with clonidine. Alpha-2b receptors are primarily located postsynaptically on blood vessels; catecholamine (norepinephrine) and sympathomimetic binding results in peripheral vasoconstriction (directly constricts vs mediation through autonomic nervous system).
- Antihypertensive effects. Clonidine is a relatively selective alpha-2 receptor agonist (weak alpha-1). Presynaptic receptor binding in the brain stem's vasomotor center ↓ SNS output and results in peripheral vasodilation, ↓ SBP, ↓ HR, and ↓ CO. However, unlike alpha-1 receptor antagonists (which block vasoconstriction but not alpha-2-mediated norepinephrine inhibition), clonidine lacks the undesirable effect of orthostatic hypotension (does not impair direct alpha-1-mediated vasoconstriction or beta-1-mediated inotropy)
- Sedation and Reduced Anesthetic Requirements. Alpha-2 receptors are also present in CNS structures that deliver SNS input to arousal centers in the forebrain. Agonism ↓ SNS input and arousal and produces the sedative, and MAC effects as well as subdues substance withdrawal symptoms.
- Analgesia. Alpha-2 receptors are present in the spinal cord's substantia gelatinosa. Neuraxial clonidine results in analgesia without the side effects seen with neuraxial opioids (itching, nausea, constipation, urinary retention, and respiratory depression).

Pharmacokinetics

- Onset: PO: anti-HTN effects in 30–60 mins, peak plasma levels: 3–5 hrs (due to rapid GI tract absorption and lipophilicity, which allows good BBB crossing). Transdermal patch: up to 48 hrs (useful when NPO and for steady-state)
- Duration of action: anti-HTN ~8 hrs
- Metabolized hepatically (50%), with metabolites and unchanged drug (50%) excreted renally.
- Elimination half-life: 6–12 hrs (up to 41 hrs with renal impairment; adjust accordingly)

Dose

- HTN: PO: 0.2–0.4 mg BID-TID;
- Preoperative sedation: PO 5 mcg/kg
- Neuraxial: 150–450 mcg; Peripheral Nerve Block 1 mcg/kg
- Shivering: 75 mcg IV
- Withdrawal Symptoms. Alcohol and opioids: PO 0.4–1.5 mg; Nicotine: transdermal patch 0.1–0.2 mgQD.
- Perioperative Ischemia: PO or transdermal patch 0.2 mg PO (apply patch night before surgery, or morning of; continue for 4 days postoperatively)
- Pheochromocytoma 0.3 mg PO (blunts normal catecholamine release)

Side Effects

- Bradycardia. Can be profound due to direct vagal effects on pacemaker cells as well as impairment of T1-T4 cardioaccelerator fibers. Treatment with antimuscarinics (atropine, glycopyrrolate) or ephedrine (effects may be pronounced)
- Rebound hypertension results from rebound in sympathetic outflow and can present with nervousness, diaphoresis, tachycardia, and headache. A gradual taper may avoid effects; treatment includes reinitiation of clonidine or alpha and beta-blockers for severe cases. Note that beta-blockers can result in unopposed alpha constriction (blocks B-2 vasodilation)
- Hypotension with perioperative and neuraxial use; effects may be compounded by anesthetic medications, blood or fluid loss.

Guanfacine (Tenex, Intuniv):

Clinical Uses/Relevance to Anesthesiology

- HTN; acute and chronic treatment
- ADHD (alternative to stimulants), insomnia

Pharmacodynamics

- HR: small ↓; contractility: ↑; SVR/PVR: ↓; cardiac output: maintained; BP: ↓
- Alpha-2a agonist. By binding to receptors in the brain stem's vasomotor center, ↓ SNS output with resultant ↓ BP and less ↓ HR and ↓ CO than clonidine. By binding to the dense concentration of receptors found in the pontine locus ceruleus, it ↓ SNS input to the arousal centers in the forebrain.

Pharmacokinetics
- Onset. Peak plasma concentrations within 1–4 hrs; good bioavailability
- Metabolism: hepatic to 3-hydroxy metabolite, but mostly cleared unchanged by the kidneys.
- Elimination half-life: 17 hrs.

Dose
- HTN: PO 1–3mg QD

Side Effects
- Cardiac: orthostatic hypotension, palpitations
- Rebound hypertension may be reduced with gradual discontinuation.
- Occasional: dizziness, depression, headache, GI disturbances (diarrhea, constipation), loss of appetite, fatigue
- Rare: blurred vision, chest pain, shortness of breath, swelling, rash, swelling of hands and feet, decreased sexual desire, impotence, dry mouth, vertigo, visual and taste changes

Methydopa (Aldomet)

Clinical Uses/Relevance to Anesthesiology
- HTN of mild to moderate severity. Has lost popularity with the advent of newer and safer alternatives
- Hypertension during pregnancy: preeclampsia, eclampsia, gestational HTN

Pharmacodynamics
- HR: normal to ↓; contractility: maintained; cardiac output: maintained; BP: ↓ (supine and standing); renal vascular resistance: ↓. Most cardiovascular reflexes remain intact.
- Methyldopa's mechanism of action is not entirely understood. It has been suggested that its metabolite, alpha-methylnorepinephrine, functions as a presynaptic alpha-2 receptor agonist and reduces norepinephrine release centrally and peripherally. Alpha-methylnorepinephrine has also been described as having a "false" neurotransmitter function whereby it substitutes for norephinephrine in presynaptic vesicles; but upon release into the synaptic cleft, has no effect on postsynaptic receptors.
- Methyldopa also inhibits DOPA decarboxylase, which converts the substrate L-DOPA to dopamine. In addition to its roles in cognition and mood, dopamine also has renal and direct sympathomimetic effects, as well as functions as a substrate for both norepinephrine and epinephrine. As a result, methyldopa depletes these neurotransmitters.
- Reductions in plasma renin activity are also demonstrated (hydralazine, NTG may have reflexive ↑ that results in tolerance of antihypertensive effects).

Pharmacokinetics
- Peak effect: 4–6 hrs after PO dose.

- Metabolism: hepatic metabolism to mono-O-sulfate conjugate, which is renally excreted along with unchanged drug (70%).
- elimination half-life 105 mins; BP returns to pretreatment levels within 12–24 hrs.
- Crosses the placental barrier, appears in cord blood and breast milk.

Dose

- Adult: 500–2000 mg Q6–12 hrs. Max daily dose 500 mg when in conjunction with other antihypertensives
- Pediatric: 10 mg/kg Q6–12 hrs. Max daily dose: 65 mg/kg or 3 g

Side Effects

- CNS. Sedation, depression, anxiety, apathy, Parkinsonism (muscle tremors, rigidity, hypokinesia), tardive dyskinesia, suicidal ideation
- Orthostatic hypotension
- Rebound HTN upon withdrawal
- Hypersensitivity: lupus erythematous, pericarditis
- Hyperprolactinemia, gynecomastia in men

Clinical Case Scenario #1

HPI: 69-year-old 80 kg male w/ a h/o CAD presenting for an elective repair of an expanding AAA. The AAA was found incidentally one year ago and measured 5.5 cm. It was being managed medically, however on recent exam was noted as 7 cm. Denies SOB, DOE, PND, orthopnea, or chest pain. Echo findings (1 month ago) showed normal LV size & function w/ an EF 65%, normal RV size & function, no valvular dysfunction. Pt lives with wife in assisted living facility, good functional status.

PMH/PSH: CAD s/p PCI w/ two DES placement 3 yrs ago in the left Cx & RCA. Currently off Plavix, on aspirin. Denies any h/o myocardial infarction, HTN, mild chronic kidney disease with baseline Cr – 1.7 (CrCl 50). Denies any prior surgeries except cardiac cath 3 yrs ago.

All: NKDA

Meds: HCTZ, toprol XL, valsartan (morning dose held), aspirin (held for 7 days)

Social Hx: Remote h/o tobacco use (40 pack year), quit 5 yrs ago, social alcohol use

Intraop: Preinduction placement of monitors was uneventful. Epidural for postop analgesia; standard monitors (ECG w/ ST segment analysis, BP cuff, pulse oximetry) and invasive monitors (arterial line, central venous line with pulmonary arterial catheter) were placed. TEE was available in room in anticipation of use.

Induction was controlled with maintenance of hemodynamic stability using close titration of IV and inhalational agents. Two large-bore peripheral IVs were placed thereafter for possible rapid fluid & blood administration.

The goal was to maintain HR & MAP within 20% of baseline for adequate organ perfusion. Prior to cross-clamping, mannitol & heparin were given. Due to significant lability in blood pressures with aortic cross-clamp (suprarenal), a sodium nitroprusside infusion was started at a rate of 0.7 mcg/kg/min & a bolus dose of 1.5 mcg/kg.

Good hemodynamic control for the initial part of the procedure but with unanticipated difficult aneurysm repair and prolonged surgical time, pt began to develop tachyphylaxis with increasing requirements of nitroprusside to maintain hemodynamic control. Infusion rate was increased to 0.9 mcg/kg/min but was finally discontinued prior to clamp removal *two hours later.*

With unclamping, pt remained hemodynamically unstable despite adequate resuscitation and prior termination of all infusions. ABGs showed worsening metabolic (lactic) acidosis with increasing MVO_2 on PAC. A diagnosis of possible impending cyanide toxicity was made considering h/o renal impairment. Administration of sodium thiosulfate infusion led to an improvement in parameters and hemodynamic status.

Pt was left intubated and monitored in the ICU. Extubated on postop day 1 with no complications.

Discussion: Treatment of cyanide toxicity consists of discontinuing the administration of sodium nitroprusside; providing a buffer for CN^- by using sodium nitrite (converts hemoglobin into methemoglobin) as the patient can safely tolerate; and then infusing sodium thiosulfate to convert the CN^- into thiocyanate. Sodium nitroprusside (>500 mcg/kg or faster than 2 mcg/kg/min) can lead to CN^- generated faster than can be eliminated. Sodium thiosulfate can ↑ the rate of cyanide processing, hence ↓ the risk of CN^- toxicity. Rarely, patients receiving >10 mg/kg of sodium nitroprusside may develop methemoglobinemia; some patients, especially those with impaired renal function may also develop thiocyanate toxicity after prolonged, rapid infusions.

Clinical Case Scenario #2

HPI: 45-year-old female w/ extensive medical hx now presenting w/ a 3-day h/o RUQ abdominal pain, nausea and vomiting. Abdominal U/S indicative of cholelithiasis, scheduled for laparoscopic cholecystectomy. Denies any fevers, chills. Denies any symptoms of chest pain, SOB, PND, orthopnea, DOE although limited physical activity due to vascular disease.

PMH/PSH: CAD, HTN, Type II DM, GERD, PVD s/p fempop bypass 3 yrs ago. Denies any surgical or anesthetic complications with prior surgery.

All: No allergies

Meds: Currently on prevacid, aspirin, lisinopril, NTG (SL) prn, carvedilol, lantus, HCTZ, metformin, plavix.

Social Hx: significant for a remote h/o tobacco use, 2 ppd X 15 yrs, occasional (social) alcohol use.In the preop area, pt's vital signs were normal with BP 132/78, HR 90, SpO$_2$ 99%. She has had nothing to eat or drink by mouth since midnight with the exception of taking her medications—prevacid & lisinopril at 5 AM with a sip of water. Metformin and plavix had been held for 7 days.

Intraop: Baseline preinduction BP was 140/92 with HR 94. Induction was uneventful. Pt was intubated and ventilated and remained hemodynamically stable for the first 30 minutes. During surgical prepping and draping (prior to insufflation), pt's BP suddenly dropped to systolic of 60s. Despite repositioning of blood pressure cuff, constant volume loading and boluses of phenylephrine, pt's BP remained suboptimal with systolic BPs of mid 70s. Vasopressin was then administered with adequate response and rebound pressures to a systolic of 130s. A low-dose vasopressin infusion was started and was weaned off prior to extubation.

Discussion: ACE inhibitors and ARBs have been shown to have an increased incidence of refractory intraoperative hypotension responsive only to Vasopressin.

References

1. Burnier M, Brunner HR. Angiotensin II receptor antagonists. *Lancet.* 2000;355(9204):637–645.

2. Calcium channel blockers. *Medicine.* 2007;35:599–602.

3. Jackson EK. Renin and angiotensin. In: Goodman LS, Gilman A, Brunton L, Lazo JS, Parker K, eds. *Goodman & Gilman's The Pharmacological Basis of Therapeutics.* 11th ed. New York: McGraw-Hill; 2006:789–821.

4. Grant v. Pharmacia & Upjohn Co. http://ca10.washburnlaw.edu/cases/2002/12/01–1509.htm. Retrieved January 17, 2009.

5. Guanfacine: official FDA information, side effects and uses. http://www.drugs.com/pro/guanfacine.html.

6. Intuniv (guanfacine) drug information. http://www.rxlist.com/intuniv-drug.html.

7. Katzung BG. *Basic and Clinical Pharmacology.* 7th ed. Stamford, CT: Appleton & Lange; 1998.

8. Parker K, Brunton L, Goodman LS, Lazo JS, Gilman A. *Goodman & Gilman's The Pharmacological Basis of Therapeutics* New York: McGraw-Hill; 2006:854–855.

9. Minoxidil official FDA information, side effects and uses. http://www.drugs.com/pro/minoxidil.html.

10. Nelson, M . Drug treatment of elevated blood pressure. *Australian Prescriber.* 2010. (33): 108–112. http://www.australianprescriber.com/magazine/33/4/108/12. Retrieved August 11, 2010.

11. Nitro. http://www.medicinenet.com/nitroglycerin/page2.html.

12. Nitropress (nitroprusside sodium) drug information: user reviews, side effects, drug interactions and dosage at RxList. Rxlist.com. Retrieved December 11, 2010.

13. Ogbru O. ACE inhibitors (angiotensin converting enzyme inhibitors). MedicineNet. com. *MedicineNet, Inc.* http://www.medicinenet.com/ace_inhibitors/article.htm. Retrieved March 20, 2010.

14. Olsen EA, Whiting D, Bergfeld W, Miller J, Hordinsky M, Wanser R, Zhang P, Kohut B (2007). A multicenter, randomized, placebo-controlled, double-blind clinical trial of a novel formulation of 5% minoxidil topical foam versus placebo in the treatment of androgenetic alopecia in men. *J Am Acad Dermatol.* 2007;57(5):767.

Chapter 8

Local Anesthetics

Nina Singh-Radcliff, MD

Role in the Practice of Anesthesiology/Relevance to Anesthesiology

- Subcutaneous infiltration, neuraxial blocks (spinal and epidural), peripheral nerve blocks (brachial plexus, femoral, sciatic, etc), IV regional blocks (Bier Block); interferes with sympathetic, sensory, and motor nerve conduction
- Lidocaine attenuates sympathetic response and laryngeal reflexes during airway manipulation (laryngoscopy, intubation, suctioning)
- Lidocaine can contribute to MAC. Can ↓ volatile anesthetic by up to 10%-28%; ↓ propofol induction and maintenance doses
- Lidocaine ↓ pain and discomfort associated with propofol injection (mix or precede as a separate injection)
- Perioperative IV lidocaine infusion may improve postoperative analgesia
- Lidocaine can treat ventricular arrhythmias
- "Lidocaine test" can be administered to aid in the diagnosis of neuropathic pain

Pharmacodynamics

- Nerve impulses are generated and then conducted in an antegrade fashion along their pathways via electrical signaling. The cell's resting membrane potential is -90mV and is maintained by the Na^+/K^+ ATPase receptor. Impulses result in slow sodium channel opening, sodium influx, and making the cell membrane positive. If the cumulative impulses result in the membrane potential reaching -55mV, cell depolarization goes on autopilot to generate an "action potential": fast voltage-gated sodium channels are triggered to open and rapid sodium influx further depolarizes the cell to +35mV. The action potential serves to "communicate" the impulse to the proceeding neuron (which in turn undergoes depolarization) or effector organ. See Figures 8.1 and 8.2.
- Local anesthetics (LA) thwart the "autopilot" segment of the action potential by reversibly blocking fast voltage-gated sodium channels on central and

peripheral nerves (as well as cardiac pacemaker cells at high concentrations). They do not change or alter the membrane resting potential, prevent slow sodium channel opening (which is responsible for depolarization up to -55mV), or cause permanent change or damage to the cell.

- Site of action: sodium channel receptors intracellularly at myelinated portions of the nerve as well as cardiac pacemaker, conduction, and myocardial cells. See Figure 8.3.

- Composed of a lipophilic benzene ring that is connected to a hydrophilic tertiary amine by an intermediate amide or ester chain. The intermediate chain determines the drug's route of metabolism. See Figure 8.4. Amides are metabolized by enzymatic biotransformation primarily in the liver; N-dealkylation and hydroxylation. Thus, liver disease or ↓ hepatic blood flow (CHF or GA) can ↓ amide metabolism. Amides have 2 "*I*s" in their name: lidocaine, etidocaine, ropivicaine, bupivacaine, mepivicaine, prilocaine. Esters are metabolized by pseudocholinesterase, found principally in plasma and are generally cleared more quickly than amides (less likely to cause systemic toxicity); pseudocholinesterase inhibitors decrease ester metabolism. One of its metabolites, para-aminobenzoic acid (PABA), can cause allergic reactions.

Pharmacokinetics

- Weak base. Exists as powdered solids that are unstable in air and poorly soluble in water. In order to store and administer LA, they are combined with hydrochloric acid; in an acidic solution, the base becomes ionized and is water soluble:

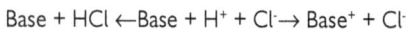

$$\text{Base} + \text{HCl} \leftarrow \text{Base} + \text{H}^+ + \text{Cl}^- \rightarrow \text{Base}^+ + \text{Cl}^-$$

- However, because the site of action is an *intracellular* sodium channel receptor, only the unprotonated, or nonionized form, is able to *cross* the lipid bilayer of the cell membrane. Furthermore, only the protonated, or ionized form, binds to the intracellular sodium channel receptor site.

- Sodium channels exist in an activated open, inactivated-closed, and rested-closed state. Local anesthetics exhibit "state-dependent" or "frequency-dependent" blockade, meaning that the drug binds more readily to the receptor in its activated, open-state (when neurons are rapidly firing)

- Potency. Mainly determined by lipid solubility. Long hydrocarbon chains facilitate drug crossing the lipid bilayer. However, in vivo, factors such as vasodilation and tissue redistribution affect potency (eg, when etidocaine, a highly lipid soluble drug, is administered epidurally, a considerable portion is sequestered and redistributed into epidural fat; there is less drug available for neural blockade).

- Cm. Term to describe the minimum concentration of LA necessary to produce conduction blockade and is a reflection of potency (analogous to utilizing MAC for volatiles). Cm is, however, ↑ by an acidic environment, ↑ nerve fiber diameter, ↓ frequency of nerve firing, ↑ blood flow or vasodilation, and motor fibers.

- Duration of action. Determined by the extent of protein binding to alpha-1 glycoprotein. LA are physiologically active, metabolized, and excreted in their free form (not bound). Protein binding functions like a "savings account." Malnourishment, liver disease, pregnancy, and chronic disease can reduce alpha-1 glycoprotein, and hence ↑ [amount of free drug]; smaller boluses and more frequent dosing should be considered. The drug's intrinsic vasodilator activity also affects duration (ie, lidocaine, a potent vasodilator, has ↑ absorption with resultant ↑ in metabolism and ↓ clinical blockade compared to drugs with similar protein binding such as prilocaine or mepivacaine).

- Onset. Determined by pKa. When the pH = pKa, 50% of the drug exists in a charged state, while the other 50% is uncharged. Thus, if the LA's pKa is close to physiologic pH, a greater % of drug is in its uncharged form and can cross the lipid bilayer. When LAs are in acidic environments (infection or fetal hypoxia) they have a pH <pKA and ↑ H+ ion binding; inhibits its ability to cross the cell lipid bilayer.

- Rate of systemic absorption/toxicity. Determined mainly by tissue blood flow. IV > tracheal > intercostals > caudal > paracervical > epidural > brachial plexus > sciatic > subcutaneous.

- first-pass pulmonary extraction occurs after entry into the venous circulation, particularly for lidocaine, bupivacaine, and prilocaine. Pulmonary extraction will limit the [drug] reaching the coronary and cerebral circulation (sites for toxicity).

- Pregnancy. ↑ LA sensitivity due to ↓ protein and ↑ epidural spread (↓ epidural space from venous engorgement). Additionally, transplacental transfer can occur between the mother and fetus (note: because protein-bound drug cannot cross the placenta, drugs with ↑ protein binding have ↓ placental transfer; bupivacaine is 95% protein bound and crosses less than lidocaine which is 65% protein bound). Esters have ↑ plasma metabolism by pseudocholinesterase and thus have ↓ placental crossing. Additionally, when the fetus is acidic from hypoxia or infection, "ion trapping" can occur; LA drug becomes protonated and charged, and ↓ return to the mother's circulation.

Additives/Adjuvants

- Vasoconstrictors. ↓ systemic absorption results in ↑ duration of action (↑ contact time between drug and nerve fiber) and ↓ toxicity (signals inadvertent vascular injection via HTN and brings the rate of metabolism closer to systemic absorption). Phenylephrine provides alpha-mediated vasoconstriction of surrounding vessels. Epinephrine provides alpha-mediated vasoconstriction *and* beta-1-mediated chronotropy; thus, can be utilized as a "test-dose" in epidural, peripheral nerve, and SQ blocks to identify accidental IV injection. A common epidural test dose consists of 3 mL lidocaine with epinephrine, often in a 1:200,000 epinephrine mixture (15 mcg of epinephrine). Epinephrine, however, is unstable in alkaline solutions; therefore, premade LA plus epinephrine solutions are markedly acidic (ph = 4). This can result in ↑ sting on injection and ↑ onset time; addition of sodium bicarbonate reduces acidicty (↑ pH).

- Narcotics. Provide an additive analgesic effect at local receptors (spinal cord when given neuraxially) and via systemic absorption. Neuraxial narcotics should be preservative free, sterile, nonpyrogenic, isobaric, and free of antioxidants and other potentially neurotoxic additives. Narcotic can cause itching, drowsiness, nausea. Sufentanil needs to be mixed with bupivacaine *prior* to neuraxial injection

- Clonidine. An alpha antagonist that when administered epidurally, can potentiate analgesia, ↑ time to first analgesic request, ↓ postoperative pain, and ↓ propofol requirements.

- Sodium bicarbonate. ↑ percentage of LA in its uncharged, lipid soluble form (LA solutions are prepared as acidic salt solutions; epinephrine mixtures reach pH of 4).

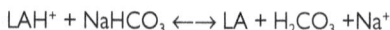

$$LAH^+ + NaHCO_3 \longleftrightarrow LA + H_2CO_3 + Na^+$$

- ↓ onset of neural blockade, ↑ depth of sensory and motor blockade, and ↑ spread of epidural blockade. 1–2cc of 8.4% $NaHCO_3$ is typically mixed with 20 cc of lidocaine with epinephrine.

- Other local anesthetics. Coadministration can harness benefits of quick onset (chloroprocaine, mepivacaine, lidocaine) with prolonged duration (bupivacaine, ropivacaine, tetracaine).

Side Effects/Adverse Reactions

- Systemic toxicity. Magnitude depends on dose administered, vascularity of the injection site, physiochemical properties of the drug, and presence of vasoconstrictors. Mixtures of LA have additive affects (50% toxic dose of lidocaine and a 50% toxic dose of ropivacaine equal 100% toxic effect of either drug)

- Central nervous system—a selective depression of inhibitory neurons results in cerebral excitation (excitatory pathways are unopposed). Toxicity has been attributed to sodium, as well as calcium, potassium, adenylyl cyclase, guanylyl cyclase, lipases, NMDA, beta-2, nicotinic acetylcholine binding. Signs begin with vertigo, tinnitus, ominous feelings, circumoral numbness, tongue paresthesia, and then progresses to tremors, myoclonic jerks, convulsions, CNS depression, and coma. Seizure treatment includes: prevention and suppression with thiopental 1–2 mg/kg, propofol, or benzodiazepines. Hyperventilation ↓ CBF (drug exposure) and causes hypokalemia (hyperpolarization).

- Cardiac—More resistant to toxic effects of LA than the CNS (3 times the blood concentration that causes seizures). LA ↓ spontaneous Phase IV depolarization and refractory period duration. ↑ the PR interval (time of atrial and ventricular depolarization), QRS complex (ventricular depolarization); smooth muscle relaxation and vasodilation (except cocaine); ↓ myocardial contractility and contraction velocity at ↑ concentrations. This can manifest as bradycardia, heart block, ventricular arrhythmias, hypotension, and eventually cardiac arrest. Treatment includes discontinuing LA administration and ACLS (substitute amiodarone for lidocaine). Intralipids may be effective in therapy of LA toxicity (bolus 1 cc/kg of 20% intralipid; repeat every 5 minutes up to a maximum of 8 cc/kg; and then start a continuous infusion of 0.25 cc/kg/min over 30 minutes).

- Allergies. May be seen with the PABA ester metabolite, preservatives in commercial preparation; rare with amides. No cross-sensitivity between classes of local anesthetics. Palpitations from epinephrine can be misconstrued by a patient as an allergy.
- Methemoglobinemia. Prilocaine, benzocaine, cetacaine; see prilocaine below
- Transient neurological symptoms. Attributed to radicular irritation. Symptoms of dysesthesia, burning pain, and aching in lower extremity or buttocks. Begins 6 to 36 hours, resolves in 1 week. Risk factors include intrathecal lidocaine, lithotomy position, obesity, outpatient status. Neurological exam is usually normal; treated with trigger point injections and NSAIDS.
- Cauda equina syndrome. Diffuse injury across the lumbosacral plexus produces varying degrees of sensory anesthesia, bowel and bladder sphincter dysfunction, and paraplegia. Risk factors include high dose LA and maldistribution or nonhomogenous distribution (microcatheters 28 g or smaller).
- Postretrobulbar apnea syndrome. Depression of medullary respiratory centers may result in ↓ hypoxemic response as well as direct paralysis of phrenic or intercostal nerves.
- Myonecrosis can result from injection into muscle. Regeneration usually takes 3–4 weeks. Worsened by steroid or epinephrine additives; ropivicaine < bupivicaine.

Dosages

dosage is expressed as percentages and milliliters. 1% = 10 mg/mL, 0.75% = 7.5 mg/mL, 0.5% = 5 mg/mL; 0.25% = 2.5 mg/mL, 0.2% = 2 mg/mL; 0.1% = 1mg/mL

Lidocaine (xylocaine)

topical (ointment, jelly, patch, aerosol), SQ infiltration, peripheral nerve block, neuraxial, and intravenous regional application. Therapeutic uses include blunting laryngeal reflexes and sympathetic response to laryngoscopy, intubation, and suctioning (1–1.5 mg/kg); ventricular arrhythmias (1–1.5 mg/kg over 3 minutes, may repeat 0.5 mg/kg over 3 minutes after 5–10 minutes for a total of 3 mg/kg; continuous infusion of 1–4 mg/minute); ↓ CMRO2; topical application may ↓ sore throat (LTA®); test dose in epidurals to rule out intrathecal injection (need ~45 mg); Bier Block (40–50 mL of 0.5%); peripheral nerve blocks. Adverse effects include direct myocardial depression, vasodilation; TNS and cauda equina syndrome

Ropivicaine (Naropin)

SQ infiltration, peripheral nerve block, neuraxial, not typically used for IV regional anesthesia. Sensory > motor blockade (differential blockade; thus intrathecal use may result in sensory without motor block); larger therapeutic index and 70% less likely to cause severe cardiac dysrhythmias than bupivicaine ($\downarrow$ lipid solubility); greater CNS tolerance.

Etidocaine (Duranest)

SQ infiltration, peripheral nerve block, epidural application. Rapid onset, long duration of action. Profound motor blockade when used epidurally

Tetracaine (Pontocaine and Dicaine)

Topical and intrathecal use. Metabolism of this ester LA requires absorption into bloodstream since no pseudocholinesterase present intrathecally.

Bupivacaine (Marcaine, Sensoricaine)

Infiltration, peripheral nerve block, neuraxial application. R isomer of bupivacaine avidly blocks cardiac sodium channels and dissociates very slowly; resuscitation can be prolonged and difficult

Mepivicaine (Carbocaine and Polocaine)

Infiltration, peripheral nerve block, neuraxial, IV regional application. Intrathecal use for short duration procedures (knee scopes, hysteroscopies); may have less urinary retention. Available in 1%, 1.5%, and 2% preservative free solutions for neuraxial use.

Chloroprocaine (Nesacaine)

Infiltration, peripheral nerve block, neuraxial, IV regional application. When administered intrathecally with morphine, may interfere with its analgesic effect. Although $\uparrow$ pKa, has quick onset due to the $\uparrow$ administered concentration (although $\uparrow$ % in ionized form, $\uparrow$ total drug available). Formulated as an acidic solution (pH 3.1), thus addition of 1 mL of $NaHCO_3$ to 30 mL of chloroprocaine may improve efficacy of the combination and subsequent bupivacaine administration. Repeat at 40–50 min intervals.

Prilocaine

Its o-toluidine metabolite oxidizes hemoglobin to methemoglobin. Methemoglobin does not bind O_2 or CO_2, and hence prevents hemoglobin's primary transport function. Typically occurs at doses >600 mg. Treatment is with methylene blue 1–2 mg/kg over 5 mins reduces methemoglobin Fe^{3+} to hemoglobin Fe^{2+}. EMLA cream is a combination of lidocaine and prilocaine.

Cocaine

Topical to mucus membranes. Vasoconstriction and local anesthetic properties; useful for nasal preparation for surgery or nasal intubation awake; drug of abuse.

Clinical Case Scenario #1

A 20-year-old healthy male underwent a repair of a right tibial fracture with epidural anesthesia with intermittent boluses of 2% lidocaine and fentanyl. Ten hours after the surgery, the patient complains of continued numbness in right lower extremity. The patient is evaluated and it is determined that this is due to transient neurologic syndrome (TNS).

Background: TNS was first described in 1993 after intrathecal injection of hyperbaric 5% lidocaine. This phenomenon is associated with pain or sensory abnormalities in the lower back, buttock, or lower extremities. The symptoms of burning pain and dysesthesia in the L5 and S1 dermatomes usually start after the effects of spinal anesthesia have concluded and may last up to hours to four days. Some reports suggest that TNS may remain for years. Not associated with sensory or motor deficits.

Incidence: More common after lithotomy position, obesity, and outpatient surgeries. Incidence is greater with use of 5% lidocaine than other local anesthetics. The incidence of TNS ranges from 0% to 37%. The following factors do not increase the risk of TNS: gender, age, history of back pain or neurologic disorder, lidocaine dose or concentration, spinal needle size, aperture, direction, or addition of epinephrine.

Pathophysiology: Unknown mechanism however often related to long duration of epidural local anesthesia.

Treatment: First-line = reassurance. Neurophysiologic evaluation in volunteers during TNS does not reveal any abnormalities in somatosensory evoked potential, electromyography, or nerve conduction studies. No treatment is required if the pain is mild. If the pain is severe, the recommended therapy for TNS is NSAIDS or oral opioid analgesic agents. TNS has become a known risk factor for spinal anesthesia. Although uncommon it should be included in discussions of the risk of spinal anesthesia to the patient along with reassurance that it is not caused by neurologic deficits and is most often mild and lasts less than four days.

Alternative: May be useful to proceed without spinal in patients in lithotomy position who are obese and going for outpatient surgery, but otherwise TNS is not a reason to change an anesthetic plan where patient safety and satisfaction involve spinal anesthesia.

References

1. Yukioka H, Hayashi M, Terai T, Fujimori M. Intravenous lidocaine as a suppressant of coughing during tracheal intubation in elderly patients. *Anesth Analg.* 1993;77(2):309–312.

2. Himes RS Jr, DiFazio CA, Burney RG. Effects of lidocaine on the anesthetic requirements for nitrous oxide and halothane. *Anesthesiology.* 1977;47(5):437–440.

3. Senturk M, Pembeci K, Menda F, Ozkan T, Gucyetmez B, Tugrul M, Camci E, Akpir K. Effects of intramuscular administration of lidocaine or bupivacaine on induction and maintenance doses of propofol evaluated by bispectral index. *Br J Anaesth.* 2002;89(6):849–852.

4. Aouad MT, Siddik-Sayyid SM, Al-Alami AA, Baraka AS. Multimodal analgesia to prevent propofol-induced pain: pretreatment with remifentanil and lidocaine versus remifentanil or lidocaine alone. *Anesth Analg.* 2007;104(6): 1540–1544.

5. McCarthy GC, Megalla SA, Habib AS. Impact of intravenous lidocaine infusion on postoperative analgesia and recovery from surgery: a systematic review of randomized controlled trials. *Drugs.* 2010;70(9):1149–1163.

6. Yardeni IZ, Beilin B, Mayburd E, Levinson Y, Bessler H. The effect of perioperative intravenous lidocaine on postoperative pain and immune function. *Anesth Analg.* 2009;109(5):1464–1469.

7. Horowitz SH. The diagnostic workup of patients with neuropathic pain. *Med Clin North Am.* 2007;91(1):21–30.

8. Butterworth JF, Strichertz GR. Molecular mechanisms of local anesthesia: a review. *Anesthesiology.* 1990; 72(4):711–734.

9. Dobrydnjov I, Axelsson K, Thorn SE, Matthiesen P, Klockhoff H, Holmstrom B, Gupta A. Clonidine combined with small-dose bupivacaine during spinal anesthesia for inguinal herniorrhaphy: a randomized double-blinded study. *Anesth Analg.* 2003;96(5):1496–1503.

10. Jang I, Shin I, Ok S, Park K, Sohn J, Lee H, Chung Y. Spinal anesthesia and intrathecal clonidine decrease the hypnotic requirement of propofol. *Reg Anesth Pain Med.* 2010;35(2):145–147.

11. Strebel S, Gurzeler JA, Schneider MC, Aeschbach A, Kindler CH. Small-dose intrathecal clonidine and isobaric bupivacaine for orthopedic surgery: a dose-response study. *Anesth Analg.* 2004;99(4):1231–1238.

12. McCartney CJ, Duggan E, Apatu E. Should we add clonidine to local anesthetic for peripheral nerve blockade? A qualitative systemic review of the literature. *Reg Anesth Pain Med.* 2007;32(4):330–3308.

13. Butterworth JF, Strichertz GR. Molecular mechanisms of local anesthesia: a review. *Anesthesiology.* 1990;72(4):711–734.

14. American Society of Regional Anesthesia and Pain Medicine. www.asra.com. Last accessed August 1, 2010.

15. Freedman JM, Li DK, Drasner K, Jaskela M, Larsen B, Wi S. Transient neurologic symptoms after spinal anesthesia: an epidemiologic study of 1,863 patients. *Anesthesiology.* 1988;29(3):633–641.

16. Lev R, Rosen P. Prophylactic lidocaine use preintubation: a review. *J Emerg Med.* 1994;12(4):499–506.

17. Evans DE, Kobrine AI. Reduction of experimental intracranial hypertension by lidocaine. *Neurosurgery.* 1987;20(4):542–547.

18. Soltani HA, Aghadavoudi O. The effect of different lidocaine application methods on postoperative cough and sore throat. *J Clin Anesth.* 2002;14(10):15–18.

19. Hogan Q. Local anesthetic toxicity: an update. *Reg Anesth.* 1996;21(6 Suppl):43–50.

20. Katzung BG. *Basic and Clinical Pharmacology.* 6th ed. New York: McGraw-Hill; 1997:395–403.

21. Kumar S. Local anesthetics. In: Duke J, ed., *Anesthesia Secrets*. 3rd ed. Philadelphia: Mosby/Elsevier; 2006.

22. Windle ML. Local anesthetic agents, infiltrative administration. www.emedicine.com

23. *Physician's Desk Reference*.

24. Pollock JE. Transient Neurologic Symptoms: Etiology, Risk Factors, and Management. *Reg Anesth Pain Med*. 2002;27(6):581–586.

Chapter 9

Antiemitics

Alissa Wilmot, MD and Sander Schlichter, MD

Role in the Practice of Anesthesiology/Relevance to Anesthesiology

- PONV may occur in ~$1/_3$ of pts undergoing GA (high-risk pts can reach 70%-80%). Emetogenic agents include volatile anesthetics, opiates, N_2O, and anesthetic duration. PONV is often ranked as being worse than postoperative pain.
- PONV frequently ↑ PACU stays and causes unanticipated admission
- PONV can result in aspiration, surgical dehiscence, electrolyte imbalances, ↑ ICP
- PONV is triggered by peripheral and/or centrally located receptors; exact etiology unknown
- The emetic center is located in the medulla oblongata and serves as a "command center"; it receives afferent input from the chemoreceptor trigger zone (CTZ), vestibular system, peripheral sensory receptors, and higher CNS centers. The CTZ is located in the area postrema at the bottom of the 4th ventricle. Because it is highly vascularized and lacks a BBB, it is capable of receiving input via direct chemical stimulation through blood or the CSF: dopamine (D2), opioid, muscarinic, serotonin (5-HT), neurokinin (NK-1), Substance P, and histamine. Emetic center efferents include motor, SNS, and PNS output that not only cause gastric contraction but also ↑ salivation, retroperistalsis, sweating, and HR.
- Vomiting/emesis: forceful expulsion of gastric contents
- Nausea: unpleasant sensation in the throat and epigastrium associated with the urge to vomit.
- Retching is the rhythmic contraction of respiratory muscles including the diaphragm and abdominal muscles without the expulsion of gastric contents
- PONV patient risk factors: Female gender, young, history of PONV or motion sickness, and nonsmoker status. Surgical risk factors: ear, breast, abdomen, gynecological surgeries

Dopamine Antagonists

Promethazine

Pharmacodynamics

- Competitively compete with dopamine, histamine, and Ach at receptors in the CTZ and emetic center.
- Alpha adrenergic receptor antagonism as well

Pharmacokinetics

- Onset: oral, IM ~20 mins, IV ~5 mins; Duration 4–6 hrs (up to 12 hrs)
- Distribution: Vd 97 L; Protein binding: 93%;
- Metabolism: primarily hepatic oxidation to inactive metabolites; Elimination half-life: 9–16 hrs;
- Excretion: primarily urine and feces (as inactive metabolites)

Dosing

- Adult: 12.5–25 mg oral, IM, IV, rectal every 4–6 hrs prn;
- Pediatric >2 yrs oral, IV, PR 0.25–1 mg/kg 4–6 times daily as needed (maximum 25 mg/dose). Do not use in <2 yrs of age (risk of respiratory depression)

Preparation

- Injection solution 25 mg/mL (1 mL) or 50 mg/mL (1 mL); rectal suppository 12.5 mg, 25 mg, or 50 mg; syrup 6.25 mg/5mL; tablet 12.5 mg, 25 mg, or 50 mg.

Cautions/Adverse reactions

- Vascular necrosis can occur with extravasation and can require plastic surgery of skin lesions and/or amputation
- Cardiac conduction may be altered
- Extrapyramidal symptoms
- Neuroleptic malignant syndrome. Fever, muscle rigidity, autonomic instability, delirium, increased CPK
- Orthostatic hypotension due to α blockade
- Sedating; avoid in pts with respiratory depression, coadministration with diphenhydramine, prochlorperazine

Metoclopramide

Pharmacodynamics

- Competitively antagonizes dopamine and serotonin receptors in the CTZ
- Cholinergic action at peripheral sites; agonism in the upper GI tract enhances motility.

Pharmacokinetics

- Onset: 1–3 min IV, 10–15 min IM; PO good absorption, low bioavailability of 50% due to hepatic first-pass metabolism
- Duration 1–2 hr; Vd ~3.5 L/kg; Protein binding ~30%;

- Elimination half-life: children ~4 hrs, adults 5–6 hrs. Excreted unchanged in the urine; hepatic metabolites are excreted in bile.

Dosing
- Adult: 10 mg IV
- Pediatric: 0.25 mg/kg, max dose 10mg

Preparation
- Injection solution 5 mg/mL, oral solution 5 mg/5mL, tablet 5 mg or 10 mg, orally disintegrating tablet (ODT) 5 or 10 mg.

Side Effects/Adverse Effects
- Tardive dyskinesia (US boxed warning) often irreversible. Duration of treatment and total cumulative dose are associated with an ↑ risk; drowsiness, hypotension, tachycardia, extrapyramidal symptoms
- Adverse effects of promotility at surgical anastamosis/closure by ↑ pressure in suture lines
- Additive dopamine-blocking properties with droperidol and promethazine may compound adverse effects

Droperidol

Pharmacodynamics
- Butyrophenone antipsychotic; blocks dopamine agonism of CTZ. Also competes with alpha binding at receptors
- Structural similarity of butyrophenone antipsychotics to GABA likely contributes to their strong sedative/tranquilizing properties
- Lacks respiratory depressant properties even at high doses.
- Historically, used for neuroleptanalgesia to create a state of reduced anxiety, motor activity, and sensitivity to painful stimuli. Can be used for sedated intubations and other procedures (does not produce anxiolysis or amnesia and should be used in conjunction with an opiate and/or benzodiazepine/GABA agonist).
- Delays repolarization of ventricular cells by blocking the potassium rectifier channel; results in QT interval prolongation on the EKG. Prevents VT in ischemia, concurrent use of epinephrine or halothane in animal models. History of use as an antiarrhythmic; not anymore.

Pharmacokinetics
- Onset: peak parenteral ~30 min; Duration: 2–4 hrs, may extend to 12 hrs
- Vd adults ~2 L/kg; Protein binding: extensive
- Metabolism: hepatic to p-fluorophenylacetic acid, benzimidazolone, p-hydroxypiperidine; elimination half-life adults 2.3 hrs; Excretion: urine 75%, feces 22%

Dosing
- Adult: 0.625–1.25 mg IV; Pediatric dosing 2–12 years: 0.05–0.075 mg/kg to a maximum of 1.25 mg IV.

Preparation
- Injection solution 2.5 mg/mL for IV or IM administration, inexpensive.

Cautions/Adverse Reactions
- QT prolongation and Torsade de Pointes; FDA "black box" warning. However, the strength of evidence behind this black box warning has been highly debated
- Dysphoria, restlessness, anxiety, EPS, dystonic reactions, pseudoparkinsonian symptoms, tardive dyskinesia, seizure, altered central temperature regulation, drowsiness, breast swelling.

Prochlorperazine
- Piperazine antipsychotic. D1, D2, anticholinergic, and weak antihistamine antagonist. Adult dosing 2.5–10 mg IV. Preparation 5 mg/mL injection. May cause extrapyramidal symptoms and drowsiness.

5-Hydroxytryptamine Type 3 Antagonists (5-HT3) Receptor Antagonists

Pharmacodynamics
- Stimulation of 5-HT$_3$ receptors in the CTZ signals the vomiting center in the lateral reticular formation of the medulla to begin the vomiting reflex
- 5-HT$_3$ receptor antagonists bind selectively and competitively to these receptors to block emetogenic signals in the vomiting center. Also bind to peripheral receptors in the GI tract

Side Effects
- Relatively safe and well tolerated.
- Dose-dependent ↑ in ECG intervals within 1–2 hrs after IV administration.
- Cardiac. Heart block or arrhythmias. QT interval prolongation and Torsades de Pointes can occur especially in conjunction with agents with similar effects (eg, Class I and III antiarrhythmics). Use with caution in patients at risk of QT prolongation and/or ventricular arrhythmia

Ondansetron
Pharmacokinetics
- Onset of action IV ~30 mins, PO peak ~2 hrs; Vd adults 2–2.5 L/kg; Protein binding 70%–76%;
- Metabolism: Hydroxylation of the indole ring followed by glucuronide or sulfate conjugation; elimination half-life 3–6 hrs in adults, 2–7 hrs in children <15 yrs

Dosing
- Adult: IV/IM 4 mg IV or IM; PO 16 mg 1 hr prior to the induction of anesthesia;

- Pediatric: IV (10–40 kg): 0.05–0.1 mg/kg; (>40 kg): 4 mg as single dose; not recommended for <10 kg

Preparation

- Infusion 32 mg/50 mL; injection solution 2 mg/mL; oral solution 4 mg/5 mL; tablet 4 mg or 8 mg, ODT 4 or 8 mg.

Cautions/Adverse Reactions

- Headache, malaise/fatigue, constipation, ECG changes as noted above.

Dolasetron

Pharmacodynamics

- Dolasetron mesylate, and its liver-converted active metabolite hydrodolasetron, are highly specific 5-HT$_3$ antagonists

Pharmacokinetics

- Peak plasma levels: IV 0.6 hrs (administer ~15 mins before cessation of anesthesia), oral 1 hr;
- Vd: 5.8 L/kg; Protein binding 69%-77%;
- Metabolism: hepatic with rapid reduction by carbonyl reductase to hydrodolasetron (active metabolite), further metabolized to inactive metabolites; Elimination half-life ~ 7 hrs

Dosing

- Adult: 12.5 mg is minimum effective dose.
- Pediatric: (2–16 yrs) 0.35 mg/kg, max of 12.5 mg. Not recommended for <2 yrs.

Preparation

- Injection 20 mg/mL (0.625, 5, or 25 mL), tablet 50 or 100 mg.

Cautions/Adverse Reactions

- Headache (7%-24%), Diarrhea (2%-12%).

Granisteron

Pharmacokinetics

- Duration: PO/IV up to 24 hrs; transdermal patch peak levels ~48 hrs
- Vd 2–4 L/kg; protein binding: 65%
- Metabolism: hepatic via N-demethylation, oxidation, and conjugation (some are active metabolites); elimination half-life PO 6 hrs, IV 9 hrs; excretion urine and feces

Dosing

- Adult: 1 mg IV;
- Pediatric (≥4 years): 20–40 mcg/kg IV as a single dose; not to exceed 1 mg

Preparation

- Injection 1 mg/mL, transdermal patch (3.1 mg/24 hr), oral solution 2 mg/10 mL, and oral tablet 1 mg.

Cautions/Adverse Reactions
- Use cautiously in pts with liver disease

Tropisetron

(Not currently available in the United States)

Pharmacokinetics
- Metabolized hepatically (oxidative hydroxylation of the indole ring followed by conjugation with glucuronic acid and sulfate); metabolites are renally excreted
- Elimination half-life ~6 hrs

Dosing
- Adult: 2 mg IV, recommended shortly before induction;
- Pediatric: 0.1 mg/kg IV, max dose 2 mg.

Preparation, Miscellaneous
- 5 mg capsule, 1 mg/mL injection solution.

Cautions/Adverse Reactions
- Headache, constipation, dizziness.

Dexamethasone

Pharmacodynamics
- ↓ inflammation; mechanism of antiemetic activity is unknown

Pharmacokinetics
- Slow antiemetic onset action; therefore, should be give prior to induction, or 2 hrs prior to emergence
- Prolonged antiemetic effect: up to 48 hrs

Dosing
- Adult: 2.5–10 mg IV for prevention of PONV, 4–8 mg IV is now commonly utilized
- Pediatric: 150 mcg/kg up to 8 mg

Preparation
- 4 mg/mL injection solution, tablets (0.5, 0.75, 1, 1.5, 2, 4, and 6 mg), oral solution 0.5 mg/5 mL or 1 mg/mL, ophthalmic drops 0.1%. Injection solution is the only form used for PONV prevention.

Cautions/Adverse Reactions
- HTN, emotional instability, adrenal suppression, hyperglycemia, and possible decreased wound healing.
- Intense rectal burning and itching can be seen in awake patients; may be reduced with dilution and slow administration

Scopolamine

Clinical Uses/Relevance to Anesthesiology
- PONV, motion sickness

- Anticholinergic uses: intestinal cramping, antisialogogue (lungs, sinuses), mydriasis (for exam, uveitis, iritis)
- Sedation: trauma cases where other sedatives or amnestics may be detrimental to hemodynamics
- Nicotine withdrawal

Pharmacodynamics

- Belladonna alkaloid; centrally, blocks cholinergic transmission from the vestibular nuclei to other higher centers as well as from the reticular formation to the emetic center
- In the periphery, competes with Ach at smooth muscle receptors and post-ganglionic muscarinic receptor sites of PNS

Pharmacokinetics

- Transdermal patch applied behind the ear (press firmly for 10–20 seconds). Provides continuous release. Onset at 4 hrs, peak levels at 24 hrs; duration of action 72 hrs. Distribution is not well understood.
- Metabolized and conjugated; less than 5% unchanged in the urine.

Preparations

- Transdermal patch 1.5 mg; film with layers that contain the viscous liquid, adhesive, and microporous membrane that controls rate of delivery
- IV, IM

Cautions/Adverse Reactions

- Anticholinergic effects: dry eyes, mouth, urinary retention; central anticholinergic syndrome ↑ in patients with dementia
- ↑ IOP from mydriasis can worsen glaucoma.
- IV and IM use for routine antiemetic prophylaxis may have large peak plasma concentration, and enhance undesirable anticholinergic effects

Aprepitant

Pharmacodynamics

- Neurokinin-1 (NK1) receptor antagonist. NK1 is found in high concentrations in the vomiting center of the brain, has a Substance P ligand, and is a G protein coupled receptor.
- Reduces vomiting, not necessarily nausea

Preparations

- Capsules 40 mg, 80 mg, 125 mg

Doses

- 40 mg PO 1–3 hrs prior to anesthetic

Cautions/Adverse Effects

- Constipation, diarrhea, fatigue

Anesthetic Technique

- Because antiemetic efficacy is not 100%, avoiding PONV triggers is key
- TIVA vs inhalational—Propofol for induction and maintenance reduces ↓PONV
- N_2O—Some evidence to suggest. Possibly via ↑ middle ear pressure, bowel distension, and/or activation of the dopaminergic system in the CTZ.
- Opiate reduction-perioperative administration ↑ PONV 2- to 4-fold. However, failure to provide adequate analgesia can also ↑ the risks of PONV
- Consider NSAIDs, regional anesthesia, and a liberal infiltration of the surgical site with local anesthetics
- Supplemental O_2: May ↓ PONV in a dose-dependent fashion
- Acupuncture: P6 acupoint stimulation may ↓ PONV

Clinical Case Scenario #1

A 45-year-old male with a history of smoking and no history of PONV or motion sickness is undergoing knee arthroscopy. On his preoperative evaluation, his QTc is 500 msec. The anesthesiologist determines that in this patient, the risks of antiemetic therapy outweigh the benefits. Background: This patient has 0 Apfel risk factors. He is not female, a smoker, or has a history of PONV or motion sickness. Recent guidelines suggest that in low-risk patients, no PONV prophylaxis is recommended unless there is risk of medical sequelae from vomiting. Given the potential for 5-HT_3 antagonists and droperidol to cause or compound QT prolongation and arrhythmia, the risks of PONV prophylaxis in this patient likely outweigh the benefits.

One should consider regional anesthesia for patients with moderate or high risk of PONV. If general anesthesia is used, patients at moderate or high risk of PONV should receive combination therapy with two or three prophylactic drugs from different classes. In general, combination therapy is superior to monotherapy for PONV prophylaxis.

Clinical Case Scenario #2

A 3-year-old girl with a PMH of infantile esotropia is scheduled for strabismus repair. She weighs 15 kg and has no other medical problems. She is treated with 2.25 mg dexamethasone (0.15 mg/kg) and 1.5 mg ondansetron (0.1 mg/kg) for PONV prophylaxis.

Background: Children are at higher risk for PONV than adults. The number needed to treat with ondansetron for PONV prophylaxis is 2 to 3 in children. The two most commonly emetogenic surgeries in children are tonsillectomies and strabismus repair. Given this patient's intrinsic higher risk coupled with a higher risk procedure, a multimodal PONV prophylaxis strategy is recommended. One could also consider anesthetic techniques such as TIVA and opiate reduction in this patient, especially if the patient had a history of PONV or motion sickness. It is important to note that scopolamine would produce mydriasis, a potentially undesirable side effect for ophthalmologic surgery.

Clinical Case Scenario #3

A 40-year-old nonsmoking female with a history of cholelithiasis presents for laparoscopic cholecystectomy. She had severe nausea and vomiting following her BTL and required inpatient admission. She also experiences significant motion sickness. The anesthesiologist gives the patient a scopolamine patch 2 hrs prior to surgery, 8 mg of dexamethasone IV at induction, a TIVA, an OG tube to decompress her stomach, minimal narcotics, 30 mg ketorolac, generous infiltration of local anesthesia, and 4 mg ondansetron IV 30 mins prior to the end of surgery.

Background: This patient is at high risk for PONV given her gender, nonsmoking status, and history of PONV and motion sickness. In this patient, a multimodal approach to PONV prophylaxis is imperative. This includes specific antiemetic medications, as well as careful attention to anesthetic technique. Options for rescue therapy in the PACU would include promethazine and droperidol.

References

1. Gan TJ. Postoperative nausea and vomiting—can it be eliminated? *JAMA*. 2002;287:1233–1236.

2. Watcha MF. Postoperative nausea and emesis. *Anesthesiol Clin N Am*. 2002;20:709–722.

3. Apfel CC, Laara E, Koivuranta M, Clemens-A G, Roewer N: A simplified risk score for predicting postoperative nausea and vomiting: Conclusions from cross-validations between two centers. *Anesthesiology*. 1999;91:693–700.

4. Apfel CC, Korttila K, Abdalla M, et al. A factorial trial of six interventions for the prevention of postoperative nausea and vomiting. *N Eng J Med*. 2004;350:2441–2451.

5. Watcha MF, White PF. Postoperative nausea and vomiting: its etiology, treatment, and prevention. *Anesthesiology*. 1992;77:162–184.

6. Kovac AL. Prevention and treatment of postoperative nausea and vomiting. *Drugs*. 2000;59:213–243.

7. Roberts GW, Bekker TB, Carlsen HH, et al. Postoperative nausea and vomiting are strongly influenced by postoperative opioid use in a dose-related manner. *Anesth Analg*. 2005;101:1343–1348.

8. Taylor G, Houston JB, Shaffer J, et al. Pharmacokinetics of promethazine and its suphoxide metabolite after intravenous and oral administration to man. *Br J Pharmacol*. 1983;15:287–293.

9. Schulze-Delrieu K. Drug therapy: metoclopramide. *N Engl J Med*. 1981;305:28–33.

10. Gan TJ, Meyer T, Apfel CC, Chung F, Davis PJ, Eubanks S, Kovac A, Philip BK, Sessler DI, Temo J, Tramer MR, Watcha M. Consensus guidelines for managing postoperative nausea and vomiting. *Anesth Analg.* 2003;97: 62–71.

11. *FDA strengthens warnings for droperidol.* Available at http://www.fda.gov/safety/medwatch/safetyinformation/safetyalertsforhumanmedicalproducts/ucm172364.htm. Last accessed November 22, 2010.

12. Ho K, Gan T. Pharmacology, pharmacogenetics, and clinical efficacy of 5-hydroxytryptamine type 3 receptor antagonists for postoperative nausea and vomiting. *Curr Opin Anaesthesiol.* 2006;19:606–611.

13. Zofran (ondansetron hydrochloride) injection premixed (prescribing information). Research Triangle Park, NC. GlaxoSmithKline, 2006. Available at http://us.gsk.com/products/assets/us_zofran.pdf. Last accessed November 22, 2010.

14. Anzemet (dolasetron mesylate) injection (prescribing information). Kansas City, MO. Aventis Pharmaceuticals Inc., 2005. Available at http://products.sanofi-aventis.us/Anzemet_Injection/anzemet_injection.html. Last accessed November 22, 2010.

15. Kytril (granisetron hydrochloride) injection premixed (prescribing information). Nutley, NJ. Roche, 2009. Available at http://www.gene.com/gene/products/information/kytril/pdf/pl_injection.pdf. Last accessed November 22, 2010.

16. Plosker GL, Goa KL. Granisetron: a review of its pharmacological properties and therapeutic use as an antiemetic. *Drugs.* 1991;42:805–824.

17. Carlisle J, Stevenson C. Drugs for preventing postoperative nausea and vomiting. *Cochrane Database Syst Rev* 2006;19:3 CD004125.

18. Emend (aprepitant) prescribing information. Whitehouse Station, NJ. Merck & Co., Inc., 2006. Available at http://www.merck.com/product/usa/pl_circulars/e/emend/emend_pi.pdf. Last accessed November 22, 2010.

19. Mraovic B, Simurina T, Sonicki Z, Skitarelic N, Gan TJ. The dose-response of nitrous oxide in postoperative nausea in patient undergoing gynecologic laparoscopic surgery: a preliminary study. *Ambulatory Anesthesiology.* 2008;107:818–23.

Chapter 10

Gastric Medications

Shanique Brown, MD and Nina Singh-Radcliff, MD

Antacids

Clinical Uses/Relevance to Anesthesiology

- Premedication to *immediately* neutralize gastric acid such that in the event of aspiration, the severity of acid pneumonitis is reduced; useful for C-sections, urgent and emergent surgical procedures
- Symptomatic treatment of duodenal, peptic ulcer, and gastric acid reflux disease; typically used as a prn medication
- Alkaline diuresis (administered to hasten renal excretion of acidic toxins and drugs as well as myoglobin); see sodium bicarbonate chapter
- Hyperphosphatemia of renal disease
- Inexpensive (compared to H2-receptor antagonists, PPI)

Pharmacodynamics

- Inorganic salts that release anions upon dissolving in acidic gastric secretions; anions combine and neutralize hydrochloric acid
- Increasing gastric fluid pH inactivates pepsin, which then has bile-chelating effects as well as stimulates gastrin release, which enhances motility and esophageal sphincter tone
- Antacids are categorized as particulate and nonparticulate. Particulates (aluminum, magnesium, calcium), if aspirated may cause a chemical pneumonitis. Nonparticulates are clear and if aspirated, cause less foreign body reaction. Mixing is more complete and rapid than particulate antacids.

Pharmacokinetics

- Tablets are less effective than liquid preparations (do not need to dissolve, more drug surface area in contact with gastric acid fluid)
- Duration of action depends on gastric emptying time; more complete neutralization occurs with increased contact time. A full stomach and opioids reduce gastric motility
- Increased urine pH can persist for >24 hours; may alter renal elimination of other drugs

Side Effects/Adverse Reactions

- Chronic alkalinization of gastric fluid may increase susceptibility to acid-sensitive bacilli
- Alkalinization of urine may predispose to UTIs; chronic use may result in urolithiasis
- The increase in gastric fluid volume with resultant stomach distention can potentially offset desirable effects of pH reduction (may increase nausea, emesis, and volume of aspirate should aspiration occur)
- Acid rebound. Unique to calcium containing antacids (marked increase in gastric acid secretion several hours following neutralization of gastric acid).
- Milk-alkali syndrome. Excessive ingestion of elemental calcium (>2 g) may result in calcification of the renal parenchyma and dysfunction. Manifests as increased BUN and Cr, systemic alkalosis, bicarbonaturia, and subsequent hypovolemia (Na^+ accompanies bicarbonate and water accompanies Na^+).
- Phosphorous depletion. Aluminum salts bind phosphate within the GI and prevent absorption (effect is harnessed in renal disease to avoid hyperphosphatemia). Symptoms may include anorexia, skeletal muscle weakness, and malaise as well as osteomalacia, osteoporosis, and fractures.
- Drug affects. Gastric alkalinization hastens gastric emptying into the small intestine (gastrin mediated); drugs requiring gastric acid exposure for activation or tablet disintegration may have impaired absorption whereas drugs absorbed in the small intestine may have quickened onset. Additionally, antacids may form complexes with drugs (ie, cimetidine, digoxin) and decrease bioavailability. pH alterations may directly increase or decrease drug solubility (by affecting ionization) and therefore onset.

Calcium Carbonate (particulate)
Potent antacid. Acid rebound may occur several hours after its ingestion; additionally can result in metabolic alkalosis, gastric distention from carbon dioxide production, a transient increase of plasma calcium (may reach toxic levels in patients with renal disease or hypercalcemia), and milk-alkali syndrome

Magnesium Hydroxide (particulate)
"Milk of magnesia." Prompt neutralization that lacks significant rebound. Side effects include a prominent laxative effect (osmotic diarrhea); and in patients with renal dysfunction, systemic absorption of magnesium may result in adverse neurologic, neuromuscular, and cardiovascular effects

Aluminum Hydroxide (particulate)
Not potent. Its ability to interfere with phosphate absorption bestows therapeutic potential for phosphate nephrolithiasis and hyperphosphatemia of renal disease. Side effects include hypophosphatemia with resultant hypercalcemia (hypercalcuria and nephrolithiasis may occur); constipating effects of aluminum; and aluminum accumulation in patients with renal insufficiency

Sodium bicarbonate (particulate)
See "Sodium Bicarbonate" chapter. Utilized for alkaline diuresis. Antacid has a high solubility that results in rapid action. Sodium load may be dangerous in patients with CHF, HTN.

Sodium citrate (nonparticulate)
Rapid and more complete mixing with gastric fluid (compared to particulate antacids). If aspirated, less foreign body reaction in the lungs. Has an unpleasant taste and may need flavoring.

Bicitra (nonparticulate)
Comprised of sodium citrate and citric acid; provides effective buffering of gastric fluid pH. Frequently used peripartum. Supplied as 30 mL of 0.3-mol solution.

Polycitra (nonparticulate)
Comprised of sodium citrate, potassium citrate, and citric acid; enhanced buffering capacity compared to bicitra.

Sucralfate

Clinical Uses/Relevance to Anesthesiology
- Symptomatic treatment of non-NSAID related duodenal and gastric ulcers as well as GERD and reflux associated with pregnancy
- Stress ulcer prophylaxis
- Prevention of nosocomial and ventilator associated pneumonia (more effective than antacids or H_2 blockers)

Pharmacodynamics
- Acid buffer with cytoprotective properties.
- Oral tablet that disintegrates in the stomach to produce sucrose sulfate and aluminum hydroxide salt. Binds with hydrochloric acid to form a cross-linking, viscous suspension that interacts with high affinity to proteins (albumin, fibrinogen) on the surface of ulcers, serving as a protective barrier. Thereby preventing further damage from acid, pepsin, and bile.

Pharmacokinetics
- Acid buffering capability for 6–8 hrs
- Poorly water soluble, minimal absorption

Side Effects
- Aluminum binds with proteins, peptides, metals, large molecules (mucin), and drugs (interferes with absorption and reduces bioavailability of tetracycline, quinolone, ciprofloxacin, phenytoin, digoxin, and amitryptyline)
- Aluminum accumulation with resultant toxicity may manifest in renal disease

- Coadministration of antacids may interfere with the efficacy of sucralfate.
- Constipation from aluminum

H2 Antagonists (cimetidine, ranitidine, famotidine, nizatidine)

Clinical Uses/Relevance to Anesthesiology

- Premedication to reduce acidity *and* volume of gastric contents; reduces incidence, amount, and damage of pulmonary aspiration. Onset ~20–30 mins, not immediate
- GERD, reflux esophagitis, and peptic and gastric ulcer disease
- Nausea
- Gastric hypersecretory states (Zollinger-Ellison syndrome, systemic mastocytosis, multiple endocrine adenomas)
- Allergic reactions; coadministration with antihistamines, steroids, and epinephrine
- Reduces incidence of stress ulcer in critically ill patients

Pharmacodynamics

- Competitive antagonist of histamine *and* inverse agonist at H_2 receptors of gastric parietal cells. Inverse agonism occurs when a competitive antagonist binds to a receptor with intrinsic activity that is independent of agonist binding and reduces the receptor's baseline function.
- Decreases baseline parietal cell acid and volume secretion as well as blunts the response to normal stimulus (ie, food, histamine, insulin, caffeine). In turn, the reduced acid and volume inactivates pepsin (inactive form is a bile-chelator) and stimulates gastrin release (increases LES pressure and gastric motility). These further reduce the incidence of and severity if pulmonary aspiration occurs.
- Minimal affect at histamine 1 receptors

Pharmacokinetics

- Metabolized by the hepatic p450 system
- Metabolites excreted via urine

Side Effects/Adverse Reactions

- Crosses placenta and can enter breast milk; consider avoiding during pregnancy and breast-feeding.
- Inhibits hepatic p450 enzymes. Drugs metabolized by this system can have prolonged duration and concentration (eg, warfarin, ethanol, lidocaine, TCA, phenytoin, propanolol, diazepam, theophylline, and phenobarbitol). This effect is more pronounced with cimetidine, less so with famotidine and nizadatidine
- Reduces the bioavailabilty of clopidegrel (subtherapeutic antiplatelet action)

Cimetidine (Tagamet)

Able to cross the BBB and cause headache, dizziness, somnolence; consider avoiding in elderly patients (lethargy, hallucinations, seizures). Long-term use can cause hepatoxicity, interstitial nephritis, granulocytopenia, and thrombocytopenia; possible gynecomastia and impotence from agonist effect at androgen receptors. Fast IV administration can cause arrhythmias, hypotension, and cardiac arrest. Potential bronchoconstriction (blocks H_2 receptor-mediated bronchodilation). Dosing: IM/IV/PO 300 mg q6 hrs, IV infusion rate of 37.5mg/hr; alternative PO dosing includes 800 mg QHS or 400 mg BID. Titrate to maintain pH >5; IV push should be done over 5 mins. Clinical half-life of 2 hrs; duration of 4–8 hrs (shortest). Protein binding 20%, oral bioavailability 60%-70%. Consider adjusting dose and frequency with hepatic and/or renal impairment; cleared with hemodialysis.

Ranitidine (Zantac)

Compared to cimetidine, more potent and with less drug interactions and crossing of the BBB (neurologic side effects still possible). Long-term therapy may result in B12 deficiency. Dosing: IV bolus 50 mg q6–8 hrs (dilute in 20 mL NS or D5W); alternatively continuous IV infusion 6.25 mg/hr. PO dose 150–300 mg (max oral dose of 6 g/day). Protein binding 15%; oral bioavailability ~50%, IM bioavailability can reach 100%; volume of distribution ~1.4L/kg.

Famotidine (Pepcid)

Compared to ranitidine, more potent and with less entry into breast milk. May cause headache, dizziness, diarrhea, and constipation. Dosage: IV/PO 20 mg q12 hrs. Protein binding 15%-20%, bioavailability 40%-45%, volume of distribution 1.0–1.3 L/kg.

Nizatidine (Axid)

Fastest H_2 blocker onset. High incidence of headaches (~16%). PO only: 300 mg qhs or 150 mg PO BID. Adjust for hepatic, renal impairment. Protein binding 35%, oral bioavailability >70%; volume of distribution 0.8–1.5 L/kg.

Proton Pump Inhibitors (omeprazole, pantoprazole, lansoprazole)

Clinical Uses/Relevance to Anesthesiology

- Active duodenal ulcers, gastric ulcers, GERD, erosive esophagitis, hypersecretory conditions, and H. pylori eradication
- Typically scheduled dosing, however can be utilized perioperatively (IV pantoprazole available)
- Stress ulcer prophylaxis in the critically ill (off-label use)
- Most potent drug available for gastric acid inhibition

Pharmacodynamics

- Binds irreversibly to and inhibits H^+/K^+ ATPase enzyme on parietal cells; inhibits "proton pump" and gastric acidity

- Terminal step of gastric acid production and irreversible; therefore, capable of inhibiting close to 100% of gastric acid secretion

Pharmacokinetics

- Metabolized by hepatic P450 system; metabolites excreted in urine
- Onset of action is rapid; maximal effect 2–6 hrs; duration of action up to 96 hrs
- Decreased dosing frequency compared to H_2 blockers can increase compliance

Adverse Effects/Side Effects:

- Reduces clopidegrol bioavailability and antiplatelet effects by inhibiting the CYP2C19 enzyme (responsible for conversion to its active metabolite).
- Enters breast milk in lactating females; consider avoiding
- Prolonged acid suppression may result in bacterial overgrowth in the GI tract and malabsorption of B12 and calcium (HCl is necessary for absorption); long-term use can cause B12 deficiency
- Headache, insomnia, diarrhea, flatulence, nausea

Omeprazole (Prilosec)
Short-term treatment for ulcers, GERD; long-term treatment for H. Pylori (as part of multidrug regimen). Dosing: PO 20–40 mg PO QD (available in 10 mg, 20 mg, and 40 mg; no IV formulation). Protein binding 95%, oral bioavailability 30%-40%. Increased bioavailability see in chronic liver disease, elderly patients, and Asian ethnicities; consider reducing dosage.

Pantoprazole (Protonix)
IV formulation makes convenient for perioperative utilization. Erosive esophagitis with GERD: IV/PO 40 mg QD (duration of therapy 7–10 days IV, 8 weeks PO). Hypersecretory disorders: IV 80 mg BID, PO 40 mg BID. Protein binding 98%, oral bioavailability 77%; no adjustment required for liver disease or kidney disease.

Lansoprazole (Prevacid)
Dosing: 15–30 mg PO QD; H. pylori eradication 15–30 mg PO BID; hypersecretory syndromes may require up to 60 mg dQD. Protein binding 97%, oral bioavailability 80%.

Clinical Case Scenario #1

73-year-old obese Caucasian male with PMHx of HTN, BMI 36, and occasional GERD presents to the ER after falling and sustaining a left lower extremity open fracture at 20:00. No other injuries identified. Last meal was at 16:00 prior to arrival and the patient now awaits anesthetic evaluation in the holding area prior to being brought in to operating room. Home Meds: HCTZ 25mg, Tums pm and baby ASA. Surgical Hx: Open Cholecystectomy, Anesthesia

Hx: Uncomplicated GA for open cholecystectomy 20 years ago. No problems with GA. Allergies: NKDA. According to the surgeon, surgical intervention will take approximately 2.5 hrs.

Anesthetic Management/ Considerations: The patient has several risk factors for aspiration: obesity, history of GERD, recent meal ingestion (4 hrs ago). Plan: Semiurgent case allows time for ranitidine 50 mg IV (onset 20–30 mL) in addition to 30 ml of bicitra (immediate gastric acid neutralization) prior to induction. The pt is placed in reverse trendelenburg position to reduce passive gastric fluid reflux (Note: head up can increase intragastric pressure). Suction is available and a RSI is performed while the nurse holds cricoid pressure until the ETT cuff is inflated and position confirmed. After induction, an OG tube is placed and suctioned to reduce gastric fluid volume (reduces incidence of aspiration and severity in the event it occurs). At the conclusion of the surgery, the pt is extubated fully awake and in the head up position.

Clinical Case Scenario #2

23-year-old unhelmeted African American female with no significant PMHx is hit by an SUV while riding her motorcycle. The patient sustains multiple rib fractures, lower extremity fractures, and a left frontal and occipital subdural hematoma that required immediate hematoma evacuation in the OR. The pt was taken to the ICU intubated. On postoperative rounds, the need for GI prophylaxis is discussed.

Anesthetic Management/ Considerations: Risk factors for the development of stress ulcers include the presence of a TBI, coagulopathy, mechanical ventilation, sepsis or severe hypotension, major burns, high dose corticosteroids, history of GI bleeding, ARF, male gender, and hepatic failure. This pt has TBI and is being mechanically ventilated. GI prophylaxis to increase gastric pH > 4 may reduce the formation of stress ulcers and thereby decrease the risk of bleeding. However, increases in nosocomial pneumonia, C. difficile infections, drug-drug interactions and accruing hospital and prescription costs necessitate balancing the risks and benefits of GI prophylaxis in the ICU setting. Generally, the presence of TBI, coagulopathy, and mechanical ventilation almost always necessitate the use of GI prophylaxis. Other risk factors lack strong evidence, but consideration should be given on an individual basis. In this pt, the ICU team decided that her benefits outweighed her risks and that either an H_2 blocker or PPI should be started and continued during her ICU stay. Upon discharge she would be reevaluated for continued administration.

References

1. Collard HR, Saint S, Matthay MA. Prevention of ventilator-associated pneumonia: an evidence-based systematic review. *Ann Intern Med.* 2003;138(6):494–501. [PubMed 12639084]

2. Katzung BG. *Basic & Clinical Pharmacology.* 7th ed. Stamford, CT: Appleton & Lange, 1998.

3. Hemstreet BA. Use of sucralfate in renal failure. *Ann Pharmacother.* 2001;35(3):360–364. [PubMed 11261535]

4. Roberts CJ. Clinical pharmacokinetics of ranitidine. *Clin Pharmacokinet.* 1984;9(3): 211–221.[PubMed 6329583]

5. Echizen H, Ishizaki T. Clinical pharmacokinetics of famotidine. *Clin Pharmacokinet.* 1991 Sep;21(3):178–94. [PubMed 1764869]

6. Mackenzie IS, Coughtrie MW, Macdonald TM, Wei L. Antiplatelet drug interactions. *J Intern Med.* 2010. doi: 10.1111/j.1365–2796.2010.02299.x. [Epub ahead of print] [PubMed 21073556]

7. Shin JM, Sachs G. Pharmacology of proton pump inhibitors. *Curr Gastroenterol Rep.* 2008;10(6):528–534. [PubMed 19006606]

8. Daily Med. 2009. November 2009. <http://dailymed.nlm.nih.gov/dailymed/drugInfo.cfm?id=31220#section-14.3>.

Chapter 11

Steroids and Antihistamines

Chapter 11.1

Steroids

Lisa Witkin, MD and Anita Gupta, DO, PharmD

Clinical Uses/Indications

- Three major classes of hormones are secreted by the adrenal cortex-androgens, glucocorticoids, and mineralocorticoids.
- Cortisol, the primary glucocorticoid secreted from the adrenal gland, is a major stress response hormone that has metabolic, anti-inflammatory, and cardiovascular properties that are vital in normal physiology.
- Glucocorticoids are the most potent and effective agents in controlling inflammation through numerous mechanisms, including effects on cytokines, inflammatory mediators, inflammatory cells, nitric oxide synthase, and adhesion molecules.
- Glucocorticoids are also important in maintaining fluid and electrolyte balance, preserving the immune system, the kidney, skeletal muscle, the endocrine system, and the nervous system.
- Cortisol is produced at a rate of 10 mg/day in normal humans but can increase 10-fold in the setting of stresses such as infection or trauma
- There are many important indications for the use of steroids in anesthesia, with the strongest evidence of support being for adrenal insufficiency, asthma, anaphylaxis, acute spinal cord injury, and increased intracranial pressure secondary to trauma, tumor, abscess, or ischemia/infarction.
- Its anti-inflammatory and immunosuppressive properties also make it very useful also in preventing transplantation rejection.
- Moreover, injections of glucocorticoids for the relief of vertebrogenic, arthritic, and radiculopathic pains are widely accepted.
- There has also been some benefit demonstrated in preventing postoperative nausea and vomiting, thyroid storm, hypothermia, airway foreign bodies, and respiratory insufficiency from fat or air embolism, ARDS or COPD.
- Equivocal evidence has been reported for the use of steroids for sepsis/septic shock, postintubation airway edema, and cardiac arrest.

Table 11.1.1 Relative Potencies and Equivalent Doses for Commonly Used Steroids

Steroids	Relative Glucocorticoid Potency	Equivalent Glucocorticoid Dose (mg)	Relative Mineralo-corticoid Potency	Half-life (hrs)
Short Acting				
Cortisol (hydrocortisone)	1.0	20.0	1.0	8
Cortisone	0.8	25.0	0.8	Oral-8, IM-18+
Prednisone	4.0	5.0	0.8	16–36
Prednisolone	4.0	5.0	0.8	16–36
Methylprednisolone	5.0	4.0	0.5	18–40
Intermediate Acting				
Triamcinolone	5.0	4.0	0	12–36
Long Acting				
Fludrocortisone	15.0	300	200	24
Betamethasone	25.0	0.60	0	36–54
Dexamethasone	30.0	0.75	0	36–54
Aldosterone	0.3	6.0	200–1,000	n/a

Pharmacodynamics

- Secretion of glucocorticoids is regulated by the hypothalamic-pituitary axis.
  - Corticotropin releasing factor (CRF) from the hypothalamus stimulates release of adrenocorticotropic hormone (ACTH), which leads to cortisol secretion.
  - Cortisol and other glucocorticoids have a negative feedback both at the pituitary and hypothalamic levels and inhibit ACTH and CRF respectively.
- Cortisol regulates carbohydrate, protein, lipid, and nucleic acid metabolism. The hormone binds to a stereospecific intracellular cytoplasmic receptor, stimulating nuclear transcription of specific mRNA molecules, which are then translated to proteins mediating its ultimate effects.
- Glucocorticoids have lympholytic and immunosuppressive properties.
  - Cortisol has negative feedback to proinflammatory cytokine production and stimulates secretion of IL-10, an anti-inflammatory cytokine.
- Glucocorticoids modulate the immune response at many levels.
  - They cause leukocytosis by enhancing the release of mature leukocytes from the bone marrow as well as inhibiting their egress from the circulation.
  - They inhibit macrophage activity by impairing phagocytosis, intracellular digestion of antigens, and the production of interleukin 1 (IL-1) and IL-6 inflammatory mediators.
  - Glucocorticoids interfere with T-cell mediated immunity.

- They inhibit the production of interferon by T lymphocytes, as well as T-cell growth factor (IL-2).
- Glucocorticoids are effective in promoting homograft survival after organ transplantation by suppressing the inflammatory response to antigen-antibody union.
- Aldosterone is the major mineralocorticoid, which causes reabsorption of sodium and secretion of potassium and hydrogen ions in the distal renal tubule as well as in salivary and sweat glands, maintaining electrolyte and volume homeostasis.
- It is regulated by the renin-angiotensin system.
  - The juxtaglomerular cells in renal arterioles sense decreased renal perfusion pressure or volume, secrete renin, which splits the precursor angiotensinogen into angiotensinogen I, which is then converted in the lung into angiotensinogen II.
  - Angiotensinogen II then binds to specific receptors to increase mineralocorticoid secretion, which is also increased by hyperkalemia and ACTH.
- Two toxic, life-threatening states may arise from either abrupt withdrawal of therapy or continued use at supraphysiologic doses.
- Withdrawal will lead to a flare of the underlying disease as well as several other complications including acute adrenal insufficiency because of prolonged therapy suppressing the HPA axis.
  - Atrophied adrenal glands cannot adequately respond to stressful situations, such as the perioperative period.
  - The time to recovery from this can vary from weeks to over one year.
  - Patients who have had 2–4 weeks of supraphysiologic doses of glucocorticoids within the last year should be treated accordingly in the setting of an acute stress.
  - In order to prevent an acute adrenal crisis, which can be fatal, aggressive treatment of hypovolemia, hyperkalemia, and hyponatremia should be achieved as well as stress dose glucocorticoids given.
- Continued use of supraphysiologic doses of glucocorticoids can cause many problems including fluid and electrolyte abnormalities, such as hypokalemic alkalosis, edema, and hypertension.
  - Metabolic changes such as hyperglycemia with glycosuria are common.
  - An increased susceptibility to infections and risk for reactivation of latent TB are also important considerations.
  - Musculoskeletal effects including osteoporosis, osteonecrosis, myopathy (particularly proximal limb muscles and respiratory muscles), and growth arrest may be seen.
  - It is also prudent to asses for peptic ulcer disease especially in patients who are concomitantly receiving NSAID therapy.

- Behavioral disturbances include insomnia, nervousness, changes in mood/psych, and overt psychosis have been reported.
- Cataracts are related to the dosage and duration of therapy and particularly children are at high risk.
- Lastly, the typical cushinoid appearance may develop (fat redistribution, striae, and ecchymoses).

Pharmacokinetics

- **Absorption:** Hydrocortisone and the synthetic analogs are orally effective, although some may be administered IV to ensure high therapeutic levels rapidly. More prolonged effects are seen with IM injection of suspensions of hydrocortisone or its analogues.

Clinical Case Scenario

A 39-year-old woman with chronic daily headaches (transformed migraine) attributed to analgesic usage had marked tenderness over both greater occipital nerves. Palpation of the nerves reproduced her headache. She received a series of six bilateral greater occipital nerve blocks over a period of 3 months with temporary benefit each time. Each injection included 1 mL of triamcinolone (40 mg), 1 mL of 2% lidocaine, and 1 mL of 0.5% bupivacaine. In all, she received a total of 480 mg of triamcinolone. Other medications employed during this period included propranolol, hydroxyzine, alprazolam, lorazepam, amitriptyline, riboflavin, sumatriptan, rizatriptan, metoclopramide, prochlorperazine, imipramine, topiramate, metaxalone, diflucan, and acyclovir.

Toward the end of the treatment period, she developed overt signs of Cushing syndrome with intermittent hypertension, severe muscle weakness, fluid retention, centripetal obesity, moon facies, a dorsal fat pad (buffalo hump), and pharyngitis that may have been due to both candida and herpes simplex.

Laboratory evaluation demonstrated suppression of the hypothalamic-pituitary-adrenal axis, indicating an exogenous source of a synthetic steroid not detected by the usual laboratory tests of adrenal function. Her plasma cortisol, adrenocorticotropic hormone, and urinary free cortisol levels were undetectable. Two weeks later, the urinary free cortisol level was still undetectable, and urinary 17-ketosteroids were low; however, the thyroid-stimulating hormone level was normal, ruling out panhypopituitarism. A week later, a cosyntropin stimulation test was performed, which showed a preserved aldosterone response, ruling out primary adrenal insufficiency; however, the cortisol response was blunted.

The apparent paradox between the clinical picture of Cushing syndrome and the laboratory picture of adrenal insufficiency was the result of the exogenous corticosteroid, triamcinolone, used in the occipital nerve block injections. The patient did not receive corticosteroids by any other route. Investigation eliminated Cushing disease, a corticosteroid-producing adrenal tumor, and an ectopic source of corticotrophin such as a neoplasm. None of the other medications she had taken are known to delay the metabolism or elimination of corticosteroids.

This patient demonstrated marked sensitivity to exogenous corticosteroids with rapid development of Cushing syndrome and secondary suppression of adrenal function. She may be a slow metabolizer of corticosteroids.

The systemic administration of exogenous corticosteroids is probably the most common cause of Cushing syndrome. Local administration of corticosteroids, such as paraspinal injections for analgesia, intradermal injection for skin disorders, intrapericardial injections, intra-urethral injection for strictures, and intra-articular injections can also induce Cushing syndrome.

Glucocorticoids may also be systemically absorbed from local sites including synovial spaces, conjunctival sac, skin, and the respiratory tract, particularly when the administration is prolonged or when an occlusive dressing is used. This may lead to systemic effects of the drugs.

- **Distribution:** After absorption, 90% or more is reversibly bound to plasma proteins. Most cortisol is bound to albumin or CBG (corticosterone-binding globulin or transcortin) but it is its unbound or free counterpart that is active. Distributes into breast milk and placenta.

- **Metabolism:** The metabolism of steroid hormones involves sequential additions of oxygen or hydrogen atoms, followed by conjugation to form water-soluble derivative. The first reduction step occurs at both hepatic and extrahepatic sites, yielding inactive compounds. The subsequent reduction occurs only in the liver. The resultant sulfate esters and glucuronides are excreted in the urine. Neither biliary nor fecal excretion is of significance in humans.

  - Synthetic steroids with an 11-keto substituent, such as cortisone and prednisone, must be enzymatically reduced to the corresponding 11Beta-hydroxy derivative before they are biologically active. This occurs mostly in the liver but also in adipocytes, bone, eyes, and skin.

  - Chemical modifications have allowed the development of steroids with greater potencies, longer durations, and less mineralocorticoid effects. This may be due to changes in affinity, specificity, and intrinsic activity at corticosteroid receptors, alterations in absorption, protein binding, rate of metabolic transformation, rate of excretion, or membrane permeability.

  - Synthetic glucocorticoids vary in their binding specificity in a dose-related manner. With supraphysiologic doses (>30 mg/day), cortisol and cortisone bind to mineralocorticoid receptors causing salt and water retention and loss of potassium and hydrogen ions. When given in maintenance replacement therapy, patients also need specific mineralocorticoid replacement for electrolyte and volume homeostasis.

Pharmacodynamics

- **Dexamethasone:** Dexamethasone is a synthetic adrenocortical steroid with potent anti-inflammatory and immunosuppressant effects, without the sodium retaining properties of hydrocortisone. It also is often used as an antiemetic (unknown mechanism) or in the management of cerebral edema and chronic swelling. It is also used off-label to accelerate fetal lung maturation in patient with preterm labor.

- **Hydrocortisone:** Hydrocortisone is a naturally occurring glucocorticoid that acts as an anti-inflammatory, antipruritic, vasoconstrictive agent and has salt-retaining properties. It is also used as replacement therapy in adrenocortical deficiency states.

- **Methylprednisolone:** Methylprednisolone is a synthetic glucocorticoid, used in the treatment of a wide variety of diseases and conditions principally for glucocorticoid effects as an anti-inflammatory and immunosuppressant agent and for its effects on blood and lymphatic systems in the palliative treatment of various diseases. Usually, inadequate alone for adrenocortical insufficiency because of minimal mineralocorticoid activity.

- **Prednisone:** Prednisone is a synthetic glucocorticoid analog with minimal mineralocorticoid activity which is mainly used for its anti-inflammatory effects in different disorders of many organ systems. It causes profound and varied metabolic effects, modifies the immune response, and can be used as replacement therapy for deficient patients.

- **Prednisolone:** Prednisolone is a synthetic glucocorticoid with minimal mineralocorticoid activity. Used to treat a wide variety of diseases and conditions, principally as an anti-inflammatory and immunosuppressant agent and for its effects on blood and lymphatic systems in the palliative treatment of various diseases

- **Fludrocortisone:** Fludrocortisone is a synthetic steroid that possesses a very potent mineralocorticoid property and high glucocorticoid activity but is only used for its mineralocorticoid effects. FDA approved for Addison's disease and adrenogenital disorders. It controls the rate of protein synthesis. In small doses, it produces marked sodium retention and increased urinary potassium excretion, while in large doses it inhibits endogenous adrenal cortical secretion, thymic activity, and pituitary corticotropin excretion.

Pharmacokinetics

- **Dexamethasone:** *onset*: prompt, *duration*: metabolic effect: 72 hours, *metabolism*: hepatic CYP3A4, *half-life* elimination: 1.8–3.5 h with normal renal function, biological half life: 36–54 h

- **Hydrocortisone:** *Absorption*: rectal—partially absorbed, 50% bioavailability; *Distribution*: corticosteroids, protein binding to plasma proteins; *Metabolism*: most tissues, but primarily hepatic; *Excretion*: inactive metabolites excreted mostly renally, with some biliary; *Half-life*: 1.5–3.5 hours; however, since it acts through intracellular receptors, its activity is not directly correlated to the serum level but instead has a well-documented prolonged end-organ effect. Duration: 1.25–1.5 days for a single 250 mg oral dose.

- **Methylprednisolone:** *Absorption-Bioavailability:* Absorption from IM injection of methylprednisolone sodium succinate is rapid. Systemic absorption of methylprednisolone acetate occurs slowly following intra-articular, intrabursal, intrasynovial, intradermal, or soft tissue injection; absorption from intra-articular injection sites usually continues for about 7 days. *Onset:* Following IM administration (80–120 mg) relief onset within 8–12 hours. Following oral administration effects may not be evident for several hours. *Duration:* about 1.25–1.5 days for a single 40-mg oral dose. *Distribution- Extent:* Most glucocorticoids are removed rapidly from the blood and distributed to muscles, liver, skin, intestines, and kidneys. Glucocorticoids appear in breast milk and the placenta. *Elimination-Metabolism:* Metabolized in most tissues, but mainly in the liver, to inactive compounds. *Half-life:* Approximately 2.5–3.5 hours following oral administration of methylprednisolone or IV or IM administration of methylprednisolone sodium succinate.

- **Prednisone**: *Absorption*: Rapid, almost complete; *Distribution*: Crosses placenta; *Metabolism*: Mainly hepatic, also renal and in the tissue. Prednisone is inactive and rapidly metabolized to active prednisolone. *Elimination*: Renal. Plasma half-life is 3.4 to 3.8 h. Peak 1 to 2 hours. Duration is 1.25 to 1.5 days.

- **Prednisolone:** *Absorption-Onset:* Following oral administration in patients with asthma, effects may not be evident for several hours. Rapidly absorbed, reaching Cmax in 1 to 2 h. *Duration*: The duration is about 1.25–1.5 days for a single 50-mg oral dose. *Distribution-Extent:* Most corticosteroids removed rapidly from blood and distributed to muscles, liver, skin, intestines, and kidneys. Distribute into breast milk and placenta. *Plasma Protein Binding:* Has a high affinity for transcortin and competes with cortisol for binding to this binding protein. Because only unbound drug is pharmacologically active, patients with low serum albumin concentrations may be more susceptible to glucocorticoid effects. *Elimination-Metabolism:* Corticosteroids metabolized in most tissues, but primarily in liver, to inactive compounds. Metabolized by CYP3A4. Excreted in the urine as sulfate and glucuronide conjugates. Half-life is 2 to 4 h

- **Fludrocortisone:** *Absorption-Bioavailability*: Readily absorbed after oral administration; *Distribution-Extent*: rapidly removed from the blood and distributed to muscles, liver, skin, intestines, and kidneys. Corticosteroids cross the placenta and are distributed into milk. *Elimination-Metabolism*: Metabolized in most tissues, but primarily in the liver, to biologically inactive compounds. *Half-life*: Plasma half-life is ≥3.5 hours. Biologic half-life is 18–36 hours.

Adult Dosing

- **Dexamethasone:** *Anti-inflammatory*: oral, IM, IV: 0.75–9 mg/day in divided doses every 6–12 hours; Intra-articular, intralesional, or soft tissue: 0.4–6 mg/day. *Extubation or airway edema*: oral, IM, IV: 0.5–2 mg/kg/day in divided doses every 6 hours beginning 24 hours prior to extubation and continuing for

4–6 doses afterward. *Antiemetic-prophylaxis*: oral, IV: 10–20 mg 15–30 minutes before treatment, or 10 mg every 12 hours by continuous infusion or 4 mg every 4–6 hours for mildly emetogenic therapy. *Antiemetic-delayed nausea/vomiting*: oral: 4–10 mg 1–2 times/day for 2–4 days or 8 mg every 12 hours for 2 days then 4 mg every 12 hours for 2 days. *Cerebral edema*: 10 mg IV stat then 4 mg IV/IM every 6 hours until response maximized, then transition to oral and reduce dosage after 2–4 days and gradually discontinue over 5–7 days. *Addisonian Crisis/Shock*: IV: 4–10 mg as single dose, repeat if necessary. *Unresponsive Shock*: IV 1–6 mg/kg single dose or up to 40 mg initially followed by repeated doses every 2–6 hours while shock persists. *Physiologic replacement*: oral, IM, IV 0.03–0.15 mg/kg/day or 0.6–0.75 mg/m2/day in divided doses every 6–12 hours

- **Hydrocortisone:** *oral*: initially 10–320 mg daily in 3 or 4 divided doses; chronic replacement is usually given twice daily with a slightly higher dose in the morning to account for normal diurnal variation. *IV/IM/Sub-Q (hydrocortisone sodium phosphate)*: 15–240 mg IV daily, *Stress dose*: 25 mg IV at the start of the case then 100 mg every 24 h after titrating down 25% per day until the normal maintenance dose can be maintained. *IV/IM (hydrocortisone sodium succinate)*: 100 mg to 8 g daily, 100–500 mg initially and every 2–10 hours after as needed; *intra-articular, intrasynovial, intrabursal, or intralesional injection or soft tissue injection (hydrocortisone acetate)*: large joints: 25–50 mg, smaller joints: 10–25 mg, repeat once every 1–4 weeks; bursae 25–50 mg may repeat once every 3–5 days; ganglia 10–25 mg, repeat as needed; soft tissues: 5–12.5 mg for tendon sheath inflammation, 25–75 mg for soft tissue infiltration, repeat as needed. *Shock IV (hydrocortisone sodium succinate)*: 50 mg/kg over a period of several minutes, repeated in 4 hours and/or every 2 hours if needed, alternatively 0.5–2 g initially and repeated at 2–6 hour intervals as needed, not to be used for more than 72 hours (if massive corticosteroid therapy is needed beyond 72 hours, use a corticosteroid with less sodium retention, ie, methylprednisolone or dexamethasone, to minimize risk of hypernatremia)

- **Methylprednisolone:** *Oral*: Initially, 2–60 mg daily, depending on disease being treated, and is usually divided into 4 doses. *IV/IM*: Methylprednisolone sodium succinate: Usually, 10–250 mg; may repeat up to 6 times daily. *IV then IV or IM*: Methylprednisolone sodium succinate: For high-dose therapy, administer 30 mg/kg over at least 30 minutes. May repeat every 4–6 hours for 48 hours. Continue high-dose therapy only until the condition stabilizes, usually ≤48–72 hours. For other conditions, 10–40 mg over several minutes. Administer subsequent doses IV or IM depending on response and clinical condition. *IM*: Methylprednisolone acetate: 10–80 mg once daily. If a prolonged effect is desired, may administer an IM dose of methylprednisolone acetate equal to 7 times the daily oral dose of methylprednisolone once weekly. *Intra-articular, intrasynovial, intralesional, or soft-tissue injection* (varies depending on location, size, and degree of inflammation): Large Joints (eg, knee): 20–80 mg of methylprednisolone acetate every 1–5 weeks as needed. Smaller Joints: 4–40 mg of methylprednisolone acetate repeated every 2–3 weeks as needed. Bursae, Ganglia, Tendinitis, Epicondylitis: 4–30 mg of methylprednisolone acetate; repeat if necessary for recurrent or chronic conditions. Soft Tissue: 4–30 mg of methylprednisolone acetate for soft tissue infiltration; repeat if necessary for recurrent or chronic conditions. *Shock:* Life-threatening shock: methyl-prednisolone as the sodium succinate such as 30 mg/kg by direct IV injection (over 3–15 minutes) initially and repeated every 4–6 hours if needed or 100–250 mg by direct IV injection (over 3–15 minutes) initially and repeated at 2- to 6-hour intervals as required. Alternatively, following the initial dose by direct IV injection, additional doses of 30 mg/kg may be administered by slow continuous IV infusion every 12 hours for 24–48 hours. Continue high-dose therapy only until the patient's condition has stabilized and usually not beyond 48–72 hours. *Acute Spinal Cord Injury:* Methylprednisolone sodium succinate: Initially, 30 mg/kg of methylprednisolone by rapid IV injection over 15 minutes, followed in 45 minutes by IV infusion of 5.4 mg/kg per hour for 23 hours (total dose administered over 24 hours)

- **Prednisone:** *Oral:* Initially, 5–60 mg daily, depending on the disease being treated, usually in 2–4 divided doses. *Allergic Conditions:* For certain conditions (eg, contact dermatitis, including poison ivy), 30 mg (6 tablets) for the first day, which is then tapered by 5 mg daily until 21 tablets have been administered
- **Prednisolone:** *Oral:* Initially, 5–60 mg daily, depending on the disease being treated; usually administered in 2–4 divided dose
- **Fludrocortisone:** 0.1mg orally 3x/week to 0.2 mg/day orally for Addison's disease, may be used as an adjunct in treating septic shock 50 mcg/day if hydrocortisone is unavailable and the substituted steroid lacks mineralocorticoid therapy. *Postural Hypotension (Oral):* 0.1–0.4 mg daily has been given to diabetic patients with postural hypotension, 0.05–0.2 mg daily has been given to patients with postural hypotension secondary to levodopa therapy

Pediatric Dosing

- ***based on severity of disease and patient response as opposed to strict adherence to dosages by weight/body surface area:**
- **Dexamethasone:** *Anti-inflammatory and/or immunosuppressant:* oral, IM, IV: 0.08–0.3 mg/kg/day or 2.5–10 mg/m2/day in divided doses every 6–12 hours. *Extubation or airway edema:* oral, IM, IV: 0.5–2 mg/kg/day in divided doses every 6 hours beginning 24 hours prior to extubation and continuing for 4–6 doses afterward. *Antiemetic-prophylaxis:* IV: 10 mg/m2 (initial dose) followed by 5 mg/m2 every 6 hours as needed or 5–20 mg 15–30 minutes before treatment. *Cerebral edema:* 1–2 mg/kg IV stat then 1–1.5 mg/kg/day (max: 16 mg/day) in divided doses every 4- 6 hours, taper off over 1–6 weeks. *Bacterial meningitis in infants and children >2 months:* IV 0.6 mg/kg/day in 4 divided doses every 6 hours for the first 4 days of antibiotic therapy. *Physiologic replacement:* oral, IM, IV 0.03–0.15 mg/kg/day or 0.6–0.75 mg/m2/day in divided doses every 6–12 hours

- **Hydrocortisone:** *oral:* 0.56–8 mg/kg daily or 16–240 mg/m2 daily administered in 3 or 4 divided doses; *IV/IM:* 0.16–1 mg/kg or 6–30 mg/m2 1 or 2 times daily
- **Methylprednisolone:** *Oral:* 0.117–1.66 mg/kg daily or 3.3–50 mg/m2 daily, administered in 3 or 4 divided doses; *IM:* Methylprednisolone sodium succinate: 0.03–0.2 mg/kg or 1–6.25 mg/m2 IM 1–2 times daily; *Croup (IV):* Methylprednisolone sodium succinate: 1–2 mg/kg, followed by 0.5 mg/kg every 6–8 hours; *Pneumocystis jiroveci Pneumonia:* Methylprednisolone sodium succinate in children >13 years of age with AIDS† and moderate to severe *Pneumocystis jiroveci* pneumonia: 30 mg twice daily for 5 days, followed by 30 mg once daily for 5 days, and then 15 mg once daily for 11 days (or until completion of the anti-infective regimen). Initiate within 24–72 hours of initial anti-pneumocystis therapy. *Acute Spinal Cord Injury:* Methylprednisolone sodium succinate: 30 mg/kg IV (administered over 15 minutes), followed after 45 minutes by a continuous IV infusion of 5–6 mg/kg per hour for 23 hours. *Lupus Nephritis:* Methylprednisolone sodium succinate: 30 mg/kg IV every other day for 6 doses.
- **Prednisone:** *Oral:* 0.14–2 mg/kg daily or 4–60 mg/m2 daily in 4 divided doses
- **Prednisolone:** *Oral* (Syrup, solution, or tablets): Initially, 0.14–2 mg/kg daily or 4–60 mg/m2 daily in 4 divided doses; *Asthma Oral:* For t refractory bronchial asthma and related bronchospasm (severe persistent asthma) not controlled with high maintenance dosages of an inhaled corticosteroid and a long-acting bronchodilator, add an oral corticosteroid (eg, prednisone, prednisolone, methylprednisolone) at a dosage of 1–2 mg/kg daily in single or divided doses. Continue a short course of oral corticosteroid therapy (usually 3–10 days) until a peak expiratory flow rate of 80% of personal best is achieved or until symptoms resolve. No evidence that tapering the dosage after improvement will prevent relapse.
- **Fludrocortisone:** not FDA approved; in infants: 0.1–0.2 mg/day orally, in children 0.05–0.1 mg/day

Preparation, Miscellaneous

- **Dexamethasone:** Oral tablets, elixir, or solution; use cautiously in elderly in the smallest possible dose; supplemental dose not required in dialysis patients; administer oral doses with food to minimize GI upset, administer IV bolus over 5–10 minutes, as rapid injection is associated with a high incidence of perineal discomfort
- **Hydrocortisone:** oral tablets or suspension; parenteral suspension for intralesional, soft tissue, or intra-articular injection; parenteral for IV, IM or SC injection
- **Methylprednisolone:** oral tablet, or parenteral for IV injection or infusion, IM, intralesional, soft tissue, intra-articular, or epidural injection. Methylprednisolone acetate formulation contains benzyl alcohol; do *not* administer intrathecally because of reports of severe adverse events with such use

- **Prednisone:** oral solution, syrup or tablet.
- **Prednisolone:** oral solution, syrup, or tablet; parenteral for soft tissue or intra-articular injection, or for IV, IM injection
- **Fludrocortisone:** oral tablet 0.1mg

Cautions/Adverse Reactions:

- Hydrocortisone (and other glucocorticoid derivatives):
  - *Neuropsychiatric*: depression, emotional instability, euphoria, headache, increased ICP, insomnia, malaise, mood swings, neuritis, personality changes, pseudotumor cerebri (usually after discontinuation), psychic disorders, seizures, vertigo
  - *Cardiovascular:* arrhythmias, bradycardia, cardiac arrest, cardiomyopathy, CHF, circulatory collapse, edema, hypertension, myocardial rupture (post-MI), syncope, thromboembolism, vasculitis
  - *Respiratory:* pulmonary edema
  - *Dermatologic:* acne, allergic dermatitis, alopecia, angioedema, bruising, dry skin, erythema, fragile skin, hirsutism, hyper/hypopigmentation, hypertrichosis, perianal pruritis (IV injection), petechiae, rash, skin atrophy, striae, urticaria, wound healing impaired
  - *Endocrine/Metabolic:* adrenal suppression, decreased carbohydrate tolerance, Cushing's syndrome, diabetes mellitus, glucose intolerance, growth suppression (children), hyperglycemia, hypokalemic alkalosis, menstrual irregularities, negative nitrogen balance, pituitary-adrenal axis suppression, protein catabolism, sodium retention
  - *Gastrointestinal:* abdominal distention, increased appetite, gastrointestinal hemorrhage or perforation, nausea, pancreatitis, peptic ulcer, ulcerative esophagitis, weight gain, hepatomegaly, elevated transaminases
  - *Musculoskeletal:* arthropathy, aseptic/avascular necrosis (femoral, humeral heads), fractures, loss of muscle mass, myopathy (particularly in conjunction with neuromuscular disease or neuromuscular blocking agents), neuropathy, osteoporosis, paresthesias, tendon rupture, vertebral compression fractures, weakness
  - *Ocular:* cataracts, exopthalmos, glaucoma, increased intraocular pressure
  - *Renal:* Gycosuria
  - *Reproductive:* altered spermatogenesis
  - *Local:* postinjection flare (intra-articular use), thrombophlebitis
  - *Miscellaneous:* abnormal fate deposition, anaphylactoid reactions, anaphylaxis, diaphoresis, hiccups, hypersensitivity, increased susceptibility to infections, Kaposi's sarcoma, moon face, secondary malignancy;
  - *Contraindications:* hypersensitivity, systemic infections, Live or live attenuated vaccines are contraindicated during therapy.

- Fludrocortisone:
  - *Cardiovascular:* Edema, cardiomegaly, CHF, hypertension, thrombophlebitis
  - *Dermatologic*: Bruising, impaired wound healing, petechiae, rash, urticaria
  - *Endocrine*: decreased body growth abnormal electrolytes, hypokalemia, hyperglycemia, secondary hypocortisolism
  - *Gastrointestinal:* Abdominal distention, peptic ulcer disease
  - *Musculoskeletal*: Drug-induced myopathy, muscle weakness
  - *Neurologic*: Headache, vertigo, increased intracranial pressure, seizures
  - *Renal*: Gycosuria
  - *Reproductive*: Irregular menses

References

1. Katzung BG. *Basic & Clinical Pharmacology*. 11th ed. New York: McGraw-Hill; 2009. via accessmedicine.com

2. Benzon H, Raj P, et al. *Raj's Practical Management of Pain*. 4th ed. Philadelphia: Mosby, 2008.

3. Brunton, LL. *Goodman & Gilman's The Pharmacological Basis of Therapeutics*. 11th ed. New York: McGraw-Hill; 2010. via accessmedicine.com

4. Wu, RS-C . Use of corticosteroids in anesthesia and critical care. *ACTA Anaesthesiol Sin*. 2002;40:53–54.

5. Han YY, Sun WZ. An Evidence-based review on the use of corticosteroids in peri-operative and critical care. *ACTA Anaesthesiol Sin*. 2002;40:71–79.

6. Miller, R, et al. *Miller's Anesthesia*, vols. 1 and 2, 7th ed. Philadelphia: Churchill Livingstone; 2009.

7. Magiakou, MA, et al. Glucocorticoid therapy and adrenal suppression. Updated: December 2007. via http://www.endotext.org/adrenal/adrenal14/ch01s02.html

8. Leung DY, Hanifin JM, Charlesworth EN, et al. Disease management of atopic dermatitis: a practice parameter. *Ann Allergy Asthma Immunol*. 1997;79(3):197–211.

9. Symreng T, Karlberg BE, et al. Physiological cortisol substitution of long-term steroid-treated patients undergoing major surgery. *Br J Anaesth*.1981;53(9):949–954.

10. Dexamethasone information. Drugs.com; c2000–10. Updated April 16, 2010. Accessed December 13, 2010.

11. Dexamethasone: drug information. Uptodate.com. c1978–2010. Lexi-Comp, Inc. Accessed December 13, 2010. Available from http://www.uptodate.com/home/index.html.

12. Dexamethasone: drugpoint summary. Micromedex.com. Accessed December 13, 2010.

13. Hydrocortisone information. Drugs.com; c2000–10. Updated April 16, 2010. Accessed December 13, 2010.

14. Hydrocortisone: drugpoint summary. Micromedex.com. Accessed December 13, 2010.

15. Methylprednisolone information. Drugs.com; c2000–10. Updated April 16, 2010. Accessed December 13, 2010.

16. Methylprednisolone: drugpoint summary. Micromedex.com. Accessed December 13, 2010.

17. Prednisone information. Drugs.com; c2000–10. Updated April 16, 2010. Accessed December 13, 2010.

18. Prednisone: drugpoint summary. Micromedex.com. Accessed December 13, 2010.

19. Prednisolone information. Drugs.com; c2000–10. Updated April 16, 2010. Accessed December 13, 2010.

20. Prednisolone: drugpoint summary. Micromedex.com. Accessed December 13, 2010.

21. Fludrocortisone information. Drugs.com; c2000–10. Updated April 16, 2010. Accessed December 13, 2010.

22. Fludrocortisone: drugpoint summary. Micromedex.com. Accessed December 13, 2010.

23. Lavin PJ, Workman R. Cushing syndrome induced by serial occipital nerve blocks containing corticosteroids. *Headache*. 2001;41:902–904. doi: 10.1111/j.1526–4610.2001.

Chapter 11.2

Antihistamines

Mona Patel, MD and Anita Gupta, DO, PharmD

Role in Practice of Anesthesiology/Relevance to Anesthesiology

- Antihistamines (1st generation H_1 receptor blockers) can be used as preoperative medication due to their sedative and antiemetic properties
- Diphenhydramine (1st generation) may be used as adjunct to H_2 blockers and steroids for prophylaxis against intraoperative allergic reactions (ie, chronic atopy, latex allergy, studies involving radiographic dye)
- Suppression of cough
- Diphenhydramine may be used as adjunct to epinephrine for laryngeal edema
- Diphenhydramine has been used as weak anxiolytic for premedication
- Diphenhydramine can be used as an antiemetic for prophylaxis against postoperative nausea and vomiting and for prophylaxis and treatment of motion-induced vomiting after middle ear and strabismus surgery.
- Diphenhydramine may be used for treatment of dystonic reactions due to parkinsonism or drug-induced (ie, phenothiazines) extrapyramidal effects
- Newer, 2nd generation H_1 receptor blockers (loratidine, fexofenadine) are used mainly for treatment of symptoms of allergic rhinitis and urticaria

Pharmacodynamics

- Reversible competitive antagonist of histamine at H_1 receptors on cells in the gastrointestinal tract, blood vessels, and respiratory system
- 1st generation H1 blockers can also antagonize muscurinic cholinergic receptors, adrenoreceptors, and serotonin receptors
- Effects of H_1 receptor blockade at various sites:
  - Smooth muscle: bronchodilation and vasoconstriction
  - Capillaries: decreased permeability and edema
  - Neural endings: decreased flare and pruritis
  - GI tract: decreased secretions and antiemetic (1st generation only)
  - CNS: sedation, antiparkinsonism effect (1st generation only)

Pharmacokinetics

- Well absorbed from GI tract with excellent bioavailability
- Extensive hepatic metabolism via cytochrome P450 enzymes
- Eliminated more slowly in those with severe liver disease.
- Eliminated more rapidly by children than by adults
- 1st generation blockers: wide distribution throughout body, including CNS
- 2nd generation blockers poorly penetrate CNS.

Side Effects/Adverse Reactions

- CNS (1st generation only): Sedation, can potentiate other CNS depressants and can delay emergence from anesthesia. Other CNS effects: dizziness, tinnitus, blurred vision, insomnia, tremors
- GI tract: loss of appetite, nausea, vomiting, constipation, or diarrhea
- Anticholinergic (1st generation): dry mouth, urinary retention
- Hypersensitivity reactions: drug allergy/fever, photosensitization (more likely with topical)
- All cross placenta regularly. Fexofenadine showed teratogenicity. 1st generation blockers may cause irritability, drowsiness, or respiratory depression in nursing infant if taken by lactating women.
- Acute overdose can result in "anticholinergic syndrome": hallucinations, excitement, ataxia, seizures, tachycardia, dilated pupils, urinary retention, dry mouth, fever. Can result in cardiopulmonary arrest if severe
- **Diphenhydramine (Benadryl)**—topical application, oral, intravenous, and intramuscular administration. Therapeutic uses include symptomatic relief of nasal allergies (oral: 25–50 mg every 6–8h, or IV 10–50 mg per dose), adjunct to epinephrine in treatment of anaphylaxis and laryngeal edema, mild sedative (up to 50 mg PO/or IV), prevention and treatment of motion sickness, antitussive (25 mg oral every 4 hours), treatment of dystonic reactions and extrapyramidal symptoms (IM or IV 50 mg single dose), topically for relief of dermatological allergies (1%-2% to affected area 3–4 times/day). For dye prophylaxis, give 50 mg PO/IV 1 hour prior to procedure. Not first-line therapy for treatment of anaphylaxis; due to other mediators, epinephrine is first choice for anaphylaxis. To prevent motion sickness, first dose should be 30 min prior to operation. Pronounced tendency to cause sedation, and may potentiate other sedatives. Significant antimuscurinic activity.
- **Loratidine (Claritin, Alavert)**—oral. Therapeutic uses include seasonal allergic rhinitis, chronic idiopathic urticaria (oral 10 mg/day). Minimal anticholinergic and sedative properties. Highly selective for H_1 receptors. Overall low incidence of side effects. Significant amounts enter breast milk. Rapid absorption from GI tract and metabolized in the liver by hepatic P450 enzymes to active metabolite with duration of action >24h. Metabolism can be affected by drugs that compete for P450 enzymes. Excreted mainly in unmetabolized form in urine.
- **Fexofenadine (Allegra)**—oral. Therapeutic uses include seasonal allergic rhinitis, chronic idiopathic urticaria (oral 60 mg twice daily or 180 mg once

Table 11.2.1 H₁ Receptor Antagonists						
Class	Drug	Route	Dose (mg)	Duration of Action (h)	Sedation	Antiemesis
1st-generation (ethanolamines)	Diphen-hydramine (Benadryl)	PO, IM, IV, topical	25–50	3–6	+	+
2nd- generation (piperidines)	Loratidine (Claritin)	PO	10	24	0	0
	Fexofenadine (Allegra)	PO	60–180	12–24	0	0

daily). Minimal anticholinergic and sedative properties. Overall low incidence of side effects. Highly selective for H₁ receptors. Nontoxic, active metabolite of terfenadine. Excreted mainly as unmetabolized form in feces. Has been shown to be teratogenic in studies.

References

1. Dotson R, Wiener-Kronish JP, Ajayi T. Preoperative evaluation and medication. In: Stoelting RK, Miller RD, eds., *Basics of Anesthesia*. 5th ed. Philadelphia: Elsevier; 2007: 168–171.

2. Hata TM, Moyers JR. Preoperative patient assessment management. In: Barash PG, Cullen BF, Stoelting RK, Calahan MK, Stock MC, eds., *Clinical Anesthesia*. 6th ed. Philadelphia: Lippincott Williams and Wilkins. 2009: 588–589.

3. Skidgel RA, Erdös EG. Chapter 24. Histamine, bradykinin, and their antagonists. In: Brunton LL, Lazo JS, Parker KL, eds., *Goodman & Gilman's The Pharmacological Basis of Therapeutics*. 11th ed. http://www.accessmedicine.com/content.aspx?aID=941777.

4. Apfel CC. Postoperative nausea and vomiting. In: Miller RD, ed., *Miller's Anesthesia* 7th ed. Philadelphia: Elsevier; 2005: 2744–2751.

5. Corre KA, Niemann JT, Bessen HA, et al. Extended therapy for acute dystonic reactions. *Ann Emerg Med*. 1984;13(3):194–197.

6. Lexi-Comp Online™. Lexi-Drugs Online™. Hudson, Ohio: Lexi-Comp, Inc.; 2010; November 28, 2010.

7. Katzung BG. Chapter 16. Histamine, serotonin, & the ergot alkaloids. In: Katzung BG, ed., *Basic & Clinical Pharmacology*, 11th ed. http://www.accessmedicine.com/content.aspx?aID=4514635.

8. Hepner DL, Castells MC. Anaphylaxis during the perioperative period. *Anesth Analg*. 2007;97:1381–1385.

9. Rinder CS. Diseases related to immune system dysfunction. In: Hines RL, Marschall KE, eds., *Stoelting's Anesthesia and Co-Existing Disease* 5th ed. Philadelphia: Elsevier; 2002: 521–532.

10. American Academy of Pediatrics Committee on Drugs. The transfer of drugs and other chemicals into human milk. *Pediatrics*. 2001;108(3):776–789.

11. Simons FE, Simons KJ. Clinical pharmacology of new histamine H1 receptor antagonists. *Clin Pharmacokinet*. 1999;36(5):329–352.

Chapter 12

Narcotic and Benzodiazepine Reversal Agents

Gaurav Bhatia, MD and Anita Gupta, DO, PharmD

Narcotic Reversal Agents: Naloxone, Naltrexone, Nalmefene

Naloxone

Role in the Practice of Anesthesiology/Relevance to Anesthesiology

- Antidote in the treatment of opioid overdose exhibited by respiratory depression, CNS depression, cardiovascular depression
- Doses should be titrated up in small increments in postoperative patients for partial reversal of opioid depression to the desired level of alertness and adequate ventilation without causing significant pain or discomfort
- IV administration can be supplemented with IM administration for longer duration (duration of action is < most opioids)
- As a secondary chemical in the drug Suboxone; mixed in a 1:4 ratio with buprenorphine in an effort to dissuade opioid abusers from grinding up the medication which is most commonly prescribed to help with opioid addiction

Pharmacodynamics

- A pure μ-opioid receptor competitive antagonist that competes and displaces narcotics at opioid receptor sites
- Also has an antagonist action at κ- and δ-opioid receptors, though with a lower affinity

Pharmacokinetics

- Onset: Dosage and route dependent. IV 45–120 seconds; IM/SQ 2–5 mins
- Distribution: crosses placenta

- Elimination: half-life 30–80 mins; Terminal 6–72 h
- Metabolism: Hepatic primarily via glucuronidation
- Excretion: Urine as metabolite naloxone-3-glucuronide

Side Effects/Adverse Reactions

- Precipitation of opioid withdrawal symptoms acutely (body aches, sweating, rhinorrhea, piloerection, nausea, vomiting, abdominal cramps, nervousness, restlessness, trembling, headache, seizures, cardiac rhythm changes, sudden chest pain)
- Postoperative use can cause dyspnea, pulmonary edema, hypotension, HTN, ventricular tachycardia, and cardiac arrest

Dosages

- Adults. Respiratory depression: 0.4 mg-2 mg IV q 2–3 mins (if no response with cumulative dose of 10 mg, other etiologies must be considered). Postoperative reversal: 0.04–2 mg IV q 2–3 mins; consider repeating IV dose in 30–60 mins or concurrent IM injection depending on amount and time from last opioid administered.
- Pediatrics. Respiratory depression: 0.1 mg/kg IV q 2–3 mins; maximum dose 2 mg for ages 0–5 yrs. Postoperative reversal: 0.01 mg/kg IV q 2–3 mins; consider repeating IV dose in 30–60 mins depending on the dosage and timing of the last opioid administered

Naltrexone

- Competitive opioid receptor antagonist (μ- and κ-opioid receptor) used primarily in the management of alcohol dependence and opioid dependence. Not commonly used in the OR for opioid overdose due to its longer-acting effect compared to naloxone. PO or IM injection for alcohol and opioid dependence; not given IV.

Nalmefene

- Competitive opioid receptor antagonist used primarily in the management of alcohol dependence and has been investigated for the treatment of other addictions (pathological gambling and shopping). Not commonly used in the OR due to its higher cost and longer-acting effect compared to naloxone. Longer half-life and greater bioavailability compared to naltrexone. Available in IV form (allows for treatment of respiratory depression in the hospital and perioperative setting; 0.5–1 mg).

Benzodiazepine Reversal

Flumazenil

Role in the Practice of Anesthesiology/Relevance to Anesthesiology

- Antidote in the treatment of benzodiazepines overdose exhibited by drowsiness, somnolence, and apnea

- Also effective in overdoses of nonbenzodiazepine sleep enhancers, such as zolpidem and zaleplon
- Does not antagonize the CNS effects of other GABA agonists (such as ethanol, barbiturates, narcotics, general anesthetics)

Pharmacodynamics

- An imidazobenzodiazepine derivative that competitively inhibits benzodiazepines at the $GABA_A$ receptor. In some animal models, it is a weak partial agonist but has little or no agonist activity in humans

Pharmacokinetics

- Onset: 1–3 mins; peak effect seen at 6–10 mins
- Elimination half-life 7–15 mins; Terminal 41–79 mins
- Metabolism: Hepatic primarily (use cautiously if hepatic dysfunction)
- Excretion: Urine 90%-95%, Feces 5%-10%. Not significantly affected by renal failure (Cl_{cr} < 10 mL/min) or HD beginning 1 hour after drug administration
- Consider repeating dosage since many benzodiazepines (including midazolam) have longer half-lives than flumazenil

Side Effects/Adverse Reactions

- Contraindicated when benzodiazepine is being utilized for control of potentially life-threatening conditions (eg, control of ICP or status epilepticus)
- Lowers seizure threshold; use cautiously in patients that use benzodiazepines chronically
- Does not consistently reverse amnesia; patient may not recall verbal instructions after procedure
- Use cautiously in pts with head injury, liver dysfunction, panic disorder, drugs/alcohol dependence, and the ICU
- GI (10%): vomiting, nausea; CV (3%): vasodilation, palpitations, altered blood pressure increase/decrease; CNS (10%): dizziness, agitation, emotional lability, headache, blurry vision; Respiratory (6%): dyspnea, hyperventilation

Dosages

- Adult.
- Pediatric. Initial dose of 0.01mg/kg IV over 15 seconds; consider repeat dose in 45 seconds, then q60 seconds to a maximum cumulative dose of 0.05mg/kg (if no response at 0.05mg/kg, other causes must be considered).

References

1. Chamberlain JM, Klein BL. A comprehensive review of naloxone for the emergency room physician. *Am J Emerg med.* 1994;12(6):650–660.
2. Chern CH, Chern TL, Hu SC, et al. Complete and partial response to flumazenil in patients with suspected benzodiazepine overdose. *Am J Emerg Med.* 1995;13(3):372–375.

3. Flomenbam NE, Goldfrank LR, Hoffman RS, Howland MA, Lewin NA, Nelson LS. *Goldfrank's Toxicologic Emergencies.* 8th ed. New York: McGraw-Hill; 2006:614–619, 1112–1117.

4. Hoffman RS, Goldfrank LR. The poisoned patient with altered consciousness. *JAMA.* 1995;274(7):562–569.

5. O'Connor PG, Kosten TR. Rapid and ultrarapid opioid detoxification techniques. *JAMA.* 1998;279(3):229–234.

6. Trujillo MH, Guerrero J, Fragachan C. Pharmacologic antidotes in critical care medicine: a practical guide for drug administration. *Crit Care Med.* 1998;26(2):377–391.

7. Wiley J, Wiley C. Benzodiazepine ingestions in children. *Clin Toxicol.* 1995;33(5):520–523.

Hematologic Agents

Chapter 13.1

Dipyridamole

Elizabeth W. Duggan, MD

Clinical Uses in Anesthesiology

- A vasodilator with mild antithrombotic effect.
- Not a first-line agent, but can be used in the management of cerebrovascular disease and cardiovascular disease.
- Used as the vasodilating agent in myocardial stress testing (trade name Persantine)
- Preventive therapy for thromboembolic events in patients with a synthetic prosthetic heart valve

Pharmacodynamics

- Dipyridamole is a pyrimidopyrimidine derivative that has both vasodilating and mild antiplatelet actions.
- Although not fully elucidated, dipyridamole's actions are likely due to its inhibition of phospodiesterase (PDE). By inhibiting PDE, cAMP degradation is limited, blocking the release of arachidonic acid. Arachidonic acid is a precursor of thromboxane A_2, a potent platelet activator. By preventing the formation of TXA_2, dipyridamole prevents platelet activation.
- Additionally, dipyridamole appears to increase concentrations of adenosine by inhibiting its breakdown by the enzyme adenosine deaminase. Adenosine is a potent coronary vasodilator.

Pharmacokinetics

- Oral administration results in maximal plasma levels within 1–3 hours of gastrointestinal absorption; bioavailability is approximately 25%-65%. Distribution half-life is 3 hours.
- When given in an intravenous formulation for stress testing, distribution time occurs within 25 minutes. Coronary vasodilation occurs within 5–10 minutes following injection.
- Systemic half-life is 10 hours
- Hepatic metabolism is followed by biliary excretion

Adult Dosing

- Oral: Available in 25 mg, 50 mg, 75 mg and 100 mg tablets.
- Thromboembolic Disease: Recommended dose is 100 mg po qid 1 hour before meals. Currently, not commonly prescribed for prevention of secondary stroke.
- Angina Prophylaxis: 50 mg PO tid 1 hour before meals
- Cardiac Valve-Associated Thrombotic Risk Reduction: 75–100 mg po qid
- Parenteral: Packaged as a 5 mg/mL preparation. Prior to use, should be diluted 1:1 with D5W.
- Myocardial Perfusion Imaging: Recommended dose is 0.142 mg/kg/minute, infused over 4 minutes. A total dose of greater than 60 mg is not recommended for use in any patient regardless of weight

Cautions and Adverse Reactions

- IV Dipyridamole should be used with caution during stress testing. It has been associated with myocardial ischemia and infarction. EKG and blood pressure monitoring should be used during myocardial stress testing due to dipyridamole associated severe arrhythmias, heart block, and hypotension.
- Care should be taken in patients with aortic stenosis; dipyridamole can cause a rapid drop in blood pressure.
- Patients with a history of bronchial hyperreactivity are at risk for developing bronchospasm (incidence 1.22 per 10,000) during myocardial perfusion imaging
- Dipyridamole used concurrently with other anticoagulants or thrombolytics may result in an increased bleeding risk
- Dipyridamole may counteract the anticholinesterase effect of cholinesterase inhibitors. Dose adjustment may be needed using reversal agents given during general anesthesia (neostigmine, eg) or for chronic drug therapy used to treat myasthenia gravis.
- Minor adverse reactions to dipyridamole include headache, flushing, dizziness, and nausea.
- As an antiplatelet agent, discontinuation of the drug prior to performing neuraxial anesthesia should follow ASRA guidelines
- If undergoing elective surgery. ACCP guidelines for stopping antiplatelet therapy should be considered to minimize the risk of surgical bleeding.

References

1. Smart S, Aragola S, Hutton P. Anti-platelet agents and anaesthesia. *Contin Educ Anaesth Crit Care Pain.* 2007;7(5):157–161.
2. Halkes PH, van Gijn J, Kappelle LJ, Koudstaal PJ, Algra A. Aspirin plus dipyridamole versus aspirin alone after cerebral ischaemia of arterial origin (ESPRIT): randomised controlled trial. *Lancet.* 2007;369(9558):1665–1673.

3. Diener HC, Sacco RL, Yusuf S, et al. Effects of aspirin plus extended-release dipyridamole versus clopidogrel and telmisartan on disability and cognitive function after recurrent stroke in patients with ischaemic stroke in the Prevention Regimen for Effectively Avoiding Second Strokes (PRoFESS) trial: a double-blind, active and placebo-controlled study. *Lancet Neurol.* 2008;7:875–888.

4. Micromedex drugpoint summary. Thompson Reuters, 2010.

5. Pharmacogenomics Knowledge Base. Dipyridamole. http://www.pharmgkb.org.

6. RxMed.com. Pharmaceutical information—persantine. http://www.rxmed.com.

7. Lette J, Tatum JL, Fraser S, Miller DD, Waters DD, Heller G, Stanton EB, Nattel S. Safety of dipyridamole testing in 73,806 patients: the multicenter dipyridamole safety study. *J Nucl Cardiol.* 1995;2(1):3–17.

8. Little SH, Massel DR. Antiplatelet and anticoagulation for patients with prosthetic heart valves. *Cochrane Database Syst Rev.* 2003;4: CD003464. Doi: 10.1002/14651858.CD003464.

9. Meyers A, Topham L, Ballow J, Totah D, Wilke R. Adverse reactions to dipyridamole in patients undergoing stress/rest cardiac perfusion testing. *J Nucl Med Technol.* 2002;30(1);21–24.

10. Horlocker T, Wedel D, Rowlingson J, Enneking FK, Kopp S, Benzon H, Brown D, Heit J, Mulroy M, Rosenquist R, Tryba M, Yuan C. Regional Anesthesia in the patient receiving antithrombotic or thrombolytic therapy: American Society of Regional Anesthesia and Pain Medicine evidence-based guidelines (third edition). *Reg Anesth Pain Med.* 2010;35(1):64–101.

11. American College of Chest Physicians. Antithrombotic and thrombolytic therapy, 8th ed: ACCP Guidelines. *Chest.* 2008;133(6 suppl).

Chapter 13.2

Adenosine Diphosphate Inhibitors

Michael J. Duggan, MD, Elizabeth W. Duggan, MD, and Jiri Horak, MD

Clinical Case Scenario

A 59-year-old male presents for an elective laparoscopic cholecystectomy. He has a PMH significant for HTN, GERD, and CAD s/p a drug-eluting stent to the left circumflex artery eight months ago. Current medications are atenolol, simvastatin, pepcid, aspirin, and plavix, all of which he took the morning of surgery. Based on the most recent ACC/AHA recommendations, the best course of action would be:

Postpone elective, nonemergent surgery for 12 months after placement of a drug-eluting stent to allow 12 months of dual antiplatelet therapy with aspirin and clopidogrel. If a surgical procedure must be performed prior to the twelve month time period, the risk of acute stent thrombosis must be weighed against the risk of increased surgical bleeding. In the case of a bare metal stent, dual antiplatelet therapy should be continued for a minimum of thirty days.

Clinical Uses/Relevance to Anesthesiology

- Acute coronary syndrome (ACS) treatment and prevention
- Drug-eluting and bare-metal coronary stents, prevention of thrombosis (duration varies)
- Post-stroke, post-MI, or established PVD to reduce thrombosis
- Caution must be exercised when stopping ADP inhibitors for elective surgery in pts with recent coronary stents. ACC/AHA recommendations are to continue ADP inhibitors for at least 12 months after a drug-eluting stent and 30 days after a bare metal stent. The risk of surgical bleeding must be weighed against the risk of stent thrombosis.

Pharmacodynamics

- Thienopyridines drug class; irreversibly inhibits the $P2Y_{12}$ platelet membrane receptor.
- $P2Y_{12}$ is an ADP receptor that is responsible for activating the glycoprotein IIb-IIIa complex (a fibrinogen receptor). ADP inhibitors prevent fibrin cross-linking and platelet aggregation for the life of the platelet (7–10 days).

Pharmacokinetics

- Prodrugs; require conversion via cytochromes to their active thiol metabolites.
- Genetic polymorphisms (pharmacogenetics) and drug interactions can reduce conversion to the active thiol metabolite

Side Effects/Adverse Reactions

- Avoid in active bleeding conditions including peptic ulcers.
- Concomitant use of aspirin or a second antiplatelet agent can lead to increased bleeding; GI tract and CNS are at highest risk
- Neutropenia and thrombocytopenia
- TTP (rare)
- Diarrhea and upset stomach

Clopidogrel

- ASRA guidelines recommend holding for 7 days prior to neuraxial block
- Genetic polymorphisms of cytochrome CYPC219 can reduce efficacy up to 40%. Affected pts have a 1.5–3 times increased risk of death, stroke, MI, or stent thrombosis after PCI or ACS.
- Nexium and Prilosec inhibit CYPC219 and render clopidogrel less effective
- Bioavailability 50%
- Duration of action: life of platelet 7–10 days
- Elimination half-life ~6 h; active thiol derivative ~30 minutes
- Loading dose for ACS or PCI: 300 or 600 mg PO—significant platelet inhibition takes 2–5 hours
- Maintenance 75 mg PO QD—significant platelet inhibition takes 5–7 days if no loading dose given

Ticlodipine

- ASRA guidelines recommend holding for 14 days prior to neuraxial block
- Bioavailability 85%
- Maintenance: 250 mg PO BID
- Elimination half-life ~29 h, up to 5 days in the elderly

References

1. Farid NA, et al. Metabolism and disposition of the thienopyridine antiplatelet drugs ticlopidine, clopidogrel, and prasugrel in humans. *J Clin Pharmacol.* 2010;50(2):126–142.

2. Horlocker TT, et al. Regional anesthesia in the patient receiving antithrombotic or thrombolytic therapy: American Society of Regional Anesthesia and Pain Medicine evidence-based guidelines (third edition). *Reg Anesth Pain Med.* 2010;35(1):64–101.

3. King SB III, et al. 2007 focused update of the ACC/AHA/SCAI 2005 guideline update for percutaneous coronary intervention. *Circulation.* 2008;117:261–295.

4. Mega JL, et al. Reduced-function CYP2C19 genotype and risk of adverse clinical outcomes among patients treated with clopidogrel predominantly for PCI. *JAMA.* 2010;304(16):1821–1830.

Chapter 13.3

Low Molecular Weight Heparin (LMWH)

Elizabeth W. Duggan, MD, Michael J. Duggan, MD, and Maurizio Cereda, MD

Clinical Uses/Relevance to Anesthesiology

- Venous thrombosis prophylaxis and treatment
- Pulmonary embolus treatment
- Unstable angina, acute non-Q wave and ST segment elevation MI treatment
- Routine lab monitoring not necessary as well as less frequent dosing; allows for reduced cost, improved convenience, and outpatient therapy
- ASRA guidelines should be followed if performing regional/neuraxial anesthesia in patients on LMWH
- Placement of central venous lines in noncompressible veins (subclavian) should be done with caution; clinicians may prefer to place venous access devices in the internal jugular or femoral veins

Pharmacodynamics

- LMWH is produced by enzymatic depolymerization of standard heparin, which causes LMWH to have a lower weight than unfractionated heparin (UH) (UH:5000–30 000 d vs LMWH: 4000–6000 d)
- LMWH has reduced size therefore has lower binding to plasma and endothelial cell proteins:
- >90% bioavailability after SQ injection
- Longer plasma half-life (4–6 h vs. 0.5–1 standard heparin)
- Predictable and reproducible dose response
- Binds to antithrombin and *accelerates* its inhibition of factor Xa (cleaves prothrombin to thrombin to enable clot formation). By inhibiting the conversion of prothrombin to thrombin, LMWH prevents thrombus formation.
- Anti-Xa Levels. Can be followed to determine appropriate dosing. Therapeutic levels range from 0.5–1.2 units/mL and prophylactic levels 0.2–0.5 units/mL; levels should be drawn 4 h following SQ injection
- Low-molecular-weight heparins currently available in the United States include enoxaparin (Lovenox), dalteparin (Fragmin) and ardeparin (Normiflo)
- No antidote (unlike protamine for heparin)

Pharmacokinetics

- Peak effect: 3–4 h after SQ
- Protein binding: none, unlike unfractionated heparin. Increases bioavailability.
- V_d is large with distribution into fat; consider dose adjustment in obese pts. Following anti-Xa levels is not necessary, but can be considered in pts >190 kg
- Renal clearance; dose adjustments need to be made in renal insufficiency (CrCl ≤ 30 mL/min). Renal failure or HD: consider UFH (in lieu of LMWH).
- Elimination half-life: 3–6 h and is dose-dependent (3–4 times > unfractionated heparin).

Dosing

- After SQ administration, a 50% anti-Xa level is achieved in 12 h; continued dosing approaches levels of 100%
- DVT PROPHYLAXIS
  - Orthopedic Surgery
    - Dalteparin: Hip replacement—2500 U SQ 4–8 h postoperatively on day of surgery, then 5000 U SQ QD for 5–10 days.
    - Enoxaparin: Hip replacement—40 mg SQ QD **OR** 30 mg SQ BID beginning 12–24 h following surgery, for 7–10 days. Knee replacement—30 mg SQ BID beginning 12–24 h following surgery, for 7–10 days
  - Abdominal Surgery
    - Dalteparin: 2500 U SQ 1–2 h postoperatively on day of surgery; if low risk, 2500 U SQ QD for 5–10 days. If high risk, 5000 U SQ QD for 5–10 days
    - Enoxaparin: 40 mg SQ QD on day of surgery followed by 40 mg SQ QD for 5–10 days
  - Restricted Mobility in Acute Medical Illness
    - Daltaparin: 5000 U SQ QD
    - Enoxaparin: 40 mg SQ QD
  - Multiple Trauma (shown to be more effective than UFH):
    - Dalteparin: 5000 U SQ QD
    - Enoxaparin: 40 mg SQ QD
- DVT TREATMENT:
  - Dalteparin: 200 U/kg (Max of 18 000 U) SQ q24 h. Initiate warfarin therapy when/if appropriate
  - Enoxaparin: Acute Inpatient Treatment: 1 mg/kg SQ BID **OR** 1.5 mg/kg SQ QD for a minimum of 5 days and until oral anticoagulant is therapeutic (INR 2.0–3.0). Outpatient Treatment: 1 mg/kg SQ BID (warfarin therapy should be started when appropriate).

- PULMONARY EMBOLUS TREATMENT:
  - Dalteparin: 200 U/kg (Max of 18 000 U) SQ q24 h
  - Enoxaparin: 1 mg/kg SQ BID **OR** 1.5 mg/kg SQ QD
- UNSTABLE ANGINA or NON-Q WAVE MI:
  - Dalteparin: 120 U/kg SQ q12 h, not to exceed 10,000 IU **AND** aspirin 75–165 mg PO QD for 5–8 days
  - Enoxaparin: 1 mg/kg SQ q12 h **AND** aspirin 100–325 mg PO QD for minimum 2 days (usual duration of 2–8 days)
- ACUTE STEMI TREATMENT:
  - Enoxaparin: <75 y.o. initial bolus of 30 mg IV **AND** 1 mg/kg SQ, followed by 1 mg/kg q12 h (max of 100 mg for the first two doses). >75 y.o. 0.75 mg/kg SQ q12 h (max 75 mg for the first two doses). No IV bolus dose.

Side Effects/Adverse Events

- Avoid in pts with hx of heparin-induced thrombocytopenia (HIT) or known hypersensitivity to pork products
- Extreme caution in pts with a high risk for bleeding, including uncontrolled HTN, bacterial endocarditis, congenital or acquired bleeding disorders, recent GI bleeding, or thrombocytopenia. Also, pts in whom a bleeding event would be catastrophic (eg, recent brain, spinal, or ophthalmological surgery).
- Neuraxial anesthesia should not be performed in pts receiving therapeutic doses of dalteparin for Non-Q wave MI, unstable angina or STEMI, due to the risk of spinal or epidural hematoma. Additionally, regional/neuraxial anesthesia is contraindicated in patients on long-term LMWH (for PE or DVT treatment).
- LMWH when compared to unfractionated heparin is less likely to cause heparin-induced thrombocytopenia
- Pts older than 65 y.o., and low-weight patients (women <45 kgs and men <57 kgs) have an increased risk of bleeding

Low-Molecular Weight Heparin and the Parturient

- Pregnancy induces a state of hypercoagulability
- Anticoagulation is required in some parturients during the antepartum period, ex. disorders of hemostasis, mechanical heart prostheses, or those at high risk of venous thromboembolism.
- LMWH does not cross the placenta
- LMWH is not teratogenic
- LMWH is unlikely to cause fetal hemorrhage

Clinical Case Scenario

A 68-year-old patient with a recently discovered left lung nodule presents for a thoracotomy and left upper lobectomy. He has a past medical history of hypertension, hyperlipidemia, and chronic low back pain. Additionally, he was diagnosed with a left lower extremity deep vein thrombosis 8 weeks ago, which is being treated with low molecular weight heparin 70 mg SQ twice daily. His other medications include aspirin, lisinopril, atorvastatin, and oxycodone. He took all of these medications the morning of surgery except for the LMWH, which was last administered at 8 pm the evening prior to surgery. During his preoperative work-up, the patient was told that he would have an epidural placed immediately prior to surgery for postoperative pain management.

Background: Case reports, small clinical series and expert experience have demonstrated an increased incidence of spinal hematoma in patients undergoing neuraxial anesthesia while concomitantly using unfractionated heparin (UFH) or LMWH, particularly with increasing use of these drugs for VTE prophylaxis following surgery. Although the actual incidence of hemorrhagic complications associated with neuraxial anesthesia is unknown, the American Society of Regional Anesthesia and Pain Medicine (ASRA) released a 2010 consensus statement on neuraxial anesthesia for patients receiving anticoagulants medications.

Treatment: According to the most recent ASRA guidelines, patients receiving higher doses of low molecular weight heparin (1 mg/kg twice daily) may require a 24-hour delay prior to undergoing neuraxial anesthesia. For patients receiving VTE prophylactic therapy (typically 30 to 40 mg SC daily), epidural placement should be postponed 10 to 12 hours after the last LWMH dose. If this patient were receiving aspirin alone, there would be no contraindication to an epidural. However, aspirin in combination with low molecular weight heparin places the patient at an increased risk of spinal hematoma.

Should the surgeon and anesthesiologist decide to pursue neuraxial anesthesia with this patient as means to control postoperative pain, the ASRA guidelines recommend waiting 24 hours from the last dose of LMWH for epidural placement. Thus, this patient's surgery should potentially be postponed for an additional 12 hours. If the surgery cannot be delayed, alternative postoperative pain management regimens should be considered including a paravertebral block, local anesthetic infiltration in the incision site and/or intravenous narcotics via patient-controlled analgesia.

References

1. Horlocker T, Wedel D, Rowlingson J, Enneking FK, Kopp SL, Benzon HT, Brown DL, Heit JA, Mulroy JA, Mulroy MF, Rosenquist RW, Tryba M, Yuan C. Regional anesthesia in the patient receiving antithrombotic or thrombolytic therapy: American Society of Regional Anesthesia and Pain Medicine evidence-based guidelines (third edition). ASRA Practice Advisory. *Reg Anesth Pain Med.* 2010;35(1):64–101.

2. Horlocker TT, Wedel DJ. Neuraxial block and low-molecular-weight heparin: balancing perioperative analgesia and thromboprophylaxis. *Reg Anesth Pain Med.* 1998;23:164–177.

Chapter 13.4

Miscellaneous Anticoagulants

Michael J. Duggan, MD, Elizabeth W. Duggan, MD, and
Jiri Horak, MD

Citrate

Clinical Uses/Relevance to Anesthesiology

- Sodium citrate is an anticoagulant added to stored blood products
- During massive transfusion, there is concern for hypocalcemia because citrate binds calcium
- It is used as an anticoagulant in blood tubes and during plasmapheresis

Pharmacodynamics

- Citrate chelates ionized calcium in blood, limiting the calcium available for coagulation
- Calcium is required for the conformational transitions of the vitamin K dependent proteins
- Calcium is also required for subunit associations of factor Va and VIIIa
- Calcium is required for platelet activation

Pharmacokinetics

- Depending on preparation, each unit of pRBC contains 3 gm of sodium citrate. The healthy adult liver metabolizes 3 gm of citrate into sodium bicarbonate in approximately 5 min.
- Patients at risk for hypocalcemia include patients receiving blood faster than 1 unit every 5 minutes and patients with impaired hepatic function

Side Effects/Adverse Reactions

- Citrate toxicity manifests with signs and symptoms of hypocalcemia including prolonged QT interval, circulatory depression, hypotension, muscle tremors, and cardiac arrhythmias.

Sodium EDTA

Clinical Uses/Relevance to Anesthesiology

- Sodium EDTA is used as an anticoagulant in blood collection tubes. It irreversibly binds calcium.
- Sodium EDTA can be used for chelation therapy in patients who are hypercalcemic and in cases of heavy metal poisoning
- EDTA chelation therapy for coronary artery disease is not FDA approved

Pharmacodynamics

- EDTA chelates calcium to form a soluble complex
- The chelation of calcium creates an anticoagulant effect as described for citrate

Pharmacokinetics

- EDTA is not metabolized
- Elimination half-life is 20–60 min, time to peak onset 24–48 hours
- Sodium EDTA undergoes renal elimination after chelation with calcium to form a water soluble complex

Adult Dosing

- Acute Hypercalcemia: 50 mcg/kg to be given over 3 or more hours with a maximum dose of 3 gm/day. Give daily for 5 days followed by a 2-day drug holiday. May repeat course for up to 15 total doses.

Side Effects/Adverse Reactions

- GI: N/V, abdominal cramps, diarrhea, electrolyte abnormalities, hypomagnesemia, hypocalcemia, hypokalemia
- CNS: Use with caution in patients with intracranial lesions and seizure disorders
- CV: Arrhythmias, hypotension
- Rapid IV infusion may cause extreme drop in serum Ca^{2+} resulting in tetany, seizures, arrhythmias, cardiac or respiratory arrest
- Use with caution in patients with renal dysfunction

References

1. Galel SA, Nguyen DD, Fontaine MJ, Goodnough LT, Viele MK. Transfusion Medicine. In: Pine JW, ed., *Wintrobe's Clinical Hematology*. 12th ed. Philadelphia: Lippincott Williams and Wilkins; 2009.

2. Sunnerhagen M, Drakenberg T, Forsen S, Stenflo J. Effect of Ca2+ on the structure of vitamin K-dependent coagulation factors. *Haemostasis*. 1996;26:45–53.

3. Esmon CT. The subunit structure of thrombin-activated factor V: isolation of activated factor V, separation of subunits, and reconstitution of biological activity. *J Biol Chem.* 1979;254:1326–1334.

4. Lowllar P, Fay PJ, Fass DN. Factor VIII and factor VIIIa. *Methods Enzymol.* 1993;222:128–143.

5. Woulfe D, Yang J, Prevost N, O' Brien JO, Brass LF. Signal transduction during the initiation, extension, and perpetuation of platelet plug formation. In: Michelson AD, ed. *Platelets.* San Diego, CA: Academic Press; 2002:197–213.

6. Sihler KC, Napolitano LM. Complications of massive transfusion. *Chest.* 2010;137(1):209–220.

7. British Society for Haematology. British committee for standardization in haematology blood transfusion task force. Guidelines for transfusion for massive blood loss. *Clin Lab Haematol.* 1988;10(3):265–273.

8. UpToDate. Sodium EDTA. Online reference : www. Uptodate.com

Chapter 13.5

Streptokinase and Tissue Plasminogen Activator (tPA)

Elizabeth W. Duggan, MD and Michael J. Duggan, MD

Streptokinase

Clinical Uses/Relevance to Anesthesiolgy

- Has fallen out of favor with the introduction of tPA
- Acute MI
- Arterial or severe deep venous thrombosis
- Multiloculated or parapneumonic pleural effusion treatment
- Pulmonary embolism
- Clearance of a blocked catheter (arteriovenous cannula, PICC line)

Pharmacology

- Fibrinolytic drug derived from beta-hemolytic streptococci
- Promotes fibrinolysis by binding to plasminogen and catalyzing its conversion to plasmin. Plasmin, a serum protease, lyses fibrin clots

Pharmacokinetics

- Onset: within 2–4 h
- Duration: up to 24 h due to the decrease in plasma fibrinogen levels
- Biphasic half-life. 1st half-life ~16–18 mins; represents the molecule forming a complex with antistreptococcal antibodies. 2nd half-life starts within 90 mins; represents elimination from hepatic degradation and renal clearance

Dosing

- Acute MI. IV: 1 500 000 IU over 60 mins (3 000 000 IU may be more effective at clot lysis). Intracoronary: 20 000 IU bolus, followed by 2000–4000 IU/minute for 30–90 mins
- Arterial Thrombosis. IV: Loading dose 250 000 IU over 30 mins, followed by 100 000 IU/hour for 24 h. Intra-arterial: 5000 IU/hour for 24 hours.
- DVT. IV: Loading dose 250 000 IU over 30 mins followed by 100 000 IU/hfor 72 h

- Infected pleural effusion. Intrapleurally via a chest tube: 250 000 IU in 100 mL of normal saline; repeated QD-BID for up to 5 days
- Pulmonary embolism. IV: Loading dose of 250 000 IU over 30 mins, followed by 10 000 IU/hour for 24 h.
- Clearance of a blocked catheter. AV cannula: 250 000 IU/2mL into each occluded line of the catheter; clamp for 2 h and then aspirate. PICC line: 10 000 IU into the catheter for 1 h and then aspirate
- Pediatric Dosing. Arterial thrombosis: IV Loading dose of 2000 U/kg over 30 mins followed by either 1000 U/kg/h for 24 h OR 2000 U/kg/h for 6–12 h

Side Effects/Adverse Events

- Contraindicated in pts with active internal bleeding, severe uncontrolled HTN, intracranial or intraspinal trauma or surgery (within past 2 months), known bleeding diasthesis, CVA within past 2 months, intracranial neoplasm, cerebral AV malformation or aneurysm
- Cautious use in pts who have received streptokinase within the last 12 months (antistreptokinase antibody can develop after the first dose), recent major surgery, recent GI bleed, subacute bacterial endocarditis, concurrent administration of anticoagulants
- Known reactions: following acute MI, the pt is at risk for dysrhythmias, hypotension, and myocardial wall rupture; major bleeding, intracranial hemorrhage, ARDS, allergic or hypersensitivity reactions (antibodies to streptococci from prior infection may reduce the efficacy of streptokinase or cause allergic reactions).

Tissue Plasminogen Activator (tPA)

Clinical Uses/Relevance to Anesthesiolgy

- Acute ischemic stroke
- Acute MI
- Arterial or severe deep venous thrombosis
- Multiloculated or parapneumonic pleural effusion treatment
- Pulmonary embolism
- Clearance of a blocked catheter (arteriovenous cannula, PICC line)

Pharmacodynamics

- Endogenous serine protease found in endothelial cells. Binds to plasminogen and catalyzes its conversion to plasmin.
- Exogenous tPA is manufactured via recombinant technology. It accelerates the conversion of plasminogen in fibrin clots to plasmin. Plasmin lyses fibrin clots. Unlike streptokinase, tPA is fibrin specific; it acts on bound fibrin but does not have any effect on circulating plasminogen.

- Available in modified forms with slightly different pharmacokinetic and dynamic properties. Reteplase (r PA), tenecteplase (TNK-tPA) and lanoteplase (n PA) are the alternative forms of tPA.

Pharmacokinetics

- Elimination half-life ~4–6 mins
- Hepatically degraded primarily; a portion is degraded by circulating plasminogen activator inhibitor-1

Dosing

- Acute MI. Total dose is based on weight and should not exceed 100 mg. Pts < 67 kg: 15 mg IV bolus, followed by 0.75 mg/kg IV over 30 mins (not to exceed 50 mg), and then 0.5 mg/kg IV over 60 mins (not to exceed 35 mg). Pts > 67kg: 15 mg IV bolus, followed by 50 mg IV over 30 mins, and then 35 mg IV over 60 mins.
- Arterial thrombosis. Intra-arterial: 1.5 mg/h via transcatheter until lysis of thrombus
- DVT. Catheter-directed infusion of 1–1.5 mg/h for 12–24 h
- Pulmonary embolism. 15 mg IV bolus, followed by 0.75 mg/kg over 30 mins (max 50 mg), and then 0.5 mg/kg over 60 mins (max 35 mg)
- Ischemic stroke. 0.9 mg/kg over 60 mins (max 90 mg); 10% of the total dose administered should be given as a bolus of 1 min. Treatment should only be initiated within 3 h after the onset of stroke symptoms, and after exclusion of intracranial hemorrhage by a cranial CT
- Clearance of a blocked catheter. 2 mg/2 mL instilled into occluded catheter; up to 2 doses may be used, separated by 120 minutes
- Pediatric dosing arterial thrombosis: 0.1 to 0.6 mg/kg/h IV for 6 h has been used, optimal doses are unknown
- Pediatric venous thrombosis: 0.03–0.6 mg/kg IV for 6 h
- Pediatric clearance of a blocked catheter. 0.25 mg/2mg instilled into the occluded catheter

Preparations

- Available in 50 mg and 100 mg vials; needs to be reconstituted with 50 mL or 100 mL of sterile water, respectively, prior to administration

Side Effects/Adverse Events

- Contraindicated in pts with SAH on pretreatment evaluation or within past 3 months, intracranial tumor, cerebral AV malformation, or aneurysm; intracranial or intraspinal trauma or surgery (within past 2 months); uncontrolled HTN, known bleeding diathesis; current use of oral anticoagulants or administration of heparin within 48 h (when tPA is being given for acute ischemic stroke); or platelet count <100 000

- Cautious use in pts with advanced age, severe hepatic dysfunction, recent major trauma or GI bleed, pregnancy
- Known reactions: following acute MI, the pt is at risk for dysrhythmias, hypotension, and myocardial wall rupture; major bleeding (doses <100 mg is 1.2%), moderate hemorrhage (<100 mg is 11%); intracranial hemorrhage, cerebral edema and herniation, and seizures

References

1. The GUSTO Investigators. An international randomized trial comparing four thrombo-lytic strategies for acute myocardial infarction. *N Engl J Med.* 1993;329:673–682.

2. Kearon C, Kahn SR, Agnelli G, Goldhaber S, Raskob GE, Comerota AJ. Antithrombotic therapy for venous thromboembolic disease: American College of Chest Physicians evidence-based clinical practice guidelines (8th edition). *Chest.* 2008;133:454S-545S.

3. Fekrazad MF, Lopes RD, Stashenko GJ, Alexander JH, Garcia D. Treatment of venous thromboembolism: guidelines translated for the clinician. *J Thromb Thrombolysis.* 2009;28:270–275.

4. Roizen MF, Fleisher LA, eds. *Essence of Anesthesia Practice.* 2nd ed. Philadelphia: Saunders; 2002: 569.

5. Ouriel, K . Comparison of safety and efficacy of the various thrombolytic agents. *Rev Cardiovasc Med.* 2002;3(Suppl 2):S 17–24.

6. http://www.activase.com/actstroke/index.jsp.

7. Baruah DB, Dash RN, Chaudhari MR, Kadam SS. Plasminogen activators: a comparison. *Vascul Pharmacol.* 2006;44:1–9.

8. Knöfler R, Dinger J, Kabus M, Müller D, Lauterbach I, Rupprecht E, Taut-Sack H, Weissbach G. Thrombolytic therapy in children: clinical experiences with recombinant tissue-plasminogen activator. *Sem Thromb Hemost.* 2001;27:169–174.

9. Horlocker T, Wedel D; Rowlingson J, Enneking FK, Kopp SL, Benzon HT, Brown DL, Heit JA, Mulroy MF, Rosenquist RW, Tryba M, Yuan C. Regional anesthesia in the patient receiving antithrombotic or thrombolytic therapy: American Society of Regional Anesthesia and Pain Medicine evidence-based guidelines (third edition), ASRA Practice Advisory. *Reg Anesth Pain Med.* 2010; 35(1): 64–101.

Chapter 13.6

Heparin and Argatroban

Crystal C. Wright, MD

Heparin

Pharmacodynamics

- Mean molecular weight of approximately 15 000 Da.
- Mechanism of Action: binds to antithrombin-III (AT-III) causing a potentiation of ATIII more than 1000-fold. Heparin therefore inhibits the action of thrombin and factor Xa predominately.
- Also causes inhibition of factors IXa, XIa, and XIIa.
- Heparin may also inhibit and activate platelets and inhibit fibrinolysis.

Pharmacokinetics

- Elimination half-life is dose dependent and temperature dependent.
- Lower doses (100–150 USP units/kg): approximately one hour for elimination half-life.
- Higher doses (300–400 USP units/kg): elimination half-life is 2 hours or more.
- Hypothermia prolongs the duration of heparin.
- Heparin is metabolized through the reticuloendothelial system.
- 50% of heparin is excreted unchanged through the kidneys.

Heparin and Cardiopulmonary Bypass

- Heparin is the most common form of anticoagulation used to allow for systemic anticoagulation for cardiopulmonary bypass.
- The initial dose of heparin for cardiopulmonary bypass is 300–400 USP units/kg
- The ACT or the heparin concentrations are monitors used to access adequate heparinization for cardiopulmonary bypass.
- ACT is most commonly used
- The ACT causes the initiation of clotting with either a celite or kaolin to activate clotting.
- Normal ACT is between 110–140.

- ACT for cardiopulmonary bypass in an elective onset of cardiopulmonary bypass is 480s
- Heparin resistance during cardiopulmonary bypass can occur secondary to: antithrombin III deficiency, unstable angina, bacterial endocarditis, pregnancy, HIT, acid glycoprotein, histidine-rich glycoprotein, immunoglobulins, or extremes of age.
- Heparin resistance is most commonly caused by inadequate antithrombin III levels.
- Preoperative heparin therapy can deplete levels of endogenous antithrombin III and further worsen antithrombin III deficiency.
- Treatment of Heparin Resistance: increase dosage of heparin or administration of ATIII either through the administration off fresh frozen plasma or antithrombin III concentrate.

Heparin Induced Thrombocytopenia and Cardiac Surgery

- There are two major types of heparin induced thrombocytopenia, HIT I and HIT II.
- HIT I thrombocytopenia is modest and usually resolves with discontinuation of heparin.
- HIT II thrombocytopenia is severe and is associated with thromboembolism, myocardial ischemia, pulmonary embolism, and cerebrovascular accidents.
- Heparin administration in HIT II is not recommended
- Administration of heparin to patients with HIT II can lead to platelet aggregation, thromboembolism, and thrombocytopenia.
- HIT II patients requiring cardiac surgery and systemic anticoagulation; unfractionated heparin is contraindicated.
- Alternative anticoagulation therapy must be considered in patients presenting with HIT II.
- Thrombin inhibitors, including argatroban, bivalirudin, and hirudin, have been used as the most common successful alternatives.

Argatroban

Pharmacokinetics and Pharmacodynamics

- Argatroban is a synthetic molecule derived from L-Arginine, $C23H36N605S.H_2O$
- Direct thrombin inhibitor that reversibly and competitively binds to the active site of thrombin.
- Exerts its anticoagulant effects by inhibiting thrombin-catalyzed or thrombin-induced reactions, including fibrin formation; activation of coagulation factors V, VIII, and XIII; activation of protein C; and platelet aggregation.
- Compound has a low volume of distribution of 180 ml/kg

- Approximately 50% of the drug is protein bound
- Elimination pathway is not temperature dependent
- Excretion is primarily hepatobiliary; minimal renal clearance
- half-life is 30 minutes

Clinical Uses

- Indicated in the United States as an anticoagulant for prophylaxis treatment of thrombosis in HIT
- Also indicated for patients with or at risk for HIT undergoing percutaneous coronary intervention.
- Used in cardiopulmonary bypass but not approved.
- There is no specific antidote to argatroban
- Clinically, argatroban increases the aPTT, ACT, PT, INR, and thrombin time

Argatroban Dosage for HIT

- Adult Initial IV dose: 2 µcg/kg/min in patients with normal hepatic function; 0.5 µcg/kg/min in patients with hepatic dysfunction
- Reduced initial dose is recommended in patients with heart failure, multiple organ system failure, severe anasarca, or after cardiac surgery.
- Therapeutic level of 1.5–3 times the baseline aPTT is recommended

Argatroban and Cardiopulmonary Bypass

- Not approved for cardiopulmonary bypass but has been successfully used during cardiac surgery.
- Recommended dosing for cardiopulmonary bypass if heparin alternative is needed:
  - Initial bolus of 0.1 mg/kg administered prior to cannulation.
  - No requirement of additional drug in the pump prime, but if chosen to do so the CPB prime should be 0.05 mg/kg.
  - Additional 2-mg IV boluses can be used to maintain appropriate levels of anticoagulation.
  - Continuous infusion of 5–10 µg/kg/minute during cardiopulmonary bypass should be instituted.
  - The infusion should be discontinued prior to the end of cardiopulmonary bypass.
- ACT can be used to monitor coagulation status intraoperatively

Contraindications

- Contraindicated in patients with overt major bleeding
- Extreme caution is advised during its use in conditions that increase the risk of hemorrhage, ie, severe hypertension, immediately following lumbar puncture, spinal anesthesia; major surgery; and hemotologic conditions associated

with increased bleeding tendencies such as congenital or acquired bleeding disorders and GI lesions.

References

1. Babuin L, Pengo V. Argatroban in the management of heparin-induced thrombocytopenia. *Vasc Health Risk Manag.* 2010;6813–6819.

2. Follis F, Filippone F, Montalbano G, Floriano M, LoBianco E, D'Ancona G, Follis M. Argatroban as a substitute of heparin during cardiopulmonary bypass: a safe alternative. *Interact Cardiovasc Thorac Surg.* 2010;10:592–596.

3. George D, Gravlee G, Filos K, Levy J. Anticoagulation monitoring during cardiac surgery. *Anesthesiology.* 1999;91:1122–1151.

4. Hurtsting M, Murray P. Argatroban anticoagulation in renal dysfunction: a literature analysis. *Nephron Clin Pract.* 2008;109:c80-c94.

5. Liu H, Fleming N, Moore P. Anticoagulation for patients with heparin-induced thrombocytopenia using recombinant hirudin during cardiopulmonary bypass. *J Clin Anesth.* 2002;14:452–455.

6. Nuttal G, Oliver W, Santrach P, McBane R, Erpelding D, Marver C, Zehr K. Patients with a history of type ii heparin-induced thrombocytopenia with thrombosis requiring cardiac surgery with cardiopulmonary bypass: a prospective observational case series. *Anesth Analg.* 2003;96:344–350.

7. Spiess, B . Treating heparin resistance with antithrombin or fresh frozen plasma. *Ann Thorac Surg.* 2008;85:2153–2160.

Chapter 13.7

Procoagulants

Peter Killoran, MD and Katherine C. Normand, MD

Aminocaproic Acid (Epsilon-Aminocaproic Acid (EACA), Amicar)

Role in the Practice of Anesthesia/Relevance to Anesthesiology

- Used for treatment hyperfibrinolysis associated with life-threatening hemorrhage. Not effective without adequate surgical hemostasis and/or vascular integrity.
- Shown to reduce intraoperative blood loss, postoperative blood loss, and transfusion requirements for cardiac surgery with cardiopulmonary bypass.
- Evidence for reduced total perioperative blood loss (reduced postoperative, but not intraoperative blood loss) associated with major orthopedic procedures without significant reduction in transfusion requirements.
- Effective for controlling hyperfibrinolysis associated with liver transplantation without statistically significant effect on transfusion requirements.
- Short-term administration for prophylaxis against recurrent subarachnoid hemorrhage when endovascular or surgical intervention is delayed.
- Treatment of bleeding when diagnosis of hyperfibrinolysis has been made. Commonly associated procedures include cardiac surgery and portacaval shunt. Commonly associated comorbidities include aplastic anemia with amegakaryocytic thrombocytopenia, acute abruptio placentae, hepatic cirrhosis, and neoplasm such as carcinoma of the prostate, lung, stomach, and cervix.
- Treatment of hematuria following prostatectomy and nephrectomy as well as nonsurgical hematuria associated with polycystic or neoplastic diseases of the genitourinary system. Successful treatment of renal papillary necrosis with massive hematuria has also been reported.
- May help reverse thrombolytic agents (eg, alteplase, antistreplase, streptokinase, urokinase) in cases of overdose or uncontrolled hemorrhage.

Pharmacodynamics

- Blood clots at the site of vascular injury are stabilized by polymers of the protein fibrin (also known as Factor Ia), formed by activation of the coagulation cascade. A natural balance between formation of fibrin at the site of hemorrhage and its degradation in areas beyond the site of injury is an essential aspect of keeping the coagulation cascade in balance.
- Fibrin is degraded by the enzyme plasmin, which is produced by the liver in an inactive form known as plasminogen. Plasminogen is converted to plasmin by tissue plasminogen activator (tPA) and urokinase. Once activated, plasmin functions as a serine protease and cleaves fibrin, allowing the clot to degrade. Plasminogen also has affinity for fibrin and is incorporated into developing clots. It is then slowly converted to plasmin and facilitates clot remodeling and breakdown.
- Aminocaproic acid is a synthetic lysine derivative that inhibits fibrinolysis primarily by preventing the conversion of plasminogen into plasmin, but may also have some direct inhibitory effect on plasmin. It may also prevent plasmin mediated degradation of platelet glycoprotein Ib receptors, thus preserving platelet function.

Pharmacokinetics

- Both parenteral and enteral forms are available. Enteral formulations are rapidly and completely absorbed by the GI tract.
- Plasma concentrations of 130 mcg/ml are necessary to maintain inhibition of systemic hyperfibrinolysis.
- Urinary concentration occurs primarily by filtration and reabsorption.
- Effective inhibitory concentrations are detectable in urine even when systemic concentrations are not detectable, so treatment of urinary tract bleeding may be possible with minimal systemic effect.
- Terminal elimination half-life is 2 hours.
- Majority of the drug is not metabolized, with 40%-65% eliminated unchanged in urine and 11% excreted as metabolite (adipic acid) within 12 hours.
- Total body clearance is reduced in renal failure but is removed by hemodialysis and may be removed by peritoneal dialysis.

Side Effects/Adverse Reactions

- Mild adverse reactions include nausea, vomiting, cramping, abdominal pain, diarrhea, dizziness, malaise, fever, conjunctival suffusion, dyspnea, nasal stuffiness, headache, pruritus, and rash.
- More serious but rare adverse reactions include edema, hemorrhage, ischemia, thrombosis, intracranial hypertension, stroke, syncope, seizures, renal failure, deafness, glaucoma, pulmonary embolism, agranulocytosis, leucopenia, and thrombocytopenia.

- Hypotension, bradycardia, and arrhythmia have been reported following rapid IV injection.
- Skeletal weakness and muscle necrosis have been reported with prolonged infusions.
- Localized pain and necrosis have been reported at the site of IV injection.
- There is a theoretical increased risk for thrombotic events due to decreased spontaneous fibrinolysis, but meta-analyses have not demonstrated a clinically significantly increased risk.
- Aminocaproic acid should not be used in treatment of disseminated intravascular coagulation (DIC) without concomitant administration of heparin

Dosages/Preparations

- Standard parenteral formulation is 250 mg/ml.
- Oral formulations available as a solution (1.25 g/5 ml) and 500 mg tablets.
- For treatment or prevention of hyperfibrinolysis—slow infusion loading dose of 4–5 g in the first hour followed by a continuous infusion of 1 g/hr. Treatment should continue for 8 hours or until the hemorrhage is under control with a daily maximum of 30 g.
- Safety and efficacy in pediatric surgery has not been established, but a 100 mg/kg (3 g/m2) loading dose followed by 33.3 mg/kg/hr (1 $g/m^2/hr$) infusion has been used with total dosage not to exceed 18 g/m^2 in 24 hours.
- Oral regimens for chronic hematologic disorders range from 5 to 30 g/day in divided doses every 3–6 hours and are titrated to the lowest possible dose to control bleeding.

Clinical Case Scenario

A 45-year-old, 80-kg man with history of end stage liver disease secondary to alcoholic cirrhosis and hepatitis C presents for liver transplant. Preoperative lab values include hemoglobin of 11.2, platelets of 65, and INR of 2.1. During initial dissection, blood loss of 1200 ml rapidly accumulates despite adequate surgical hemostasis and administration of 12 units of platelets and 4 units of fresh frozen plasma. Oozing is noted throughout the surgical field and at the site of the central venous catheter. Thromboelastography is performed and is consistent with fibrinolysis.

Background: The patient is undergoing liver transplantation, which is associated with a significant risk for hyperfibrinolysis. Although evidence to support routine use of aminocaproic acid to reduce blood loss in liver transplantation is lacking, it has been shown to effectively control hyperfibrinolysis as measured by thromboelastography.

Pathophysiology: Hyperfibrinolysis is frequently noted during liver transplantation and results from imbalances between activators and inhibitors of the fibrinolytic system. The result is inappropriate degradation of fibrin leading to increased blood loss and increased transfusion requirements.

Treatment: A loading dose of 5 g aminocaproic acid slowly administered followed by a maintenance infusion of 1 g/hr. Repeat thromboelastograms should be obtained to confirm improvement in fibrinolysis and guide further administration of blood products including packed red blood cells, fresh frozen plasma, platelets, and cryoprecipitate. Additional laboratory studies including PT/PTT, platelet count, fibrinogen, hemoglobin, and hematocrit may also be helpful to guide both correction of coagulopathy and fluid resuscitation.

Alternative Treatments: Tranexamic acid works by a similar mechanism to prevent fibrinolysis and has also been successfully used to control hyperfibrinolysis in liver transplantation. Aprotinin is also effective, but was removed from the general US market in 2008 after evidence for increased mortality associated with its use emerged.

References

1. Henry DA, Carless PA, Moxey AJ, O'Connell D, Stokes BJ, Fergusson DA, Ker K. Anti-fibrinolytic use for minimising perioperative allogeneic blood transfusion. *Cochrane Database Syst Rev.* 2011;1: CD001886. doi: 10.1002/14651858.CD001886.pub3.

2. Zuffery P, Merquiol F, Laporte S, Decousus H, Mismetti P, Auboyer C, Samama CM, Molliex S. Do antifibrinolytics reduce allogeneic blood transfusions in orthopedic surgery? *Anesthesiology.* 2006;105:1034–1046.

3. Makwana J, Paranjape S, Goswami J. Antifibrinolytics in liver surgery. *Indian J Anaesth.* 2010;54(6):489–495.

4. Kang Y, Lewis JH, Navalgund A, Russell MW, Bontempo FA, Niren LS, Sarzi TE. Epsilon-aminocaproic acid for treatment of fibrinolysis during liver transplantation. *Anesthesiology.* 1987;66:766–773.

5. Xia VW, Steadman RH. Antifibrinolytics in orthotopic liver transplantation: current status and controversies. *Liver Transpl.* 2005;11(1):10–18.

6. Harrigan MR, Rajneesh KF, Ardelt AA, Fisher WS. Short term antifibrinolytic therapy before early aneurysm treatment in subarachnoid hemorrhage: effects on rehemorrhage, cerebral ischemia, and hydrocephalus. *Neurosurgery.* 2010;67:935–940.

7. Amicar Package insert.

8. Gabrovsky A, Aderinto A, Spevak M, Vichinsky E, Resar L. Low-dose, oral epsilon aminocaproic acid for renal papillary necrosis and massive hemorrhage in hemoglobin SC disease. *Pediatr Blood Cancer.* 2010;54:148–150.

9. Marder VJ. Comparison of thrombolytic agents: selected hematologic, vascular, and clinical events. *Am J Cardiol.* 1989;64:2A-7A.

10. Wells P. Safety and efficacy of methods for reducing perioperative allogentic transfusion: a critical review of the literature. *Am J Ther.* 2002;9:377–388.

11. McEvoy G, Snow E, Miller J, Kester L, Welsh O, Heydorn J, Le T, Mendham N, O'Rourke A, eds. *AHFS Drug Information 2011.* Bethesda, MD: American Society of Health-System Pharmacists; 2011.

12. Brown J, Birkmeyer N, O'Connor G. Meta-analysis comparing the effectiveness and adverse outcomes of antifibrinolytic agents in cardiac surgery. *Circulation.* 2007;115:2801–2813.

13. Edmunds L. Managing fibrinolysis without aprotinin. *Ann Thorac Surg*. 2010:324–331.

14. Furgusson D, Hebert P, Mazer C, Fremes S, MacAdams C, Murkin J, Teoh K, Duke P, Arellano R, Blajchman M, Bussieres J, Cote D, Karski J, Martineau R, Robblee J, Rodger M, Wells G, Clinch J, Pretorius R, for the BART investigators. A comparison of aprotinin and lysine analogues in high-risk cardiac surgery. *N Engl J Med*. 2010;358(22):2319–2331.

Aprotinin

Relevance to Anesthesia

- Used to treat or prevent hyperfibrinolysis associated with life-threatening hemorrhage. Not effective without adequate surgical hemostasis and/or vascular integrity.

- Removed from the US market by the manufacturer in 2008 after publication of data showing an increased risk of cardiovascular complications and death associated with its use.

- Currently only available through the manufacturer as an investigational drug under a special treatment protocol.

- More effective at reducing blood loss, transfusion requirements, and reoperation due to bleeding than other available antifibrinolytics (ie, tranexamic acid, aminocaproic acid).

- Significant increase in risk of death when compared directly to tranexamic acid and aminocaproic acid, but not associated with increased risk of myocardial infarction, stroke, deep vein thrombosis, pulmonary embolus, renal dysfunction, or overall mortality when compared to no treatement.

- General consensus that other fibrinolytics are safe and effective, but use of aprotinin may be appropriate in situations where the specific risk bleeding might outweigh a generally higher mortality rate.

Pharmacodynamics

- Aprotinin is a naturally occurring protease inhibitor isolated from bovine lung tissue that is a potent inhibitor of fibrinolysis.

- Blood clots at the site of vascular injury are stabilized by polymers of the protein fibrin (also known as Factor Ia), formed by activation of the coagulation cascade. A natural balance between formation of fibrin at the site of hemorrhage and its degradation in areas beyond the site of injury is an essential aspect of keeping the coagulation cascade in balance.

- Fibrin is degraded by the enzyme plasmin, which is produced by the liver in an inactive form known as plasminogen. Plasminogen is converted to plasmin by tissue plasminogen activator (tPA) and urokinase. Once activated, plasmin functions as a serine protease and cleaves fibrin, allowing the clot to degrade. Plasminogen also has affinity for fibrin and is incorporated into developing clots, which is then slowly converted to plasmin and facilitates clot remodeling and breakdown.

- The precise mechanism of action by which aprotinin reduces blood loss during cardiopulmonary bypass (CPB) is not clear, but likely involves effects on platelet function, coagulation, and fibrinolysis. As a broad-spectrum protease inhibitor, it modulates the response to CBP, thus attenuating the resulting inflammatory response, fibrinolysis, and thrombin generation. Its inhibitory effects are concentration dependent, with the greatest effect on trypsin, followed by plasmin and then kallikrein. By inhibiting proinflammatory cytokine release, it reduces loss of platelet glycoprotein receptors (ie, GPIb, GpIIb/IIIa) and prevents expression of granulocyte adhesive glycoproteins (ie, CD11b).

Pharmacokinetics

- Linear pharmacokinetics over dose ranges from 50 000 to 2 million kallikrein inactivator units (KIU).
- Rapid redistribution into the total extracellular space followed by plasma half-life of about 150 minutes
- After more than 5 hours from dosing, half-life during the terminal elimination phase is about 10 hours.
- Filtered by glomeruli and actively reabsorbed by proximal tubule, then metabolized by lysosomal enzymes. Approximately 25%-40% of metabolites and 2%-9% of the unchanged drug are excreted in urine over 48 hours.

Side Effects/Adverse Reactions

- Anaphylactic or anaphylactoid reactions have been documented on first exposure, but risk is higher with subsequent administration. Use is contraindicated in patients with known or suspected previous exposure during the prior 12 months. Aprotinin is a component of some fibrin sealant products, and exposure from this source should be considered.
- Rapid administration is associated with hypotension.
- Should only be administered after intubation in a setting where immediate resuscitation is available and cardiopulmonary bypass can be rapidly initiated.
- Associated with increased risk of renal dysfunction and perioperative dialysis. The risk is especially increased in patients with preexisting renal impairment or those who receive aminoglycoside antibiotics.
- Prolongs the activated clotting time (ACT) independently from concurrent use of heparin, and may lead to a false overestimation of the degree of anticoagulation. Kaolin-based ACT assays are not increased as much as celite-based ACT assays.
- If ACTs are being used to monitor anticoagulation in the presence of aprotinin, a minimum kaolin-based ACT of 480 seconds or a celite-based ACT of 750 seconds is recommended during CPB. Specific recommendations of the assay manufacturer should also be consulted.

- If a fixed heparin dosing schedule is being used, it should total at least 350 IU/kg should be administered prior to cannulation with additional doses administered based on patient weight and duration of CPB.
- Titration of heparin dosing based on a protamine titration method may also be used during CPB. A heparin dose response should be performed prior to aprotinin administration to determine the heparin loading dose with additional doses administered based on heparin levels as measured by protamine titration. Heparin levels during bypass should not drop below 2.7 U/ml (2.0 mg/kg) or the level indicated by the initial heparin dose response testing.

Dosages/Preparations

- Potency is typically expressed in kallikrein inactivator units (KIU). There are approximately 7143 KIU per milligram of drug.
- Standard concentration is 10 000 KIU or 1.4 mg/ml.
- A test dose of 10 000 KIU should always be administered at least 10 minutes prior to the loading dose.
- The loading dose should be slowly administered with the patient in a supine position over 20–30 minutes.
- Should be administered only through a dedicated central line port. Heparin and aprotinin should be added to the bypass circuit prime volume while it is recirculating to assure adequate dilution and avoid physical incompatibility.
- Two dosing regimens were investigated during clinical trials. Regimen A includes a 2 million KIU loading dose, 2 million KIU in the pump prime volume, and a 500 000 KIU per hour continuous infusion. Regimen B is a half dose or a 1 million KIU loading dose, 1 million KIU in the pump prime, and a 250 000 KIU per hour continuous infusion. Regimen A was used in the BART trial that resulted in removal of aprotinin from the US market.
- Maximum daily dosage has not been established, but dosages up to 17.5 million KIU in a 24-hour period have been safely administered without apparent toxicity.
- Manufacturer states no dose reduction is necessary in renal failure although some clinicians have recommended reduced dosing regimens. Other risk factors for renal dysfunction and potential concurrent administration of nephrotoxins (eg, aminoglycoside antibiotics) should be considered.

Clinical Case Scenario

A 68-year-old, 65-kg woman with history of coronary artery disease status post 3 vessel CABG 3 years ago, angina, hypertension, hyperlipidemia, and type 2 diabetes mellitus presents for repeat coronary artery bypass surgery. She is a Jehovah's Witness and has agreed to the use of cell-saver and coronary artery bypass during her operation, but states that she "would rather die" than receive any blood products including packed red blood cells, fresh frozen plasma, platelets, and cryoprecipitate. Her cardiologist has referred her for surgery because her disease is progressing and is not amenable to less invasive therapies.

Background: This patient is undergoing repeat coronary artery bypass surgery and is at high risk for significant blood loss, but she is unable to receive blood products due to her religious convictions. Aprotinin has been shown to more effectively reduce blood loss and transfusion requirements than other available antifibrinolytics, but is also associated with a higher mortality rate. For this patient, aprotinin use may be appropriate because the specific risk of bleeding may outweigh the generally higher mortality rate. Since this is an elective case, there is time to discuss potential use with the patient and surgical team and obtain drug from the manufacturer under the special treatment protocol.

Pathophysiology: Cardiopulmonary bypass increases activation of fibrinolysis by increasing the concentration of tissue plasminogen activator without concomitant increases in its inhibitor plasminogen activator inhibitor 1. Thrombin production is also accelerated by CPB, leading to consumptive coagulopathy where both thrombin and plasmin are produced in excess. Coagulopathy following separation from CPB is further worsened by platelet dysfunction, hypothermia, and residual heparin effect.

Treatment: After induction of anesthesia and placement of a central line, she is given a 10 000 KIU test dose, which she tolerates well. After ten minutes, a 2 million KIU loading dose is slowly infused over 30 minutes during sternotomy and scar dissection. Once complete, a 500 000 KIU/hr infusion is started and 2 million KIU are added to the CPB prime volume.

Alternative Treatments: Aminocaproic acid and tranexamic acid are also effective inhibitors of fibrinolysis during cardiac surgery and are generally considered safer alternatives. However, aprotinin has the greatest impact on reducing blood loss, transfusion requirements, and reoperation rates during cardiac surgery compared to alternatives, but is associated with a higher mortality rate. Therefore, aminocaproic acid and tranexamic acid are the preferred drugs for routine use, except in cases where the specific risk of bleeding might outweigh a the risk of higher general mortality rate.

References

1. Furgusson D, Hebert P, Mazer C, Fremes S, MacAdams C, Murkin J, Teoh K, Duke P, Arellano R, Blajchman M, Bussieres J, Cote D, Karski J, Martineau R, Robblee J, Rodger M, Wells G, Clinch J, Pretorius R, for the BART investigators. A comparison of aprotinin and lysine analogues in high-risk cardiac surgery. *N Engl J Med*. 2010;358(22):2319–2331.

2. United States Food and Drug Administration. www.fda.gov. Last Accessed January 18, 2010.

3. Henry DA, Carless PA, Moxey AJ, O'Connell D, Stokes BJ, Fergusson DA, Ker K. Anti-fibrinolytic use for minimising perioperative allogeneic blood transfusion. *Cochrane Database Syst Rev*. 2011;1: CD001886. doi: 10.1002/14651858.CD001886.pub3.

4. McEvoy G, Snow E, Miller J, Kester L, Welsh O, Heydorn J, Le T, Mendham N, O'Rourke A, eds. *AHFS Drug Information 2011*. Bethesda, MD: American Society of Health-System Pharmacists; 2011.

5. Trasylol Package insert. Bayer Pharmaceuticals. Available at www.trasylol.com.

6. Xia VW, Steadman RH. Antifibrinolytics in orthotopic liver transplantation: current status and controversies. *Liver Transpl*. 2005;11(1):10–18.

7. Edmunds L. Managing fibrinolysis without aprotinin. *Ann Thorac Surg*. 2010:324–331.

Protamine

Relevance to Anesthesia

- Used in cardiac and vascular surgery to reverse the anticoagulant effects of heparin.
- Used to reverse toxicity associated with continuous heparin therapy where there is significant bleeding.
- Used to reverse anticoagulation in pregnant women receiving continuous heparin therapy who go into spontaneous labor.
- Contained in certain preparations of subcutaneous insulin to slow absorption and prolong the duration of action.
- Prior exposure increases risk of anaphylactic reaction on subsequent exposures, so a history of use should be obtained from all patients undergoing cardiac or vascular surgery where use of protamine is anticipated. There is also some limited evidence for an increased risk of anaphylaxis in men who have undergone vasectomy.
- There is no convincing evidence that protamine reverses clinical bleeding associated with low molecular weight heparin (LMWH) administration, although it does neutralize the anti-IIa and a variable portion of the anti-Xa activity of LMWH and will normalize the activated partial thromboplastin time and thrombin time.
- If administered in the absence of heparin or in excess of amount needed to neutralize circulating heparin, protamine has a weak anticoagulant effect.

Pharmacodynamics

- Protamine sulfate is an arginine-rich, basic, polycationic protein derived from salmon sperm used to reverse anticoagulant effects of heparin. It is also used in long-acting formulations of insulin to slow absorption and prolong the effect of insulin.
- Protamine binds to heparin to form a stable, inactive salt compound which does not have any anticoagulant effects, thus reversing anticoagulation associated with heparin and removing it from circulation.
- In vitro studies have demonstrated an intrinsic anticoagulant effect when protamine is administered in excess of the amount necessary to neutralize circulating heparin through decreased thrombin activity, decreased activation of factor VII by tissue factor, enhanced tissue-type plasminogen activator-mediated fibrinolysis, decreased factor V activation by activated

factor X or thrombin, and attenuated platelet function by inhibition of glyco-protein Ib-von Willebrand factor activity.

Pharmacokinetics

- Onset of action is rapid, with effective neutralization of heparin within 5 minutes of administration.
- Half-life of protamine administered in the absence of heparin is about 7 minutes. In patients who received heparin during cardiopulmonary bypass, the half-life has been reported to be 4.5 minutes.
- Metabolism of heparin-protamine complexes is not clear, but it may be partially metabolized by fibrinolysin, which may result in regeneration of free heparin.
- Rebound anticoagulation and bleeding have been documented following complete neutralization of heparin with protamine. Release of heparin from the heparin-protamine complex and mobilization of heparin from extravascular compartments are the most likely contributors to this effect.

Side Effects/Adverse Reactions

- Significant adverse reactions range from mild hypotension to profound hemodynamic instability. A variety of different reactions have been reported including type 1 anaphylactic reactions and both immediate and delayed anaphylactoid responses. Mechanisms to explain different reactions are also variable and include mast cell degranulation (at high concentrations), complement activation, and antibody formation. Complement activation by either protamine-heparin complexes or antiprotamine antibodies has been implicated in severe reactions associated with C5a-mediated thromboxane generation leading to pulmonary hypertension, right heart failure, and circulatory collapse.
- Isolated hypotension, with normal to low filling pressures and normal airway pressures, generally responds to volume resuscitation, vasopressors, and slowing of the protamine infusion rate.
- Hypotension associated with increased airway pressure, bronchoconstriction, elevated PA pressures, and evidence of right ventricular failure may quickly progress to circulatory collapse and requires aggressive treatment including inotropic support and potential initiation of cardiopulmonary bypass.
- Slow administration over 5–10 minutes is generally advised to reduce the risk of adverse reaction.
- Bradycardia, urticaria, edema, dyspnea, nausea, vomiting, lassitude, and back pain have also been reported.
- Protamine has an anticoagulant effect when administered in the absence of heparin or in excess of the amount needed to neutralize circulating heparin through a variety of effects on the coagulation cascade, fibrinolysis, and platelet function.

Dosages/Preparations

- Available only for parenteral use. Standard concentration is 10 mg/mL. May be administered without further dilution or mixed with 5% dextrose or normal saline to the desired concentration.

- For reversal of heparin following cardiopulmonary bypass, either give 1.5 mg/100 units of heparin administered or determine the residual heparin concentration using sequential ACTs and a dose response curve.

- Reversal of heparin during vascular procedures is variable and depends on patient temperature, time since last administration, total dose administered, and practitioner preferences. After a short period of heparinization in a euthermic patient, slow administration of 1 mg protamine/100 units heparin is typically administered.

- For reversal of anticoagulation in a patient on continuous heparin therapy a few minutes following the last dose, slowly administer 1 mg/100 units heparin. If the last dose was >30 minutes prior, administer 0.5 mg/100 units heparin. If the dose was >2 hours prior, administer 0.25–0.375 mg/100 units heparin.

- For severe bleeding following administration of subcutaneous heparin, several different dosing schemes have been reported. Some clinicians have recommend administering 1–1.5 mg/100 units as a prolonged infusion. Others recommend a loading dose of 25–50 mg followed by a continuous infusion the remaining calculated dose over 8–16 hours.

- For reversal of low molecular weight heparin (LMWH) within 8 hours of the last dose, administer 1 mg/100 anti-Xa units. If the aPTT 2–4 hours later remains prolonged or bleeding continues, a second dose of 0.5 mg/100 anti-Xa units may be administered. For severe bleeding >8 hours after administration of LMWH, administer 0.5 mg/100 anti-Xa units administered. There are no convincing human studies to confirm or refute the clinical benefit of protamine for reversal of anticoagulation associated with LMWH.

Clinical Case Scenario

A 48-year-old 70-kg man with a history of aortic stenosis presents for aortic valve replacement. After induction of anesthesia an arterial line and central venous catheter are placed. Following sternotomy and prior to placement of the cardiopulmonary bypass cannulas, 21 000 units of heparin (300 units/kg) are administered. The ACT drawn 3 minutes later is 490 seconds and cardiopulmonary bypass is initiated followed by uneventful valve replacement. Once the venous cannula is clamped and the patient successfully weaned from CPB, 315 mg protamine (1.5 mg/100 units heparin) is slowly administered. Blood pressure decreases from 105/65 to 85/45 after the first minute of infusion. The rate of infusion is slowed and a small bolus of phenylephrine is given with 250 ml of crystalloid. The blood pressure returns to 108/50 and the remainder of the protamine dose is slowly infused over the next 10 minutes without complication. A repeat ACT drawn after 5 minutes is 105 seconds.

Background: This patient is undergoing cardiac surgery with cardiopulmonary bypass and therefore requires heparinization. Once separated from CPB, the heparin should be neutralized to reduce hemorrhage.

Pathophysiology: Protamine binds to heparin to form an inactive salt, which is then rapidly removed from circulation and reverses anticoagulation. Hypotension is a common adverse reaction associated with protamine and occurs by a variety of mechanisms. Slowing the rate of infusion, vasopressors, and administration of volume are often sufficient. However, severe reactions associated with pulmonary hypertension, right ventricular failure, systemic hypotension, and circulatory collapse are also possible and should prompt aggressive treatment including inotropes and possible reinitiation of CPB.

Alternative Treatments: In patients with a documented protamine allergy, alternatives to anticoagulation with heparin (as done for patients with heparin induced thrombocytopenia) should be considered to avoid the use of protamine. Nonprotamine heparin reversal agents have also been used including PF4 and heparinase I, but these are not commercially available and do not have favorable safety profiles.

References

1. Nybo M, Madsen J. Serious anaphylactic reactions due to protamine sulfate: A systematic literature review. *Basic Clin Pharmacol Toxicol.* 2008;103:192–196.

2. Levy J, Adkinson N. Anaphylaxis during cardiac surgery: Implications for clinicians. *Anesth Analg.* 2008;106:392–403.

3. Miller, RD. Chapter 60: Anesthesia for cardiac surgical procedures. In: *Miller's Anesthesia.* New York: Elsevier; 2005.

4. Hirsh J, Bauer K, Donati M, Gould M, Samama M, Weitz J. Parenteral anticoagulants: American College of Chest Physicians evidence-based clinical practice guidelines (8th edition). *Chest.* 2008;133:141S-159S.

5. Nielsen V, Malayaman S. Protamine sulfate: crouching clot or hidden hemorrhage? *Anesth Analg.* 2010;11 (3):593–594.

6. McEvoy G, Snow E, Miller J, Kester L, Welsh O, Heydorn J, Le T, Mendham N, O'Rourke A, eds. *AHFS Drug Information 2011.* Bethesda, MD: American Society of Health-System Pharmacists; 2011.

7. Barash PG. Chapter 41: Anesthesia for cardiac surgery. In: Barash PG et al., eds. *Clinical Anesthesia.* Philadelphia: Lippincott Williams and Wilkins; 2006.

8. Stafford-Smit, M, Lefrak E, Qazi A, Welsby I, Barber L, Hoeft AA, Dorenbaum A, Mathias J, Rochon J, Newman M. Efficacy and safety of heparinase I versus PROTAMINE in patients undergoing coronary artery bypass grafting with and without cardiopulmonary bypass. *Anesthesiology.* 2005;103(2):229–240.

Tranexemic Acid (TEA)

Relevance to Anesthesia

- Used for treatment hyperfibrinolysis associated with life-threatening hemorrhage. Not effective without adequate surgical hemostasis and/or vascular integrity.
- Evidence supporting use to reduce blood loss and transfusion requirements for cardiac, major vascular, and major orthopedic surgery.
- Conflicting evidence to support reduction in blood loss and transfusion requirements in liver transplantation, but effective if diagnosis of hyperfibrinolysis is made.
- Evidence for reduced mortality in trauma patients, but without associated reductions in transfusion rates, transfusion volumes, or surgical interventions.
- Short-term (2–8 day) use indicated for patients with hemophilia to reduce blood loss and replacement therapy during and following tooth extraction.
- Oral preparations approved for treatment of heavy menstrual bleeding.
- May help reverse thrombolytic agents (eg, alteplase, antistreplase, streptokinase, urokinase) in cases of overdose or uncontrolled hemorrhage.

Pharmacodynamics

- Blood clots at the site of vascular injury are stabilized by polymers of the protein fibrin (also known as Factor la), formed by activation of the coagulation cascade. A natural balance between formation of fibrin at the site of hemorrhage and its degradation in areas beyond the site of injury is an essential aspect of keeping the coagulation cascade in balance.
- Fibrin is degraded by the enzyme plasmin, which is produced by the liver in an inactive form known as plasminogen. Plasminogen is converted to plasmin by tissue plasminogen activator (tPA) and urokinase. Once activated, plasmin functions as a serine protease and cleaves fibrin, allowing the clot to degrade. Plasminogen also has affinity for fibrin and is incorporated into developing clots, which is then slowly converted to plasmin and facilitates clot remodeling and breakdown.
- Tranexamic acid is a synthetic lysine derivative that inhibits fibrinolysis by competitive inhibition of plasminogen conversion into the active enzyme plasmin. At high concentrations, it also acts as a noncompetitive inhibitor of plasmin. It may also prevent plasmin mediated degradation of platelet glycoprotein lb receptors, thus preserving platelet function.

Pharmacokinetics

- Available in both parenteral and enteral formulations. Approximately 45% of the oral dose is absorbed by the GI tract. Bioavailability is not affected by food intake.
- Elimination half-life is about 2 hours.
- Primarily eliminated via urinary excretion via glomerular filtration, >95% of administered dose is excreted unchanged.

- Urinary excretion decreases as renal function declines. Dose adjustments are necessary in patients with renal insufficiency.
- Approximately 1.5% of drug is metabolized and excreted as dicarboxylic acid and an acetylated metabolite. No dose adjustment is necessary in hepatic failure.
- 3% bound to plasma proteins with no apparent binding to albumin
- Crosses the placenta, into CSF, and into the aqueous humor.

Side Effects/Adverse reactions

- Adverse reactions noted during clinical trials included headache, sinus/nasal symptoms, back pain, abdominal pain, musculoskeletal pain, joint pain, muscle cramps, migraine, anemia, and fatigue.
- Additional reported side effects and adverse reactions include nausea, vomiting, diarrhea, rash, anaphylaxis, thromboembolism, impaired color vision, visual disturbances, and dizziness.
- Increased risk of postoperative seizures has been reported primarily following valve, redo CABG, and aorta surgery.
- Hypotension has been reported associated with rapid IV infusion.
- Contraindicated in patients with active thromboembolic disease, history of thrombosis/thromboembolic disease, or suspected increased risk of thrombosis/thromboembolism.
- Use of hormonal contraceptives increases risk of thromboembolism and are therefore a relative contraindication.
- Should not be administered concomitantly with factor IX complex concentrates or anti-inhibitor coagulant concentrates.
- Retinal venous and arterial occlusions have been reported. If any visual changes are noted, the drug should be promptly discontinued and ophthalmological consultation obtained.
- Should not be used in treatment of subarachnoid hemorrhage due to increased risk of cerebral edema and infarction.
- Hematuria from the upper urinary tract poses a risk of intrarenal obstruction due to clot. Intravascular precipitation of fibrin may also occur associated with renal parenchymal disease, which may exacerbate existing disease.

Dosages/Preparations

- Standard parenteral formulation is 100 mg/ml, most commonly supplied in 10 ml ampules.
- For hemophilia patients undergoing tooth extraction, administer 10 ml/kg IV with replacement therapy. Redose 10 mg/kg 3–4 times per day for 2–8 days. Limited data suggests 10 mg/kg is appropriate for pediatric patients.
- Maximum effective regimen for cardiac surgery reported in BART trial: 30 mg/kg loading dose followed by 16 mg/kg/hr infusion with additional 2 mg/kg added to CPB prime.

- For orthopedic surgery, typical dosing regimens reported in the literature range from 10–20 mg/kg loading dose followed by 1–10 mg/kg/hr infusion.
- For liver transplantation, the most common regimen is a 10 mg/kg/hr infusion, but reported doses range from 2 to 40 mg/kg/hr.
- Improved mortality in trauma patients reported after 1 g infused over 10 minutes followed by 1g infused over 8 hours.
- Oral formulation available in 650 mg tablets and is used for treatment of heavy cyclical menstrual bleeding. Typical dose is 1300 mg three times per day for a maximum of 5 days during menstruation.
- Dosing should be reduced in renal failure.

Clinical Case Study

A 72-year-old man, 90 kg, with history of coronary artery disease, hypertension, hyperlipidemia, and type 2 diabetes presents for 3 vessel coronary artery bypass graft with cardiopulmonary bypass. After induction of anesthesia and placement of a central line, a test dose of 5 mg/kg tranexamic acid is administered followed by slow administration of an additional 25 mg/kg. Once complete, a maintenance infusion of 16 g/hr is continued throughout the remainder of the case. An additional 2 mg/kg is added to the CPB prime.

Background: The patient is undergoing coronary artery bypass with cardiopulmonary bypass, which is associated with a significant risk for blood transfusion. Evidence supports the prophylactic use of an antifibrinolytic agent to reduce blood loss and transfusion requirements and is not associated with a significant increased risk for thromboembolic event.

Pathophysiology: Cardiopulmonary bypass (CPB) increases activation of fibrinolysis by increasing the concentration of tissue plasminogen activator without concomitant increases in its inhibitor plasminogen activator inhibitor 1. Thrombin production is also accelerated by CPB, leading to a consumptive coagulopathy where both thrombin and plasmin are produced in excess. Coagulopathy following separation for CPB is further worsened by platelet dysfunction, hypothermia, and residual heparin effect.

Alternative Treatments: Aminocaproic acid works by a similar mechanism to prevent fibrinolysis and is widely used in cardiovascular surgery. Aprotinin has been shown to have the greatest clinical effect in reducing blood loss and transfusion requirements, but was removed from the general US market in 2008 after evidence for increased mortality associated with its use emerged.

References

1. Henry DA, Carless PA, Moxey AJ, O'Connell D, Stokes BJ, Fergusson DA, Ker K. Anti-fibrinolytic use for minimising perioperative allogeneic blood transfusion. *Cochrane Database Syst Rev.* 2011;1: CD001886. Doi: 10.1002/14651858.CD001886.pub3.

2. Zuffery P, Merquiol F, Laporte S, Decousus H, Mismetti P, Auboyer C, Samama CM, Molliex S. Do antifibrinolytics reduce allogentic blood transfusions in orthopedic surgery? *Anesthesiology.* 2006;105:1034–1046.

3. Brown J, Birkmeyer N, O'Connor G. Meta-analysis comparing the effectiveness and adverse outcomes of antifibrinolytic agents in cardiac surgery. *Circulation.* 2007;115:2801–2813.

4. Xia VW, Steadman RH. Antifibrinolytics in orthotopic liver transplantation: current status and controversies. *Liver Transpl.* 2005;11(1):10–18.

5. The CRASH-2 trial collaborators. Effects of tranexamic acid on death, vascular occlusive events, and blood transfusion in trauma patients with significant hemorrhage (CRASH-2): a randomized, placebo-controlled trial. *Lancet.* 2010;376:23–32.

6. Cyklokapron Package insert.

7. Lysteda package insert.

8. Marder VJ. Comparison of thrombolytic agents: selected hematologic, vascular, and clinical events. *Am J Cardiol.* 1989;64:2A-7A.

9. Wells P. Safety and efficacy of methods for reducing perioperative allogentic transfusion: a critical review of the literature. *Am J Ther.* 2002;9:377–388.

10. Martin K, Wiesner G, Breuer T, Lange R, Tassani P. The risks of aprotinin and transexamic acid in cardiac surgery: A one-year follow-up of 1188 consecutive patients. *Anesth Analg.* 2008;107(6):1783–1790.

11. Furgusson D, Hebert P, Mazer C, Fremes S, MacAdams C, Murkin J, Teoh K, Duke P, Arellano R, Blajchman M, Bussieres J, Cote D, Karski J, Martineau R, Robblee J, Rodger M, Wells G, Clinch J, Pretorius R, for the BART investigators. A comparison of aprotinin and lysine analogues in high-risk cardiac surgery. *N Engl J Med.* 2010;358(22):2319–2331.

12. Molenaar I, Warnaar N, Groen H, TenVergert E, Slooff M, Porte R. Efficacy and safety of antifibrinolytic drugs in liver transplantation: a systematic review and meta-analysis. *Am J Transplant.* 2007;7:185–194.

13. Edmunds L. Managing fibrinolysis without aprotinin. *Ann Thorac Surg.* 2010:324–331.

Chapter 14

Obstetrics

Chapter 14.1

Prostaglandins (Carboprost, Misoprostol, Alprostadil)

Cristianna Vallera, MD

Clinical Uses/Relevance to Anesthesiology

- Endogenous concentration of prostaglandins increases during labor, peaking at placental separation (Stage 3); uterine atony may be secondary to failure of increased prostaglandin concentration
- Refractory uterine atony not responsive to oxytocin infusion
- Specific agents have alternate uses for obstetrics, urology, pediatrics, and gastroenterology
- Carboprost is contraindicated in reactive airway disease, pulmonary hypertension, or hypoxemia. Misoprostol is a safe alternative in this setting.

Cautions/Adverse Reactions

- Common side effects include chills, fever, malaise, nausea, vomiting, and explosive diarrhea
- Patients with chorioamniomitis may have decreased response to prostaglandin therapy

Carboprost (15-methyl prostaglandin F2alpha, Hemabate)

Clinical Uses/Relevance to Anesthesiology

- Refractory uterine atony

Pharmacodynamics

- Increases myometrial free Ca^{++} concentration; results in increased myosin light-chain kinase activity and smooth muscle contraction (uterus, bronchioles)

Pharmacokinetics

- Onset within minutes
- Metabolized in the liver and lung; excreted in the urine; half-life unknown

Adult Dosing

- 250 micrograms IM or IU; may repeat q15 mins (not to exceed a total dose of 2 mg)

Cautions/Adverse Reactions

- Bronchospasm increases intrapulmonary shunting and hypoxemia via V/Q mismatching

Misoprostol (Cytotec)

Clinical Uses/Relevance to Anesthesiology

- Refractory uterine atony via rectal administration; off-label use for patients with contraindications to carboprost or methylergonovine
- Cervical priming and induction of labor for term pregnancy

Pharmacodynamics

- Increases myometrial free Ca^{++} concentration, leading to increased myosin light-chain kinase activity, and smooth muscle contraction

Pharmacokinetics

- Onset within minutes
- Metabolized partially by gut parietal cells; 80% excreted in the urine; half-life 20–40 mins

Adult Dosing

- Uterine atony: 800–1000 micrograms per rectum

Cautions/Adverse Reactions

- May be safely used in place of carboprost or methylergonovine in pts with pulmonary HTN or reactive airway disease

Alprostadil (Prostaglandin E1, Prostin)

Clinical Uses/Relevance to Anesthesiology

- Patent ductus arteriosis in neonates prior to surgical repair

Pharmacodynamics

- Relaxes arterial smooth muscle and inhibits platelet aggregation

Pharmacokinetics

- Metabolized in the lung, primarily excreted in the urine. Half-life of 5–10 minutes

Cautions/Adverse Reactions

- Approximately 10% of neonates with congenital heart disease experience apnea with alprostadil administration

Clinical Case Scenario

Background: A 39-year-old G1P0 woman at 41 weeks gestational age has had labor induced with oxytocin. The pregnancy was uneventful, and her past medical history is notable only for essential hypertension, which has been well controlled with Labetolol throughout this pregnancy. Five hours into the induction, a lumbar epidural was placed for pain control, with good effect. After 18 hours, a c-section is called for failure to progress. The epidural is used for operative anesthesia with good results. Following uneventful delivery of the neonate, an oxytocin infusion is started, but the uterus remains atonic, even after increasing the concentration of the oxytocin infusion.

Pathophysiology: The use of oxytocin for induction of labor has led to tachyphylaxis to further doses. Methergine is contraindicated by the patient's essential hypertension.

Treatment: Hemabate 250 micrograms IM is given. Five minutes later the obstetrician notes that the uterus has begun to develop acceptable tone. The surgery is completed, estimated blood loss is 1000 ml, and the patient is taken to the PACU is stable condition. One hour later an emergency page calls you to the PACU, where the patient has lost approximately 500 ml of blood and the uterus is again noted to be atonic. Cytotec 1000 micrograms rectally is given, with restoration of uterine tone. The remainder of the patient's clinical course is uneventful, although she does complain of nausea and has diarrhea on postoperative day one.

Alternatives: Hemabate could be given repeatedly every 15 minutes up to a total dose of 2 mg.

References

1. Fuchs AR, Husslein P, Sumulong L, Fuchs F. The origins of circulating 13,14-dihydro-15-keto-prostaglandin F2 alpha during delivery. *Prostaglandins*. 1982;24:715–722.

2. Noort WA, van Bulck B, Vereecken A, et al. Changes in plasma levels of PGF2 alpha and PGI2 metabolites at and after delivery at term. *Prostaglandins*. 1989;37:3–12.

3. Mayer DC, Smith KA. Antepartum and postpartum hemorrhage. In: Chestnut DH, Polley LS, Tsen LC, Wong CA, eds. *Chestnut's Obstetric Anesthesia Principles and Practice*. 4th ed. Philadelphia: Mosby Elsevier; 2009: 820–821.

4. Hayashi RH, Castillo MS, Noah ML. Management of severe postpartum hemorrhage with a prostaglandin F2 alpha analogue. *Obstet Gynecol*. 1984;63:806–808.

5. Izumi H, Garfield RE, Morshita F, Shirakawa K. Some mechanical properties of skinned fibres of pregnant human myometrium. *Eur J Obstet Gynecol Reprod Biol*. 1994;56:55–62.

6. Blum J, Alfirevic Z, Walraven G, et al. Treatment of postpartum hemorrhage with misoprostol. *Int J Gynaecol Obstet*. 2007;99:S202-S205.

Chapter 14.2

Ergots (Methylergonovine Maleate)

Emily Baird, MD

Role in the Practice of Anesthesiology/Relevance to Anesthesiology

- Uterotonic agent for postpartum hemorrhage or subinvolution of the uterus. The uterine stimulant properties of ergots have been described as early as the 1500s. Methylergonovine maleate (Methergine) is the only ergot preparation currently used as a stimulant for uterine contractions. It is considered a second-line therapy when oxytocin fails to produce adequate uterine activity. Unlike oxytocin, prophylactic administration of methylergonovine does not decrease the risk of postpartum hemorrhage. Administration prior to delivery of the placenta may cause captivation of the placenta.
- Historic use in induction of labor. The use of ergots for induction and augmentation of labor ended in the early 1800s. The tetanic contractions produced by ergots often resulted in significant decreases in uterine blood flow and fetal distress.

Pharmacodynamics

- Ergots interact with adrenergic, dopaminergic, and tryptaminergic receptors. Stimulation of α-adrenergic and serotonin receptors leads to vasoconstriction. Central nervous system (CNS) effects are mediated by interaction with serotonin and dopamine receptors. The effect of ergot administration depends on the dosage, tissue interaction, and physiologic condition of the patient.
- Methylergonovine directly stimulates uterine smooth muscle producing an increase in amplitude and frequency of contractions. The increase in uterine tone compresses myometrial blood vessels and reduces maternal hemorrhage.

Pharmacokinetics

- Onset of action: po ~ 5 to 10 min; IM ~ 2 to 5 min; IV ~ 30 sec.
- Duration of action: po ~ 3 h; IM ~ 3 h; IV ~ 45 min (although rhythmic contractions may persist for up to 3 h).
- Primarily hepatic biotransformation and renal excretion.
- Methylergonovine does not appear to accumulate after multiple doses.

Adult Dosing

- Oral dosage (Methylergonovine Maleate Tablets): 0.2 mg every 6 to 12 h until uterine tone is sufficient. Recommended for short-term use only, usually no more than 2 to 3 days, with a maximum of 1 week.
- IM dosage (Methylergonovine Maleate Injection): 0.2 mg repeated in 2 to 4 h if necessary, up to 5 doses.
- IV administration used only in cases of life-threatening hemorrhage. Methylergonovine Maleate Injection: 0.2 mg diluted in 250 mL of normal saline and infused with close attention paid to blood pressure.

Preparation

- Rapidly deteriorates with exposure to light, heat, and humidity.
- Tablets: Store in tight, light-resistant container at below 25°C.
- Ampules: Refrigerate in light-resistant container at 2°C-8°C. Administer only if solution is clear and colorless.

Adverse Reactions

- Ergot administration may be associated with minor CNS side effects including nausea, vomiting, tinnitus, and headache.
- Methylergonovine may cause intense vasoconstriction leading to severe hypertension, myocardial ischemia, and/or cerebral vascular accident. Coadministration of sympathomimetic agents, including ephedrine and phenylephrine, can accentuate the hemodynamic effect of ergots. Ergot-induced vasoconstriction may require administration of a potent vasodilator, such as nitroglycerine or sodium nitroprusside.
- Relative maternal contraindications include preeclampsia or eclampsia, history of cerebral or coronary vascular disease, and peripheral vascular disease or Raynaud's phenomenon.
- Rare reports of vasospasm leading to cerebral ischemia and ischemia of the extremities with the coadministration of certain ergots and potent CYP 3A4 inhibitors, including macrolide antibiotics, HIV protease or reverse transcriptase inhibitors, and azole antifungals.

Clinical Case Scenario

A 34-year old gravida 6, para 5 parturient at 38 weeks gestation presents for cesarean deliver. The obstetrician is concerned about chorioamnionitis after 16 h of oxytocin-augmented labor. Following an uneventful delivery of the infant and placenta, the obstetrician notes uterine atony. The anesthesiologist rapidly infuses 40 U of oxytocin diluted in 1000 mL of normal saline. A few minutes later, the obstetrician reports no improvement in uterine tone. The maternal heart rate has increased from 88 bpm to 112 bpm and the blood pressure has decreased from 112/68 to 92/54. Methylergonovine (0.2 mg) is given into the patient's deltoid muscle. Two minutes later, palpation of the uterus confirms appropriate uterine tone. The maternal heart rate and blood pressure normalize following further infusion of intravascular fluid.

The most common cause of postpartum hemorrhage is uterine atony. Predisposing factors include prolonged oxytocin infusion, protracted delivery, tocolysis, overdistention of the uterus, high parity, chorioamnionitis, and retained placenta. Atony is initially treated with uterine massage and infusion of oxytocin. If initial efforts are unsuccessful, second-line defenses include methylergonovine, 15-methyl prostaglandin F2α, and/or misoprostol. The appropriate combination of uterotonic agents depends on the patient's comorbidities. Methylergonovine can cause severe hypertension and should be avoided in patients with a history of preeclampsia/eclampsia, cerebral or coronary vascular disease, and Raynaud's phenomenon.

References

1. de Groot A, van Dongen P, Vree TB et al. Ergot alkaloids: current status and review of clinical pharmacology and therapeutic use compared with other oxytocics in obstetrics and gynaecology. *Drugs.* 1998;56:523–535.

2. Payton RG, Brucker MC. Drugs and uterine motility. *JOGNN.* 1999;28:628–638.

3. Rajan PV, Wing DA. Postpartum hemorrhage: evidence-based medical interventions from prevention and treatment. *Clin Obstet and Gynecol.* 2010; 53: 165–181.

Chapter 14.3

Oxytocin (Pitocin)

Emily Baird, MD

Role in the Practice of Anesthesiology/Relevance to Anesthesiology

- Induction or augmentation of labor.
- Uterotonic agent for postpartum hemorrhage. Most effective agent in stimulating uterine contractions. The risk of postpartum hemorrhage is decreased by > 60% with prophylactic use of oxytocin.
- Adjunctive therapy in the management of incomplete or inevitable abortion in the late 2nd or 3rd trimester. Ineffective in evacuating the uterus in the 1st or early 2nd trimester because of relative myometrial unresponsiveness.

Pharmacodynamics

- Endogenous oxytocin is released from the posterior hypothalamus in response to nipple stimulation, cervical stretch, or manipulation of the lower genital tract.
- Uterine responsiveness depends on the concentration of specific oxytocin receptors within the myometrium. The number of uterine oxytocin receptors increases dramatically during pregnancy, with the greatest increase occurring during the 3rd trimester.
- Interaction of oxytocin with its receptor promotes uterine contractions by increasing the concentration of free calcium within myometrial cells. The influx of calcium facilitates formation of the contractile protein actomyosin.

Pharmacokinetics

- Onset of action: IM ~ 3 to 5 min; IV ~ 30 sec.
- Duration of action: IM ~ 2 to 3 h; IV ~ 1 h.
- Metabolized by oxytocinase enzyme and rapid renal and hepatic removal from plasma.

Adult Dosing

- Wide variability in dosing requirements given the dependence of uterine responsiveness on oxytocin receptor concentration.

- Augmentation of labor: Initial dose 1 to 4 mU/min. Dose increased in incre-ments of 1 to 4 mU/min at 30 to 60 min intervals until establishment of the desired contraction pattern. Maximum dose of 40 mU/min.
- Control of postpartum bleeding: Oxytocin infusion begun immediately after umbilical cord clamping at cesarean delivery and placental delivery at vaginal delivery. Infusion prepared with 10 to 40 U of oxytocin diluted in 1000 mL of normal saline or lactated ringers. Infused at a rate of 200 mU/min until the uterus remains firmly contracted. After bleeding is controlled, infusion rate reduced to 10 to 20 mU/min and continued until transfer to the postpartum unit.
- Treatment of incomplete or inevitable abortion: Dilute 10 U of oxytocin into 500 mL of normal saline. Infuse at a rate of 200 mU/min following suction or sharp curettage until achievement of adequate uterine contraction.

Preparation

- Store at 15°–25°C.
- Oxytocin strength expressed in US Pharmacopoeia (USP) units. Each unit is equivalent to ~ 2 µg of pure hormone.
- Oxytocin should not be administered in a hypotonic solution. Cross-reactivity with renal antidiuretic hormone (ADH) receptors may lead to dilutional hyponatremia.

Adverse Reactions

- Hypotension. When given as a rapid IV bolus, oxytocin exhibits a direct relax-ing effect on the vascular smooth muscle.
- Water intoxication or hyponatremia. Oxytocin is chemically similar to ADH and can promote fluid retention when used in large doses. Oxytocin may lead to reduced urine production at doses >20 mU/min.
- Fetal distress secondary to uterine hyperstimulation and decreased fetal oxygenation.
- Uterine atony with protracted use of oxytocin for labor augmentation.
- Uterine rupture. 20% of cases of uterine rupture are attributed to inappro-priate administration of oxytocin.

Clinical Case Scenario

A 32-year old parturient at 39 weeks gestation with breech presentation pres-ents for an elective cesarean delivery. The delivery is performed under spinal anesthesia using 12.5 mg bupivicaine with 100 µg morphine. Following um-bilical cord clamping, the anesthesiologist rapidly infuses 10 U of oxytocin in 500 mL of normal saline. Although adequate uterine tone is achieved after delivery of the placenta, the patient's blood pressure drops from 106/74 to 85/48. The oxytocin infusion is decreased to 20 U/min and 100 µg of phenyl-ephrine is given. The patient's blood pressure remains stable at 100s/70s for the remainder of the procedure.

Oxytocin is the most commonly administered uterotonic agent. It has been shown to prevent postpartum hemorrhage in >60% of cases when given prophylactically. Given its structural similarity to antidiuretic hormone, it is essential to administer oxytocin in an isotonic solution. Failure to do so may result in water intoxication or hyponatremia. A rapid intravascular bolus of oxytocin causes direct relaxation of the vascular smooth muscle leading to a decreased systemic vascular resistance, hypotension, and tachycardia.

References

1. Payton RG, Brucker MC. Drugs and uterine motility. *JOGNN.* 1999;28:628–638.

2. Rajan PV, Wing DA. Postpartum hemorrhage: evidence-based medical interventions from prevention and treatment. *Clin Obstet Gynecol.* 2010;53:165–181.

3. Wei SQ, Luo ZC, Qi HP, et al. High-dose vs low-dose oxytocin for labor augmentation: a systematic review. *Am J Obstet Gynecol.* 2010;203:296–304.

Chapter 14.4

Magnesium

Robert Gaiser, MD

Role in the Practice of Anesthesiology/Relevance to Anesthesiology

- Seizure prophylaxis in parturients with preeclampsia
- Cerebral palsy prophylaxis for neonates in parturients with preterm labor
- Previously used in the treatment of preterm labor, however randomized clinical outcome trials did not support this use.
- Torsades de Pointes
- Hypomagnesemia
- Asthma, severe exacerbations (not routine for acute attack but effective for patients who fail first-line initial therapy)

Pharmacodynamics

- Mg is ubiquitous and involved in various biochemical processes with over 300 enzyme systems being involved (functions as a cofactor as well as a role in neurochemical transmission and muscular excitability)
- It is the 4th most prevalent mineral in the body; 50% found in bone, 50% intracellularly (<1% found in the plasma and RBCs). Normal serum Mg concentration is 1.5–2 mEq/L. In the body, Mg exists as a cation, or bound to albumin. It is physiologically active in its ionized form and able to pass rapidly through cell membranes (therefore, extracellular levels reflect intracellular levels).
- Magnesium sulfate ($MgSO_4$) is a chemical compound that contains sulfur, oxygen, and magnesium. Administration of exogenous Mg is done to maintain adequate levels and normal physiologic function; additionally, it functions as a Ca^{++} antagonist and blunts the release of catecholamines.
- Preeclampsia. Preeclamptic seizures are believed to be due to the excessive release of the excitatory neurotransmitter glutamate, which activates the NMDA receptor and leads to massive neural activity. Mg competitively antagonizes glutamate at the NMDA receptor in the CNS.
- Cerebral palsy. Administration of Mg to women at risk for preterm delivery may reduce the incidence of cerebral palsy in infants that survive. The neuroprotective effect of Mg is believed to be from its ability to oppose

the movement of solutes, in particular Ca^{++}, through the tight junctions of endothelial cells.

- Tocolysis. Although Mg blocks Ca^{++} entry into smooth muscle and inhibits contraction, it is not utilized as a tocolytic. A Cochrane Review concluded that it did not differ from placebo in regard to preventing preterm birth.

Pharmacokinetics

- Lab values are a measure of serum ionized Mg, which can be used to estimate intracellular levels.
- Renal system regulation. Increased Mg levels result in receptor activation and diuresis along with ion elimination. Parturients with renal disease or renal insufficiency from preeclampsia are at ↑ risk for the development of Mg toxicity

Side Effects/Adverse Reaction

- Flushing, sweating, nausea, vomiting, pain at site of infusion are the most common adverse effects. Vasodilation produces flushing (direct action on arterial blood vessels; ↓ SVR).
- Respiratory weakness is the major risk of Mg overdosage. ↓ muscle strength results in a ↓ in respiratory volumes (↓ in FEV_1 and FVC).
- At high levels, cardiac arrest is possible (note: does not affect myocardial contractility)
- ↑ sensitivity to both nondepolarizing (clinically significant) and depolarizing (not clinically significant) muscle relaxants in parturients. Mg inhibits the presynaptic release of acetylcholine at the motor end plate, thus ↑ increasing the sensitivity of the motor end plate to NDNMB.
- May be contraindicated in pts with neuromuscular disorders such as myasthenia gravis or Eaton-Lambert syndrome; risk of paralysis.
- The antidote to Mg toxicity is calcium. Calcium gluconate should be readily available to treat cases of Mg toxicity whenever IV Mg is being administered

Dosage

- $MgSO_4$ 1 gram = 4 mmol, 8 mEq, or 98 mg of elemental magnesium.
- Preeclampsia. IV bolus loading dose: 4–6 g over 15–20 mins, followed by maintenance: 1–4 g/hr. Therapeutic range is a serum level of 4–7 mEq/L. Mg levels are followed via physical examination (monitoring of deep tendon reflexes) and laboratory testing. Deep tendon reflexes ↓ well before respiratory depression and cardiac arrest; they provide immediate information, are easy to perform, and are noninvasive.
- IM administration is possible, but results in significant pain at the injection site.

Clinical Case Scenario

A 17-year-old primigravid parturient presents with elevated blood pressure (BP 160/110 mmHg) and proteinuria at 34 weeks gestation. She is diagnosed with severe preeclampsia and is scheduled for induction of labor. She receives a magnesium load of 4 gm intravenously and then a maintenance of 1 gm/hr. Following the bolus, she feels flushed and weak. Due to profound fetal bradycardia, she requires urgent cesarean delivery during general anesthesia. She receives rapid sequence induction with propofol 200 mg and succinyl choline 100 mg. Five minutes following the succinylcholine, the provider gives the patient 4 mg vecuronium to maintain muscle relaxation. At the end of the 45-minute procedure, the patient was unable to be extubated as she had no evident twitches on the train-of-four monitor.

Magnesium increases the sensitivity of the postjunctional motor end plate while decreasing the presynaptic release of acetylcholine. As such, magnesium significantly potentiates muscle relaxants, requiring careful monitoring of neuromuscular function with a nerve stimulator in any parturient who is receiving magnesium. The administration of muscle relaxants must be carefully titrated for the desired effect.

References

1. Euser AG, Cipolla MJ. Magnesium sulfate for the treatment of eclampsia: A brief review. *Stroke.* 2009;40:1169–1175.

2. Cahill AG, Stout MJ, Caughey AB. Intrapartum magnesium for prevention of cerebral palsy: continuing controversy? *Curr Opin Obstet Gynecol.* 2010;22:122–127.

3. Han S, Crowther CA, Moore V. Magnesium maintenance therapy for preventing preterm birth after threatened preterm labour. *Cochrane Database Syst Rev.* 2010;7: CD000940.

4. James MFM. Magnesium in obstetrics. *Best Pract Res Clin Obstet Gynaecol.* 2010;24:327–337.

5. Yoshida M, Matsuda Y, Akizawa Y, Ono E, Ohta H. Serum ionized magnesium during magnesium sulfate administration for preterm labor and preeclampsia. *Eur J Obstet Gynecol.* 2006;128:125–8.

Chapter 14.5

Beta-2 Adrenergic Agonists (Terbutaline)

Robert Gaiser, MD

Role in the Practice of Anesthesiology/Relevance to Anesthesiology

- Tocolysis for preterm labor. Ritodrine was the only medication approved by the FDA for this use; however terbutaline became widely used due to its lower cost. In 1988, the manufacturer of ritodrine withdrew it from the American market, leaving terbutaline as the only β-adrenergic agonist for tocolysis. Effective for short-term tocolysis (no benefit beyond 48 hours); chronic administration is extremely rare.
- Uterine tetany (sustained uterine contraction).
- Asthma

Pharmacodynamics

- Specific agonist to B-2 receptors, located on smooth muscles (uterine, vascular, bronchial, sphincters). Terbutaline B-2 receptor agonism ↑ intracellular production of cAMP resulting in ↓ intracellular calcium and myometrial relaxation. Actin and myosin are contractile proteins that are inhibited by ↓ calcium levels.
- Capable of up to 48 h of prolonged labor. Prolonged or continuous exposure to these medications results in desensitization/down-regulation of myometrial B-2 receptors. Therefore, cannot provide long-term tocolysis.
- Additionally, pharmacogenetics of the B-2 receptor may also explain the failure to prolong pregnancy beyond 48 hours. An arginine to glycine substitution in the receptor has been shown to improve receptor desensitization in response to exposure. Homozygosity for arginine improves pregnancy outcome after β-2 adrenergic agonist tocolysis.

Pharmacokinetics

- Mean peak plasma concentration time: SQ administration 30 mins. Peak plasma concentration following 0.25 mg SQ: 5.2 ng/mL.
- Elimination half-life: 2.9 h. Excreted unchanged in the urine

Side Effects/Adverse Reactions

- Relative maternal contraindications include advanced cervical dilation, maternal cardiac disease, hyperthyroidism, and uncontrolled DM. Fetal contraindications include placental abruption and preeclampsia.
- Maternal side effects from chronic administration include hyperglycemia (pancreas secretes glucagon, resulting in gluconeogenesis and glyconeolysis), hypokalemia (B-2 effects of H^+/K^+ ATPase shift K^+ intracellularly; does not change total body K^+), and ↑ risk of pulmonary edema (estimated incidence of 1:350–1:400 treated patients; ↑ risk with multiple gestations and maternal infection).
- Flushing, tachycardia, and palpitations. Cross-reactivity to B-1 receptors (seen even with a single dose) is responsible for ↑ HR and ↑ SV; vasodilation is the result of B-2 agonism (often undesirable).
- Fetal tachycardia; able to cross the placenta
- Neurotoxicity to the neonatal brain is seen in the animal model. Elicits alterations and structural damage in the immature brain during a critical time period.

Dose

- IV/SQ: 0.25 mg q 1–6 h. SQ administration is an advantage in pts lacking IV line.
- Pump delivery: basal IV rate with scheduled SQ boluses of 0.25 mg (max of 3–4 mg/day).

Clinical Case Scenario

A 26-year-old parturient at 38 weeks gestation presents in active labor at 6 cm cervical dilation. She rates her pain as a 10 on a scale From 1 to 10. She consents for regional analgesia and the anesthesiologist plans a combined spinal/epidural analgesic using 2.5 mg bupivacaine/25 μg fentanyl. Following the intrathecal injection, a prolonged fetal heart rate deceleration occurs to a rate of 80 bpm. The obstetrician palpates the abdomen and notes uterine tetany. The parturient is given 0.25 mg terbutaline intravenously to relax the uterus. Following the injection, the sustained contraction is interrupted and the fetal heart rate returns to normal. The maternal heart rate, which was previously 88 bpm, increased to 112 bpm, and the blood pressure increased from 113/76 mm Hg to 128/82 mm Hg.

Prolonged fetal decelerations frequently accompany the intrathecal administration of fentanyl or sufentanil. The deceleration is frequently due to uterine tetany. The etiology of the uterine tetany is unclear but appears to be related to the dose of the intrathecal opioid or to the stage of labor. Beta 2 adrenergic agonist medications are frequently administered to induce rapid uterine relaxation in cases of uterine tetany. They have also been used for the treatment of preterm labor with variable results. The major side effects are maternal with the drugs affecting the maternal cardiovascular system.

References

1. Lam F, Gill P. β-Agonist tocolytic therapy. *Obstet Gynecol Clin N Am*. 2005;32:457–484.

2. The Canadian Preterm Labor Investigators Group. Treatment of preterm labor with the beta-adrenergic agonist ritodrine. *N Eng J Med*. 1992;327:308–312.

3. Landau R, Morales MA, Antonarakis SE, Blouin JL, Smiley RM. Arg16 homozygosity of the β-2 adrenergic receptor improves the outcome after the β-2agonist tocolysis for preterm labor. *Clin Pharmacol Ther*. 2005;78:656–663.

4. Nanda K, Cook LA, Gallo MF, Grimes DA. Terbutaline pump maintenance therapy after threatened preterm labor for preventing preterm birth. *Cochrane Database Syst Rev*. 2002;4:CD003933.

Chapter 15

Antiepileptic Drugs

Emily E. Peoples, MD

Carbamazepine (Tegretol, Tegretol-XR [ER], Carbatrol [ER])

Clinical Uses/Relevance to Anesthesiology

- Epilepsy (partial, generalized, and mixed seizures)
- Neuropathic pain (trigeminal neuralgia, herpes zoster); provides analgesia
- ADHD, schizophrenia, phantom limb syndrome, PTSD; off-label use
- Induction of P450 may accelerate metabolism and excretion of some perioperative medications, making them subtherapeutic, resistant, or requiring higher dosages. Nondepolarizing neuromuscular blockers are relatively resistant; alfentanil
- Should be continued perioperatively as appropriate; long half-life allows a degree of leeway in the event of a missed dose
- Preoperative assessment of LFTs, Hg, and WBC should be considered

Pharmacodynamics

- Metabolite, carbamazepine-10,11-epoxide, stabilizes membrane voltage-gated Na^+ ion channels in their inactive state, preventing subsequent depolarization and action potential generation. Reduces polysynaptic input into neurons and blocks posttetanic potentiation.
- Also potentiates GABA receptors

Pharmacokinetics

- Absorption: 4.5–7.7 h depending on preparation
- Vd: large; protein binding ~76%
- Metabolism: hepatic cytochrome P450; elimination half-life: initially 26–65 h, then decreases to 12–17 h (due to enzyme autoinduction). Renally excreted

Preparations

- Available in oral chewable tablets (100 mg), suspension (100 mg/5 mL), ER tablets (100, 200, 400 mg)

Cautions/Adverse Reactions

- Neurologic: dizziness, sedation, impaired coordination; Psychiatric: increased risk of suicidal ideation or behavior, worsening of depression
- Cardiac: arrhythmias, AV block (including 2nd and 3rd degree), CHF, edema
- GI: nausea and vomiting
- Endocrine: exacerbation of preexisting hypothyroidism; SIADH (potentiates ADH release and excessive retention of free water and hyponatremia)
- Dermatologic: Stevens-Johnson and toxic epidermal necrolysis occur in 1–6/10 000 new users; higher in Asian ancestry (due to HLA-B* allelic variant)
- Hematologic: Blood dyscrasia (aplastic anemia, agranulocytosis, pancytopenia). Acute intermittent porphyria
- Autoinduction.   Increases cytochrome P450 metabolic effect and may reduce therapeutic levels of several drugs (eg, oral contraception).
- Acute toxicity result in respiratory depression, tachycardia, conduction disorders, coma; treat with forced emesis and diuresis, consider HD

Oxcarbazepine (Trileptal)

Clinical Uses/Relevance to Anesthesiology

- Epilepsy (partial seizures); monotherapy or adjunct
- Anxiety, bipolar disorder, benign motor tics;
- Induction of P450 may accelerate metabolism and excretion of some perioperative medications, making them subtherapeutic, resistant, or requiring higher dosages. Nondepolarizing neuromuscular blockers are relatively resistant
- Initiation preoperatively may reduce postoperative seizures; able to be titrated rapidly and does not require dose plasma concentration monitoring. Less adverse effects (hyponatremia) compared to other antiepileptics make this an attractive choice.

Pharmacodynamics

- Prodrug; eslicarbazepine metabolite stabilizes membrane voltage-gated Na^+ ion channels in their inactive state, preventing subsequent depolarization and action potential generation. Reduces polysynaptic input into neurons and blocks posttetanic potentiation
- May also affect membrane K^+ and Ca^{++} ion channels
- Derivative of carbamazepine with a ketone substitution on dibenzazepine ring

Pharmacokinetics

- Vd large; protein binding 40%
- Prodrug is hepatically metabolized to active metabolite; renally excreted. Elimination See Table 15.1life of the parent drug ~2 h and active metabolite ~9 h

Dosing

- Renal impairment (Cr clearance <30 mL/min) should have reduced dosing

Preparations

- Oral tablets (150, 300, 600 mg) or suspension (300 mg/5 mL); equivalent

Adverse Reactions

- Ketone substitution reduces adverse effects (eg, less blood dyscrasias, sedation, and cytochrome interactions)
- CNS: sedation, dizziness, psychomotor slowing; Psychiatric: suicidal ideation and behavior are increased.
- Dermatologic: Stevens-Johnson syndrome (30% of pts who have had reaction to carbamazepine will also experience)
- Endocrine: clinically significant hyponatremia; up to 2.5% of treated pts develop Na^+ <125 mEq/L (usually within first 3 months of therapy); lab monitoring should be considered when drug is initiated

Eslicarbazepine acetate (BIA 2–093)

- Produced by Sunovion (under the supervision of Bial) to be marketed under the trade name Stedesa in America

Clinical Uses/Relevance to Anesthesiology

- Epilepsy (partial seizures); FDA-approved in 2009 as adjunctive therapy
- Other forms of epilepsy as an adjunct or monotherapy, bipolar disorder, and trigeminal neuralgia are other potential clinical uses

Pharmacodynamics

- The active metabolite eslicarbazepine (also the active metabolite of the prodrug oxcarbazepine) stabilizes membrane voltage-gated Na^+ ion channels in their inactive state, preventing subsequent depolarization and action potential generation. Reduces polysynaptic input into neurons and blocks posttetanic potentiation.
- Prodrug, with eslicarbazepine being the active metabolite (same as the prodrug oxcarbazepine). However structural differences from oxcarbazepine produce differences in metabolism without the formation of toxic epoxide metabolites.

Pharmacokinetics

- Does not induce its own metabolism

Adult Dosing

- 800–1200 mg PO QD
- Dose reduction recommended for Cr clearance < 60 mL/min

Pediatric Dosing

- Under investigation

Preparations

- Oral

Adverse Reactions

- More favorable than carbamazepine and oxcarbazepine
- Dizziness, sedation, headache, nausea

Valproic Acid (Depakene, Stavzor)

Clinical Uses/Relevance to Anesthesiology

- Epilepsy (multiple seizure types, status epilepticus, and posttraumatic), bipolar disorder, major depression, migraine headache prophylaxis, schizophrenia, myoclonus
- Cancer and HIV potential treatment due to inhibition of histone deacetylase-1
- Neuropathic pain treatment, including herpes zoster
- May be coagulopathic
- Affects drug metabolism and clearance;

Pharmacodynamics

- Principal mechanism of action likely involves inhibition of GABA transamination
- May also block voltage-gated Na+ channels in a manner similar to other antiepileptics; may block T-type calcium channels

Pharmacokinetics

- Metabolized by hepatic mitochondrial -oxidation; elimination half-life 9–16 h
- Age effects. Infants up to 2 months have decreased elimination; children (3 mo-10 yrs) have 50% greater clearance expressed on weight basis compared to adults; elderly (>68 yrs) have reduced elimination

Dosing

- Epilepsy dosing: max dose 60 mg/kg/day.

Preparations

- Oral as capsules (250 mg), extended release capsules (125, 250, 500 mg) and syrup (250 mg/5 mL)

Adverse Reactions

- Constitutional: alopecia, acne, peripheral edema; Endocrine: weight gain, hyperammonemia; GI: hepatic failure (increased risk in children < 2 yrs), pancreatitis, dyspepsia; Hematologic: thrombocytopenia, prolonged coagulation times; Neurologic: dizziness, sedation, headache, tremors
- Drug interactions. Inhibits enzyme responsible for breakdown of active epoxide metabolite of carbamazepine, prolonging its effects. Decreases clearance of amitriptyline, nortriptyline, and lamotrigine. Reduces or inhibits metabolism of diazepam, ethosuximide, phenobarbital, phenytoin. Increases unbound fraction of warfarin.

Phenytoin/Fosphenytoin (Dilantin, Cerebyx)

Clinical Uses/Relevance to Anesthesiology

- Epilepsy; prevention and treatment of perioperative seizures related to neurosurgery
- Trigeminal neuralgia analgesia (phenytoin only)
- Herpes zoster
- Chronic use induces hepatic enzymes. By increasing the metabolism and elimination of some perioperative drugs, can be subtherapeutic. Nondepolarizing muscle relaxants (also has mild blocking action at the NMJ, which can lead to up-regulation of the AchR), benzodiazepines, warfarin.
- Reduces local anesthetic toxicity threshold; consider test-dosing with epinephrine to rule out intravascular injection, and reduce dosing.

Pharmacodynamics

- Modulates voltage-gated Na^+ and Ca^{++} channels to make neurons less excitable
- Fosphenytoin is a water-soluble prodrug hydrolyzed to phenytoin, phosphate, and formaldehyde

Pharmacokinetics

- Hepatic metabolism; elimination half-life 22 h

Dosing

- Fosphenytoin prescribing and dosing is expressed as phenytoin equivalents (PE); avoids the need for dose conversion from phenytoin
- Divided dosage: 100 mg PO/IV TID, titrate to clinical effect, up to 300 mg TID
- Once daily dosage: equivalent total daily divided dose taken as single dose in extended-release capsule

- Loading dose (rapid levels): 15–20 mg/kg IV bolus followed by maintenance dosing 12 h later
- Pediatric dosing: 5 mg/kg/day divided to BID or TID, titrate to clinical effect, up to max 300 mg daily

Preparations

- Oral (100 mg capsule and 125 mg/5 mL suspension); IM/IV
- Fosphenytoin is available in IV form only

Side Effects/Adverse Reactions

- Neurologic: nystagmus, peripheral neuropathy, paresthesias (greater with fosphenytoin), sedation. TCAs can precipitate seizures in susceptible patients.
- Cardiac: hypotension with IV loading dose (less with fosphenytoin
- GI: nausea, vomiting, gingival hyperplasia
- Renal: hyperphosphaemia in ESRD receiving phosphenytoin
- Musculoskeletal: osteomalacia (interferes with Vitamin D metabolism)
- Drug-induced lupus, megaloblastic anemia, thrombocytopenia; toxic epidermal necrolysis and Stevens-Johnson syndrome

Ethosuximide (Zarontin)

Clinical Uses/Relevance to Anesthesiology

- Epilepsy (mainly absence seizures)

Pharmacodynamics

- Blocks T-type Ca^{++} channels and enhances GABA-mediated inhibition

Pharmacokinetics

- Hepatic metabolism by CYP3A4; elimination half-life 53 h

Dosing

- 3–6 yrs: 250 mg PO QD, and increased 250 mg weekly until clinical response achieved; optimal dose 20 mg/kg/day
- >6 yrs: 500 mg PO QD initially, and increased 250 mg weekly until clinical response achieved

Preparations

- Oral as 250 mg capsule or 250 mg/5 mL syrup

Side Effects/Adverse Reactions

- Neurologic: headache, sedation
- GI: anorexia, nausea, gingival hyperplasia

- Hematologic: pancytopenia, agranulocytosis
- Drug-induced lupus, Stevens-Johnson syndrome

Lamotrigine (Lamictal)

Clinical Uses/Relevance to Anesthesiology

- Epilepsy
- Bipolar disorder
- Peripheral neuropathy, trigeminal neuralgia, cluster headaches, migraines, neuropathic pain; off-label uses
- Induction of P450 may accelerate metabolism and excretion of some perioperative medications, making them subtherapeutic, resistant, or requiring higher dosages. Nondepolarizing neuromuscular blockers are relatively resistant

Pharmacodynamics

- Exact mechanism unknown; believed to act as Na+ channel blocker

Pharmacokinetics

- Hepatically metabolized; elimination half-life 13 h

Preparations:

- Oral as tablets (25, 100, 150, 200 mg), chewable tablets (2, 5, 25 mg) and orally disintegrating tablets (25, 50, 100, 200 mg)

Side Effects/Adverse Reactions

- Dry mouth, night sweats, nausea
- Anticonvulsant hypersensitivity syndrome. Triad of fever, skin rash, and internal organ involvement; start 2–8 weeks after initiation. Skin rash can progress to Stevens-Johnson syndrome.

Topiramate (Topamax)

Clinical Uses/Relevance to Anesthesiology

- Epilepsy
- Migraine prevention
- Bipolar disorder, infantile spasms, PTSD, essential tremor, OCD, neuropathic pain, cluster headache, obesity, smoking cessation, alcoholism; off-label uses
- Induction of P450 may accelerate metabolism and excretion of some perioperative medications, making them subtherapeutic, resistant, or requiring higher dosages. Nondepolarizing neuromuscular blockers are relatively resistant

Pharmacodynamics

- Exact mechanism unknown; believed to block voltage-gated Na+ channels and glutamate receptors; enhance GABA neurotransmitter activity at GABA receptors; and inhibit carbonic anhydrase

Pharmacokinetics

- Hepatic metabolism via hydroxylation, hydrolysis, and glucuronidation

Dosing

- Epilepsy monotherapy. 10 yrs to adult: 25–200 mg PO BID
- Epilepsy adjunct therapy: 2–16 yrs 5–19 mg/kg/day PO; adult 100–200 mg PO BID
- Migraine Prophylaxis: 25–200 mg PO QD

Preparations

- Oral as tablets (25, 50, 100, 200 mg) and sprinkle capsules (15, 25 mg)

Side Effects/Adverse Reactions

- Memory problems, sedation, neurocognitive dysfunction (greatest among the newer anticonvulsants); nausea, diarrhea; URI;
- Central neurogenic hyperventilation can result from the hyperchloremic non-gap metabolic acidosis (due to carbonic anhydrase-inhibiting diuretic effect). Can result in CSF acidosis; treatment includes discontinuation of topiramate.

Gabapentin (Neurontin)

Clinical Uses/Relevance to Anesthesiology

- Epilepsy (partial seizures)
- Post-herpetic neuralgia
- Neuropathic pain, migraine prevention, postoperative chronic pain, CRPS, fibromyalgia; off-label use
- Continue perioperatively to avoid withdrawal syndrome
- Compounds morphine analgesic effects

Pharmacodynamics

- GABA analogue; increases synaptic release of GABA and glutamate decarboxylase function (converts glutamate to GABA). However, does not appear to act at GABA receptors.
- Exact mechanism unknown; therapeutic action for neuropathic pain thought to involve voltage-gated N-type Ca^{++} channels and NMDA receptor.

Pharmacokinetics

- Excreted 100% unchanged in urine; elimination half-life 5–7 h; consider dosage adjustment in pts with impaired renal function (CrCl <60 mL/min)

Dosing

- Post-herpatic neuralgia: up to 600 mg PO TID
- Neuropathic pain: up to 1200 mg PO TID
- Epilepsy. Adults: up to 600 mg PO TID; Pediatric: 35–40 mg/kg/day PO divided TID

Preparations

- oral as capsules (100, 300, 400 mg), tablets (600, 800 mg) and syrup (250 mg/5 mL)

Side Effects/Adverse Reactions

- Peripheral edema, hepatotoxicity, dizziness, sedation

Clinical Case Scenario #1

A 71-year-old man presented to preoperative surgery clinic prior to a microscopic lumbar discectomy due to low back pain associated with a vertebral disc protrusion. His history also included hypertension, and diabetes mellitus type 2 complicated by peripheral neuropathy and hypothyroidism. His medications included lisinopril, metformin, carbamazepine, and levothyroxine. In his review of symptoms, the patient reported new onset of peripheral edema following the recent addition of carbamazepine for his peripheral neuropathy. The patient's wife reported that her husband also seemed to be confused. Preoperative labs revealed a sodium of 130 mmol/L. The patient followed up with his primary physician. His carbamazepine was discontinued with resolution of symptoms and normalization of serum sodium level.

Clinical Case Scenario #2

A 28-year-old man with a history of migraine headaches was being treated with gabapentin 800 mg TID for migraine prophylaxis. He experienced good results for 6 weeks. He abruptly stopped his gabapentin 2 days prior to a planned inguinal hernia repair. He presented on the day of surgery with irritability, diaphoresis, and a headache. Physical exam, vital signs, and laboratory values were all within normal limits. The man's symptoms resolved within hours following reinitiation of gabapentin. A diagnosis of gabapentin withdrawal was made and the patient was counseled to taper his gabapentin over at least a week before discontinuing in the future.

Clinical Case Scenario #3

A 4-year-old Chinese girl was started on oxcarbazepine for partial seizures. Three weeks after initiation of therapy, the child complained of fever, sore throat, and fatigue. This was followed by ulcerations of her mucous membranes, conjunctivitis, and a diffuse rash. A diagnosis of Stevens-Johnson syndrome was made in the emergency department. Her oxcarbazepine was stopped immediately and she was admitted for supportive care of her condition.

Chapter 16

Bronchodilators

Anita Gupta, DO, PharmD and Amna Mehdi, BS

Clinical Uses/Indications

- Inhaled Beta-2 agonist drugs are the most effective bronchodilators available for clinical use in symptomatic antiasthma therapy and obstructive lung disease.
- Inhaled, short-acting, selective beta-2 adrenergic agonists are the mainstay of acute asthma therapy, while inhaled, long-acting, selective beta-2 adrenergic agonists (in combination with inhaled glucocorticoids) play a role in long-term control of moderate to severe asthma.
- Albuterol, levalbuterol, and pirbuterol are bronchodilators that relax smooth muscle. Short-acting beta-2 agonists are therapy of choice for relief of acute symptoms and prevention of exercise-induced bronchoconstriction.
- Salmeterol and formoterol are bronchodilators that have a duration of at least 12 hours after a single dose. Long-acting beta-2 agonists are not used as monotherapy for long-term control of asthma and are to be used in combination with inhaled glucocorticoids to control and prevent moderate to severe persistent asthma.

Pharmacodynamics

- Beta adrenoceptors have been classified into B_1, B_2, and B_3 subgroups, with B_2-receptors being widely distributed in the respiratory tract, particularly in airway smooth muscle.
- Intracellular signaling following B_2-receptor activation by agonist is largely affected through a trimeric Gs protein coupled to adenylate cyclase-cAMP-PKA pathway, resulting in bronchial smooth muscle relaxation through phosphorylation of muscle regulatory proteins and lowering of cellular Ca^{2+} concentrations.
- The mechanism by which cAMP induces airway smooth muscle cell relaxation is by catalyzing the activation of protein kinase A, which in turn phosphorylates key regulatory proteins involved in the control of muscle tone. cAMP also results in inhibition of calcium ion release from intracellular stores, reduction

of membrane Ca^{2+} entry, and sequestration of intracellular Ca^{2+} leading to relaxation of the airway smooth muscle.

- B_2 agonist induces acute inhibition of the PLC-IP_3 pathway and its mobilization of cellular Ca^{2+}
- Inhibition of myosin light chain kinase activation
- Activation of myosin light chain phosphatase
- Opening of a large conductance of Ca^{2+} -activated-K^+ channel (K_{ca}), which repolarizes the smooth muscle cell and may stimulate the sequestration of Ca^{2+} into intracellular stores. B_2 receptors may also couple to K_{ca} via G_s so that relaxation of airway smooth muscle may occur independently of an increase in cAMP.

Pharmacokinetics

- The molecular size and structure of a B_2-agonist determines the manner in which it interacts with the B_2-adrenoceptor in airway smooth muscle.
- β_2-Agonists have been characterized as those that directly activate the receptor (albuterol), those that are taken up into a membrane depot (formoterol), and those that interact with a receptor-specific auxiliary binding site (salmeterol). These differences in mechanism of action are reflected in the kinetics of airway smooth muscle relaxation and bronchodilation in patients with asthma.
- The albuterol molecule accesses the active site of the B_2-adrenoceptor directly from the extracellular compartment. There is therefore a rapid onset of airway tissue relaxation and of bronchodilation in patients. However, the drug rapidly reequilibrates, its residency time at the active site is limited, and the resulting duration of action short (4–6 h).
- Formoterol is moderately lipophilic in nature. It is taken up into the cell membrane in the form of a depot, from where it progressively leaches out to interact with the active site of the B_2-receptor. The size of the depot is determined by the concentration or dose of formoterol applied. In airway preparations, the onset of action of formoterol is somewhat delayed compared with albuterol, and the duration of relaxant activity, although longer, is concentration-dependent.
- The mechanism of action of salmeterol involves the interaction of the side chain with an auxiliary binding site (exosite), a domain of highly hydrophobic amino acids within the fourth domain of the B_2-adrenoceptor. When the side chain is in association with the exosite, the molecule is prevented from dissociating from the B_2-adrenoceptor. The onset of action of salmeterol on airway smooth muscle is therefore slower than that of other B_2-agonists, such as albuterol and formoterol.

Side Effects/Adverse Effects

- Beta agonists are associated with several side effects.
- Tremor is the most frequent acute side effect and is more noticeable with oral therapy than with inhaled agents. Muscle tremor is the direct effect on skeletal muscle B_2 receptors
- Tachycardia-increased heart rate and palpitations are dose dependent and are less common with the selective beta-2 agonists (such as albuterol) than with nonselective agents (such as metaproterenol).
- Metabolic disturbances, such as hyperglycemia and hypokalemia, which is a direct B_2 effect on skeletal muscle uptake of K^+.
- Hypoxemia-increased V/Q mismatch due to reversal of hypoxic pulmonary vasoconstriction.
- Stress-induced (takotsubo) cardiomyopathy has been associated with treatment of status asthmaticus in case reports.
- Use of a spacer or chamber device reduces these side effects by reducing oral deposition of medication, which contributes to side effects but not bronchodilation.

Preparation and Dose

- **Albuterol:** Short-acting, inhaled beta-2 agonists
  - ≥4 years old: MDI 90 mcg/puff : Adult and Pediatric dosage: 2 puffs every 4–6 h, PRN
  - ≥2 years old: Nebulizer solutions 0.021 percent (0.63 mg/3 mL), 0.042 percent (1.25 mg/3 mL), 0.083 percent (2.5 mg/3 mL), 0.5 percent (0.5 mg/20 mL): Adult dosage 2.5 mg every 4–6 h, PRN: Pediatric dosage 0.1–0.15 mg/kg every 4–6 h, PRN
- **Levalbuterol:** Short-acting, inhaled beta-2 agonists
  - ≥6 years old: 45 mcg/puff: Adult dosage 2 puffs every 4–6 h, PRN: Pediatric dosage 1–2 puffs every 4–6 h, PRN
  - ≥6 years old: Nebulizer solution 0.31, 0.63 or 1.25 mg/3 mL: Adult dosage 0.63 to 1.25 mg, 2 to 4 times daily, PRN: Pediatric dosage 0.31 mg, 2 to 4 times daily, PRN
- **Pirbuterol:** Short-acting, inhaled beta-2 agonists
  - ≥12 years old: Breath-actuated MDI: 200 mcg/puff: Adult dosage 2 puffs every 4–6 h, PRN: Pediatric dosage 2 puffs every 4–6 h, PRN
- **Salmeterol:** Long-acting, beta-2 agonists
  - >4 years old: DPI 50 mcg/inhalation: Adult and Pediatric dosage 1 inhalation every 12 h
- **Formoterol:** Long-acting, beta-2 agonists
  - ≥5 years old: DPI 12 mcg/inhalation: Adult and Pediatric dosage 1 inhalation every 12 h

References

1. Goodman LS, Brunton LL, Chabner B, Knollmann BC. *Goodman & Gilman's The Pharmacological Basis of Therapeutics.* New York: McGraw-Hill Medical, 2011. Print.

2. Johnson M. The B-adrenoceptor. *Am J Respir Crit Care Med.* 1998;158(5):146–153.

3. Lemanske RF. Beta agonists in asthma: acute administration and prophylactic use. *UpToDate.* Bochner BS, ed. May-June 2011. Web.

IV Fluids

Chapter 17.1

Crystalloids

Katherine Chuy, MD and Nina Singh-Radcliff, MD

Clinical Uses/Relevance to Anesthesiology

- Fluid replacement
- Correct electrolyte imbalances
- Deliver medications
- Dilute blood products during transfusion to ↓ viscosity
- Perioperative administration ↓ dizziness, drowsiness, thirst, headache in ambulatory surgery patients
- Inexpensive, easy storage, long shelf-life, readily available, few adverse reactions, variety of formulations, no special compatibility testing, no religious objections to use

Pharmacology

- Solution of sterile water with added electrolytes (ie, K^+, Ca^{++}, Mg, lactate) to approximate the mineral content of human plasma
- Ranges from hypotonic, isotonic, or hypertonic in relation to plasma
- "Balanced" or "physiological" solutions contain a chloride concentration close to that of plasma; unbalanced fluids have a proportionally high chloride concentration
- Generally provides 20%-30% expansion in plasma volume after equilibration
- Adequate intravascular volume is essential for stable hemodynamics and perfusion to vital organs.
- IV fluid administration is based on several factors: NPO status, maintenance, insensible losses, third spacing, and blood loss. Maintenance rate(4–2-1 rule): 4 mL/kg/hr for first 10 kg of body weight; 2 mL/kg/hr for second 10 kg of body weight; 1 mL for each kg afterward of body weight over 20 kg. The initial fluid deficit can be replaced in the following manner: ½ during 1st hour of surgery, ¼ during 2nd hour of surgery, ¼ during 3rd hour of surgery. Estimated blood loss (EBL): 3:1 ratio of crystalloid administration to blood loss to maintain intravascular volume, 1:1 ratio for colloid or blood product administration. Insensible losses/third spacing: Minimal tissue trauma (laparoscopy): ~ 0–4mL/kg/hr; Moderate

tissue trauma (ie, thoracic procedures): ~ 5–7.5 mL/kg/h; Large tissue trauma (ie, exploratory laparotomy): ~ 10–15 mL/kg/h
- Total body water (TBW) for 75 kg individual.

Pharmacokinetics

- $1/3$ to $1/4$ remain intravascular, remaining enters extravascular space

Adverse Events

- Volume overload, edema, electrolyte abnormalities, pH disturbances
- Interstitial edema can impair wound healing, gas exchange in lungs; ↓ cardiac compliance and absorption from the gut; ↑ bacterial translocation in gut and in extremities; obtund consciousness

Normal Saline

Clinical Uses/Relevance to Anesthesiology

- Hyperkalemic states (does not contain K^+)
- Dilution of blood products (does not contain Ca^{++})

Pharmacology

- NS has 9 g/L of NaCl and MW = 58 g/mole; thus ([9 g/L]/ [58g/mole] = 0.154 moles/Liter. NaCl dissociates into 2 ions (Na+, Cl^-), thus NS = 154 x 2 = 308 osmoles.
- Na^+ = 154 mEq/L, Cl^- = 154 mEq/L; thus although called "physiological saline" or "isotonic saline," this is inaccurate (plasma Na^+ = 135–145, plasma osmolarity = 275–299).

Adverse Effects

- Non-anion gap **hyperchloremic metabolic acidosis:** $NaCl + H_2O \longleftrightarrow HCl + NaOH$. The strong acid, HCl, and strong base, NaOH, should cancel each other out with no effect on pH. However, the ↑ Cl^- in 0.9% NaCl (154 mEq/L) tips the acid-base balance toward HCl ($NaCl + H_2O \longleftrightarrow\rightarrow\rightarrow HCl + NaOH$), causing metabolic acidosis. Normal saline lacks buffering salt, such as lactate or acetate. Additionally, excessive renal bicarbonate elimination exacerbates metabolic acidosis. Another way of describing this phenomenon is that electrical neutrality has to be restored, and the dissociation of H_2O produces H^+ that electrically balances Cl^-. "Dilutional acidosis" implied that plasma bicarbonate was diluted, however, this is not the principle mechanism
- Hyperchloremic acidosis: (1) ↓ gastric mucosal perfusion, (2) profoundly affects eicosanoid release in renal tissue, leading to vasoconstriction and ↓ GFR, (3) inactivates membrane Ca^{++} channels and inhibits norepinephrine release from sympathetic nerve fibers resulting in redistribution of cardiac output away from internal organs.

- Attempted correction of the abnormality may actually be the main adverse effect. Acidosis is often seen as a reflection of poor organ perfusion or poor myocardial function. A negative base excess may prompt more saline boluses containing fluids that exacerbate acidosis, the use of blood products, escalation of inotrope support and initiation of ventilator support. Furthermore, when coupled with acidosis from a different source (ie, lactic acidosis from tissue hypoperfusion) can complicate management of patient care.
- Renal blood flow and GFR may be ↓. Hyperchloremia affects afferent arteriolar tone through Ca^{++} activated Cl^- channels and modulates release of renin.

Lactated Ringers

Clinical Uses/Relevance to Anesthesiology

- Electrolyte and fluid replacement, with more physiological sodium, chloride, and pH values compared to NS
- Lactate anion functions as an alternate source of bicarbonate
- Contains calcium; do not coadminister with blood products

Pharmacology

- NaCl 6g/L; $NaC_3H_5O_3$ 3.1 g/L (sodium lactate), $CaCl_2$ 0.2 g/L, and KCl 0.3 g/L. Isotonic with blood; pH 6.5, Na^+ = 130 mEq/L, Cl^-=109 mEq/L, K^+ = 4 mEq/L, Ca^{++} = 3 mEq/L, lactate = 28 mEq/L; osmolarity = 275
- Lactate is hepatically metabolized to glycogen, which is oxidatively metabolized to CO_2, H_2O. CO_2 accepts a H^+ ion to yield bicarbonate (alternate source of bicarbonate). Conversion (1–2 h) depends on integrity of cellular oxidative processes, thus less effective source of bicarbonate in lactic acidosis, shock, or ↓ perfusion states.

Adverse Effects

- Caution in acidotic and anoxic states (affects lactate metabolism); Hyperkalemia, renal disease, and in conditions in which potassium retention is present (contains K+); cannot be administered with blood products (Ca^{++} in solution clots blood products); may cause respiratory acidosis (CO_2 production; mild hyponatremia (thus not suitable for maintenance therapy)
- May be associated with panic attacks secondary to complexing of Ca^{++} despite absence of serum levels or symptoms of hypocalcemia.

Normosol

- Electrolyte and fluid replacement, with more physiological Na^+, Cl^-, Mg^{++}, K^+, and pH values compared to NS
- Acetate and gluconate function as an alternate source of bicarbonate

- Does not contain calcium; therefore, can be coadministered with blood products

Pharmacology

- NaCl 5.26 g/L, sodium acetate 2.26 g/L, sodium gluconate 5 g/L, KCl 0.37 g/L, MgCl and hexhydrate 0.3 mg/L; Na^+ 140 mEq, K^+ = 5 mEq/L, Mg^{++} = 3 mEq/L, Cl^- = 98 mEq/L, acetate = 27 mEq/L, gluconate = 23 mEq/L; isotonic with blood; pH 7.4, 295 mOsm
- May contain HCl and/or sodium hydroxide for pH adjustment.
- Mg is the second most plentiful cation of intracellular fluid; plays important role as cofactor for enzymatic reactions and in neurochemical transmission and muscular excitability.
- Sodium acetate provides sodium and acetate (CH_3COO^-) ions. Acetate serves as a source of H^+ acceptors, and is an alternate source of bicarbonate (HCO_3^-) by metabolic conversion in the liver, even with severe liver disease. Thus, acetate anion exerts a mild systemic antiacidotic action that may be advantageous during fluid and electrolyte replacement therapy.
- Sodium gluconate provides sodium and gluconate ($C_6H_{11}O_7^-$) ions. Although gluconate is a theoretical alternate metabolic source of bicarbonate anion, a significant antiacidotic action has not been established. Thus the gluconate anion serves primarily to complete the cation-anion balance of the solutions.

Adverse Effects

- Use cautiously in hyperkalemia, renal disease, and in conditions in which K^+ retention is present; metabolic or respiratory alkalosis (bicarbonate alternates: acetate and gluconate ions); severe hepatic insufficiency; dilutional hyponatremia

Plasmalyte

Clinical Uses/Relevance to Anesthesiology

- Electrolyte and fluid replacement, with more physiological Na^+, Cl^-, Mg^{++}, and pH values compared to NS
- Acetate and gluconate functions as alternate sources of bicarbonate
- Does not contain calcium; therefore can be coadministered with blood products

Pharmacology

- NaCl 5.26 g/L, sodium gluconate 5.02 g/L ($C_6H_{11}NaO_7$); sodium acetate trihydrate 3.68 g/L ($C_2H_3NaO_2 \times 3H_2O$); KCl 0.37 g/L; magnesium chloride 0.3 g/L; Na^+ 140 mEq/L, K^+ 5 mEq/L, Mg^{++} 3 mEq/L, Cl^- 98 mEq/L, acetate 27 mEq/L, gluconate 23 mEq/L; osmolarity 294 mOsmol/L.

- Acetate and gluconate serve as bicarbonate alternatives/precursors; these anions are the conjugate base to the corresponding acid (lactic acid) and do not contribute to development of an acidosis as they are administered with Na^+ rather than H^+ as the cation. Produces a metabolic alkalinizing effect; acetate and lactate ions are ultimately metabolized to CO_2 and H_2O, which requires the consumption of H^+

Adverse Effects

- Used cautiously with hyperkalemia, renal disease, and in conditions in which potassium retention is present; Metabolic or respiratory alkalosis (bicarbonate alternates: acetate and lactate ions); Severe hepatic insufficiency, or impaired utilization of these ions

D5W (Dextrose 5% in Water)

Clinical Uses/Relevance to Anesthesiology

- Dextrose source; provides calories and avoids hypoglycemia and protein and nitrogen catabolism
- Maintenance or water replacement to replenish ICW without electrolytes

Pharmacology

- Dextrose = 50 g/ L; approximate to 2 cookies, or a candy bar. Promotes glycogen deposition and $\downarrow$ or prevents ketosis if sufficient doses are provided.
- pH 4.5; osmotically inactive. ~14% plasma expansion.
- No Na^+, thus net effect is equivalent to giving **pure water** that is distributed throughout TBW with each compartment receiving fluid in proportion to TBW. Thus a large percent moves **intracellularly**.

Adverse Effects

- Hyperglycemia
- Hypotonicity can develop and affect intracellular volume (may lyse)

D5 in NaCl, Lactated Ringers, etc

- 50 g/L of dextrose can be coadministered with a crystalloid; several dextrose formulations are available from 2.5% (25 g/L) to 10% (100 g/L)
- Provides calories, hydration, and electrolytes
- D5 ½ NS is hypertonic (77 mEq Na^+, and Cl^-)

Hypertonic Saline 3% (HTS)

Clinical Uses/Relevance to Anesthesiology

- Severe hyponatremia; TURP Syndrome, SIADH with symptomatic hyponatremia (coma, seizures, lethargy, confusion)
- Volume resuscitation due to osmotic property
- Trauma
- Burn injuries
- Potential benefit after SAH (increased blood flow can counteract cerebral vasospasm)
- Traumatic brain injury (TBI)/cerebral edema (effective in cases refractory to mannitol, hyperventilation)
- Trials are looking at outcomes; currently no clear protocol regarding concentration, timing of administration, or infusion rate (intermittent versus continuous infusion) for acute resuscitation in field or in the ICU.

Pharmacology

- Osmolarity = 1027 mOsm/L; Na^+ = 513 mEq/L, Cl^- = 513 mEq/L; pH 4.5–7
- Hypertonicity creates an osmotic gradient for fluid to shift from the intracellular to interstitial/intravascular space; results in ↑ preload. It also results in vasodilation from direct vascular smooth muscle relaxation and improved capillary blood flow. Furthermore, hypertonicity ↓ endothelial cell volume (intracellular to extracellular flow) which ↑ capillary diameter and ↓ vascular resistance. Increased regional blood flow has been demonstrated in virtually all areas of microcirculation. May counteract cerebral vasospasm seen after SAH
- Cerebral edema. ↑ serum osmolarity draws fluid from brain cells into the intravascular space; ↓ cerebral water content, edema formation, and ICP. ↑ intravascular volume may lead to an autoregulatory ↓ in intracerebral blood volume (assuming autoregulation remains intact). Studies have demonstrated improved survival in TBI with HTS infusion.
- Burn injuries. HTS has physiochemical interaction with glycocalyx and may be less prone to cause "leaky" vascular endothelium. Studies have shown that severe burns have a ↓ incidence of abdominal compartment syndrome, possibly from ↓ capillary leak (less bowel wall, intra-abdominal fluid accumulation).
- Trauma. Can ↑ BP with small volume resuscitation; may ↑ survival. Attributed to avoidance of hemodilution seen with excess amounts of isotonic fluids, hypothermia, acidosis, coagulopathy, sustained hyperosmolar state.

Adverse Effects

- Rapid ↑ in Na^+ can result in osmotic demyelination syndrome or central pontine myelinolysis. To avoid, Na^+ should ↑ at a maximum rate of 0.5 mEq/L/hour and should not exceed 10–12 mEq/Liter in 24 h
- Higher incidence of renal insufficiency/failure than other crystalloids

- Hemorrhage secondary to excessive fluid resuscitation
- Can ↓ afterload (from ↓ PVR, SVR); can result in transient hypotension often seen after boluses are administered
- Dilution of plasma constituents with rapid intravascular volume expansion
- Hypokalemia or hyperchloremic acidosis
- Rebound ↑ ICP after bolus or when continuous infusions are stopped
- Phlebitis, tissue necrosis from hypertonicity (central line preferable)

Clinical Case Scenario

52-year-old female is undergoing an open cholecystectomy. She was NPO since 10 pm the night prior to surgery. She was wheeled into the OR and an IV was started at 7 am. Incision was made at 8 am. It is currently 9 am and the patient is currently 1 hour into the surgery. Estimated blood loss is 10 mL so far. The patient is 60 kg. What is the patient's maintenance fluid rate? What is her fluid deficit from being NPO? How do you estimate the amount of fluids she should be getting?

Maintenance rate for 60 kg patient: 4 mL x first 10 kg = 40 mL. 2 mL x second 10 kg = 20 mL. 1 mL x remaining 40 kg = 40 mL. Maintenance rate = 40 mL + 20 mL + 40 mL = 100mL/hr

Fluid deficit: 100 cc/hr x 9 hours (10 pm-7 am). This is amount of time patient has been NPO without additional fluids) = 900 mL

Replacement of fluid deficit: Replace ½ of deficit in first hour, ¼ of deficit in second hour, ¼ of deficit in third hour. Thus give additional 450 mL in first hour, 225 mL in second hour, 225 mL in third hour in addition to maintenance rate.

Fluids to replace estimated blood loss: 10 mL x 3 = 30 mL

Small-moderate cavity exposure: ~3 mL/kg/hr = 3 x 60 = 180 mL/hr additional

References

1. Skellett S, Mayer A, Durward A, Tibby SM, Murdoch IA. Chasing the base deficit: hyperchloremic acidosis following 0.9% saline fluid resuscitation. *Arch Dis Child.* 2000;83:514–516.
2. Wilcox CS. Regulation of renal blood flow by plasma chloride. *J Clin Invest.* 1983; 71:726–735.
3. Hansen PB, et al. Chloride regulates afferent arteriolar contraction in response to depolarization. *Hypertension.* 1998;32:1066–1070.
4. Strandvik GF. Hypertonic saline in critical care: a review of the literature and guidelines for use in hypotensive states and raised intracranial pressure. *Anaesthesia.* 2009;64;990–1003.
5. Tyagi R, Donaldson K, Loftus Cm, Jallo J. Hypertonic saline: a clinical review. *Neurosurg Rev.* 2007;30:277–290.

Chapter 17.2

Colloids

Katherine Chuy, MD and Nina Singh-Radcliff, MD

Clinical Uses/Relevance to Anesthesiology

- Volume expansion
- ↑ oncotic pressure
- However, studies have not shown a benefit in morbidity and mortality over crystalloids in burns, traumas, perioperative patients.

Pharmacology

- Often based in crystalloid solutions (contains water and electrolytes), with added component of colloidal substances that do not freely diffuse across a semipermeable membrane.
- Able to generate vascular oncotic pressure similar to plasma proteins and expand vascular volume by drawing fluid from extracellular and intracellular spaces
- Maintains intravascular volume over longer period than crystalloids
- Natural (albumin) or synthetic (dextrans, gelatins, hydroxyethyl starches, or HES) generally, offer 60%-100% plasma expansion.

Albumin

Clinical Uses/Anesthetic Implications

- Emergency treatment of shock due to loss of plasma
- Acute burn management
- ICU fluid resuscitation
- Hypo-albuminemia (following paracentesis, liver transplantation, spontaneous bacterial peritonitis, acute lung injury, cirrhosis, extracorporeal albumin dialysis)

Pharmacology

- 5% solution can produce up to 80% initial volume expansion; 25% solution can produce up to 200%-400% volume expansion in 30 mins.

- Endogenous albumin is synthesized hepatically. Largest component of colloid osmotic pressure in human blood (50% of all plasma proteins, thus contributing ~80% of oncotic pressure in a healthy patient).
- Albumin is a monomer (all molecules have the same size)
- Exogenously administered albumin is in the form of FFP, whole blood transfusions, or human albumin solutions (5% or 25%). It is a natural colloid with less side effects (pruritus, anaphylaxis, coagulopathies) compared to synthetic colloids
- 5% albumin has similar expansion to hetastarch but greater than gelatins and dextrans

Pharmacokinetics

- Endogenous albumin has an elimination half-life ~20 days (thus not indicative of liver function in acute disease like hepatitis)
- Exogenous albumin has volume expanding effects that last 16–24 h.

Dosages/Preparations

- 5% solution is iso-oncotic; 25% solution is hyperoncotic

Adverse Effects

- Volume overload
- During septic shock states, inflammatory mediators that are released result in "leaky" vascular endothelium that can cause interstitial edema; colloidal administration may worsen this by now adding an oncotic driving force toward extracellular fluid
- Expensive
- Component of blood plasma and therefore some Jehovah's Witnesses may refuse administration; should be clarified during time of consent

Dextrans

Pharmacology

- Capable of 100%-150% volume expansion (greater than HES and 5% albumin)
- Highly branched polysaccharide molecules produced by bacteria containing enzyme dextran sucrase that grows on sucrose medium
- Dextran 40 can improve microcirculatory flow during microsurgical reimplantation, CPB (likely due to hemodilution and inhibition of erythrocyte aggregation)
- Can affect normal coagulation, worsen coagulopathy, and interfere with cross-matching
- Not contraindicated in Jehovah's Witnesses

Pharmacokinetics

- Colloidal/volume expansion effect: ~6–12 h
- Primarily renal excretion
- Smaller molecules excreted in 15 mins; larger molecules remain in circulation several days

Dosages

- Dextran 40 (MW 40,000) is 10% solution; Dextran 70 (MW 70,000) is a 6% solution

Side Effects

- Anaphylaxis. Dextran antibodies trigger release of vasoactive mediators. Incidence may be reduced by pretreatment with hapten (Dextran 1)
- Coagulopathy from ↓ platelet adhesiveness, factor VIII, and ↑ fibrinolysis
- Interferes with ability to cross-match; coats RBC surface. Inform blood bank if used
- ARF due to accumulation of dextran molecules in renal tubules

Hydroxyethyl Starches (HES)

Clinical Uses/Relevance to Anesthesiology

- Stabilization of systemic hemodynamics
- Anti-inflammatory properties (preserves intestinal microvascular perfusion in endotoxemia)
- Cost-effective (similar volume expansion, less expensive than albumin)
- Coagulation: does not appear to affect with doses of <50 mL/kg

Pharmacology

- Volume expansion ~100%
- Preparations are characterized by concentration (low 6% HES solutions iso-oncotic so 1 L replaces 1 L blood loss; high 10% solutions are hyperoncotic with volume effect exceeding infused volume by about 145%)
- Composed of starches (polysaccharides) of varying molecular weights. Derived from amylopectin (complex carbohydrate similar to glycogen) with hydroxyethyl groups substituted at C_2 and C_6 positions for ↑ stability.

Pharmacokinetics

- Duration of volume expansion ~8–12 h.
- Plasma amylase cleaves glucose moieties from large polymers. Small HES molecules (<60kDa) rapidly excreted by kidneys. Medium sized molecules excreted into bile and feces. Some taken up by reticuloendothelial system, where molecules are broken down slowly.
- Molar substitution (low 0.45–0.58; high 0.62–0.7) by addition of hydroxyethyl groups ↑ resistance to degradation and prolongs intravascular volume effect

Dosages/Preparation

- Hetastarch. 6% solution in isotonic saline; most commonly used. MW 10 000–3 400 000 kDa; average MW 600 000 kDa. Polydisperse, so small molecules are rapidly excreted while larger molecules are retained in circulation longer. Osmotic effectiveness dependent on number of particles, not molecular size. Thus as smaller particles are excreted, osmotic effectiveness slowly declines (however, compensated for by breakdown of larger molecules).
- Pentastarch similar to hetastarch except MW smaller (mean MW 200 000 kDa)

Side Effects

- Coagulopathy ($\downarrow$ circulating factor VIII and von Willebrand factor levels, impairs platelet function, prolongs PTT and aPTT)
- Pruritis associated with accumulation of high molecular weight HES
- Higher degree of anaphylaxis compared to other synthetic colloids and albumin
- Renal impairment; associated with higher creatinine levels, oliguria, and acute renal failure in patients who were critically ill with existing renal impairment
- $\uparrow$ amylase levels but not clinically significant

Chapter 17.3

Transfusion Products

Nina Singh Radcliff, MD

Whole Blood (WB)

Clinical Uses/Relevance to Anesthesiology

- Increases O_2-carrying capacity, provides coagulation factors/colloidal volume; however, blood is a scarce resource, component therapy should be implemented for goal-directed treatment
- Autologous blood transfusion; transfusion indications may be more liberal than that with allogenic transfusion
- Rapid, life-threatening hemorrhage where component therapy is not readily available
- When component therapy is inadequately correcting coagulopathy; obviates the need to determine ratio and timing of blood products to each other
- "Damage Control Resuscitation" in massive hemorrhage; warm WB is an alternative to the 1:1:1 pRBC:platelet:FFP ratio. Goal is to avoid the "lethal triad" (coagulopathy, acidosis, hypothermia)
- Neonatal transfusion. Blood is reconstituted from pRBC and FFP to produce a specific Hct with Type O pRBC and Type AB plasma; reduces complications.
- Cardiac surgery. Studies suggest that may reduce EBL, transfusion requirements, donor exposure
- Exchange transfusions for sickle cell anemia with organ- or life-threatening conditions (acute chest syndrome, progressive splenic sequestration, priapism), preoperatively for major surgery or eye surgery. Needs to be irradiated and leukocyte-reduced
- Military operations requiring massive transfusion; warm, convenient, contains coagulation factors
- Used in the developing world, where preparation of component therapy not affordable

Pharmacodynamics

- Unmodified, collected blood; containing RBCs, coagulation factors, platelets, proteins, leukocytes

Pharmacokinetics

- Anticoagulant is added (see pRBCs)
- Needs to be Typed and Crossed to recipient
- 450–500 mL/unit; Hct 30%-40%
- Platelets, granulocytes, labile clotting factors decline with storage. Lymphocytes remain viable.
- Can be irradiated, leukocyte-reduced, and tested for CMV

Adverse Events/Reactions

- Transfusion associated circulatory overload (TACO); each unit administered adds 450–500 mL of colloidal load to the intravascular space
- Dilutional thrombocytopenia. Platelets decline with storage time; if frozen, will be damaged
- TRALI, infectious transmission, acute hemolytic transfusion reaction, delayed transfusion reaction (see pRBCs)

References

1. Spinella PC. Warm fresh whole blood transfusion for severe hemorrhage: U.S. military and potential civilian applications. *Crit Care Med*. 2008;36(7 Suppl):S340-S345.

2. Jobes D, Wolfe Y, O'Neill D, Calder J, Jones L, Sesok-Pizzini D, Zheng XL. Toward a definition of "fresh" whole blood: an in vitro characterization of coagulation properties in refrigerated whole blood for transfusion. *Transfusion*. 2011;51:43–51.

3. Damage control resuscitation: a sensible approach to the exsanguinating surgical patient. *Crit Care Med*. 2008l;36(7 Suppl):S267-S274.

Packed Red Blood Cells (pRBCs)

Clinical Uses/Relevance to Anesthesiology

- Increases O_2-carrying capacity; component therapy, allows to conserve un-needed components.
- Almost always indicated for a EUVOLEMIC Hg < 6 mg/dL, almost never indicated for a EUVOLEMIC Hg >10 mg/dL
- Hg of 6–10 mg/dL. Avoid arbitrary "transfusion trigger." Assess adequate oxygenation to tissues and clinical picture: continued bleeding, end organ disease (cerebral, cardiac, pulmonary, renal), presence of lactic acidosis (anaerobic metabolism), vasopressors to support BP, reduced MVO_2, or hypoxia to heart or brain (angina, AMS in awake; EKG abnormalities in asleep).
- Transfusion is strongly discouraged for uses such as to enhance the general sense of well-being, promote wound healing, expand intravascular volume in the absence of inadequate O_2-carrying capacity or delivery (effects of anemia must be separated from those of hypovolemia), or serve as prophylaxis

against low O_2-carrying capacity. Incidence of inappropriate transfusions as high as 18%-57%

- Sepsis; maybe ineffective at reducing lactate, or improving MVO_2 or O_2 deficits in organ systems

Pharmacodynamics

- O_2 content (mL of O_2/dL blood) = [Hg x O_2 saturation x 1.39] + [pO_2 x 0.003]. O_2 is carried in blood in 2 forms: Hg (efficient) and gas form (undissolved, inefficient). Thus, a small increase in Hg level can significantly increase blood O_2 content.
- Hg/Hct needs to be assessed EACH AND EVERY TIME in relation to volume status: hyper-, hypo-, euvolemia. Blood loss is "whole blood" loss (plasma and red blood cells). Therefore, Hg/Hct measurements after blood loss may not reflect total RBC loss *unless* fluid restoration has occurred (crystalloids and colloids will contribute to plasma volume, and unmask the change in RBCs).
- Hct contributes to whole blood viscosity; viscosity affects PVR. Resistance ~ $(n_* L)/ r^4$, where n = viscosity, L = length, r = radius. Therefore, Hct affects blood pressure (Pressure = Cardiac Output * Resistance).
- Furthermore, microvascular perfusion and functional capillary density are impaired by low viscosity. Tissue survival may be jeopardized due to local microscopic maldistribution of blood flow.

Pharmacokinetics

- Whole blood is centrifuged to separate plasma from platelets and RBCs
- 1 unit of pRBCS has a volume of ~300 mL, Hct 70%-80% (contains a small amount of plasma and anticoagulant); and needs to be stored at 1–6° C to slow metabolism, increase storage life, and reduce incidence of bacterial growth
- Federal regulations require that >70% of transfused pRBCs survive >24 h posttransfusion
- CPD (21 days)—citrate is an anticoagulant (binds Ca^+), phosphate is a buffer, dextrose provides energy to red cells and allows glycolysis to continue during storage
- CPDA-1 (35 days)—CPD + adenosine, a precursor for ATP synthesis.
- Adsol (42 days)—CPD + adenosine, glucose is an energy source, mannitol is a free radical scavenger, NaCl; 100 mL (increases total volume in unit, while reducing Hct)
- Deglycerolized—Allows prolonged storage of rare blood types, Rh(-), autologous blood, and for patients with antibodies to high-incidence antigens, multiple allo-antibodies, IgA deficiency (plasma free). RBCs are incubated in 40% glycerol solution ("antifreeze" within the cells), then deep freezed to -60° C in sterile containers. Prior to use, thaw, wash free of glycerol, and resuspend in saline. Use within 2–4 h to limit bacterial contamination. The process depletes the unit of plasma and leukocytes.

- "Washing" with NaCl removes up to 99% of plasma proteins, electrolytes, platelets, leukocytes, and antibodies. Utilized in patients with allergic or febrile reactions to plasma components of the blood product or hyperkalemia. However, reduces shelf life; 10%-20% loss of RBCs

- "Leukocyte reduced." Filtration process that separates leukocytes from other blood components; reduces risk of nonhemolytic febrile transfusion reactions, CMV and HTLV-I/II transmission (virus is carried in leukocytes), development of HLA antibodies; used for pediatric patients, immune-compromised. Results in 10%-15% loss of RBCs

- "Irradiated." Gamma irradiation inactivates any lymphocytes present; however, increases efflux of intracellular K^+ (mean 44.7 mEq/L) and reduces post-transfusion red cell recovery. Utilized in immunosuppressed pts (premature infants, GVHD, immune-deficiencies, aggressively treated cancers).

- CMV (-). Tests for CMV (50%-80% prevalence). Important in severely immune-suppressed pts who are CMV seronegative (bone marrow, organ transplants; premature infants)

- pRBCs can be reconstituted in crystalloid solutions (NaCl, normosol) or albumin to make less viscous, which facilitates transfusion. Avoid hypotonic solutions (hemolysis; water flows into RBC down osmotic gradient) or Ca^+ containing solutions (clotting; overwhelms anticoagulants that bind Ca^+)

- 170 micrometer filter traps clot and debris

- Electrolyte and substrate content of stored blood depends on: the addition of anticoagulant preservative solution (increases Na^+ and glucose); metabolism of stored RBCs (even at 4°C, anaerobic metabolism occurs, lactate produced, K^+ increases, pH reduces); the volume and plasma constituents of donor blood.

Adult Dosing

- 1 unit typically raises Hg by 1 g/dL, Hct 3%-4%

Pediatric Dosing

- "Pedi-pack" is a divided unit used to minimize wasting blood (small volume transfusion required); may reduce donor exposure if more than 1 unit needed (same donor). Practices vary; typically leukocyte reduced, HbS (-), often irradiated. Typed and Crossed to pt. However, Type O can be requested for fetus where ABO Type is unknown, exchange transfusions in neonates used when fetal-maternal ABO incompatibility may be involved, or in case of an emergency. Usual dose 10–15 mL/kg

Adverse Events/Reactions

- TRALI—Transfusion Related Acute Lung Injury. 1:1500 to 1:10 000; 5%-15% are fatal (leading cause of transfusion related deaths). Results from donor neutrophil-specific antibodies and HLA antibodies reacting with the recipient's white cells; antibodies aggregate in the pulmonary circulation and release mediators that damage alveolar/capillary membranes; pulmonary edema develops in the absence of circulatory overload; 1–2 h posttransfusion. Results in decreased O_2 saturation/pO_2, hyperthermia, fluid in ETT.

- Acute hemolytic reactions—1:33 000. ABO incompatibility results in immediate intravascular hemolysis (host antibodies to ABO of recipient). Severity depends on amount of incompatible blood given (can result from as little as 10 mL). Signs and symptoms in anesthetized pt include tachycardia, hypotension, hyperthermia, hemoglobinuria, diffuse oozing in the field. DIC, shock, and renal failure can occur.

- Delayed hemolytic reaction. 1%-5% of all transfusions. Mild; sensitization to Rh and Kidd antigens from a prior blood transfusion or pregnancy. Antibody levels during initial transfusion are too low to cause destruction. Upon re-exposure with subsequent transfusion, recipient antibodies coat transfused RBCs and are destroyed in the reticuloendothelial system 2–21 days later. Signs and symptoms include malaise, jaundice, and fever; Hct drops

- Febrile nonhemolytic reactions. Occur 1–6 h posttransfusion. Donor white cells cause increase in temperature, dyspnea; benign and resolves without therapy.

- Urticarial reactions. Signs and symptoms: erythema, hives, and itching due to sensitization to donor plasma proteins. Steroids and antihistamines can reduce occurrence.

- Transfusion-associated Graft-vs-Host Disease (GVHD). Immune attack by transfused cells against the recipient. Occurs in severely immunosuppressed patients and carries a high mortality. Irradiation may prevent.

- Metabolic derangements. K+: intracellular potassium shifts extracellularly and increases with storage time; can result in serious cardiac arrhythmias. Na+: anticoagulants have a high sodium load; effect is transient and distributes throughout ECF, expanding it at the expense of ICF; may reduce brain cell volume and ICP. Glucose: anticoagulants may contain; hyperglycemia interferes with platelet function, neurological recovery from cerebral ischemia. Lactate: increased production; a byproduct of cell metabolism.

- Acid-base abnormality. Accumulation of lactic acid and production of CO_2 from glycolysis and metabolism can result in a pH of 6.9 at day 21 of storage.

- Hypothermia if products are not warmed. Can cause coagulopathy, arrhythmias, cardiac arrest, delayed awakening.

- Citrate toxicity. Citrate binds to Ca^+. With massive transfusion (1 unit q5–10 m) clinically significant hypocalcemia can result and manifests as cardiac depression, hypotension.

- Reduced 2,3 DPG (with storage time). Causes a left-shift of Hb-O_2 dissociation curve; increases O_2 affinity to Hg, reduces off-loading at tissue level (tissue hypoxia)

- Increased storage time can result in reduced RBC deformability, adhesiveness, viability. Can also reduce tissue oxygenation, pH and increase K+, lactate, and the release of substances that can elicit adverse systemic responses

(fever, cellular injury, alterations in regional and global blood flow, organ dysfunction)

- Transfusion-associated immunomodulation. Some evidence that perioperative allogenic transfusion may result in earlier recurrence and lower survival rates in pts with colorectal, breast, prostate, and certain other cancers
- CMV 50%-90% of some pt populations; Hepatitis C 1:100 000 to 1:200 000; Hepatitis B 1:200 000. HIV 1:2 000 000. Parasitic and bacterial clinically significant disease 1:2 000 000.

References

Ratcliffe JM, Elliott MJ, Wyse RKH, Hunter S, Alberti KGMM. The metabolic load of stored blood: implications for major transfusions in infants. *Arch Dis Child.* 1986;61:1208–1214.

The Task Force on Blood Component Therapy. Practice guidelines for blood component therapy: A Report by the American Society of Anesthesiologists Task Force on Blood Component Therapy. *Anesthesiology.* 1996;84(3):732–747.

Fresh Frozen Plasma (FFP)

Clinical Uses/Relevance to Anesthesiology

- Little evidence exists to inform best therapeutic plasma transfusion practice
- Abnormal coagulation screening tests, therapeutically in the face of bleeding, or prophylactically in nonbleeding subjects prior to invasive procedures or surgery
- Correction of microvascular bleeding in the presence of PT, PTT >1.5 times normal. Believed to correspond to factor levels <30% normal. However, the relationship between clinical coagulopathy, laboratory tests of coagulation, and need for FFP remain unclear based on existing data.
- Thromboelastogram. Reduced maximal amplitude suggests qualitative or quantitative deficiency
- Massive transfusion may require "component therapy" with FFP for microvascular bleeding. Urgent situations may not afford time to wait for lab results. Abnormalities are often seen after infusing >4 units of pRBCs.
- "Damage control resuscitation." pRBC:FFP:platelets are administered in a 1:1:1 ratio
- Urgent reversal of warfarin; otherwise consider vitamin K if time permits
- Disseminated intravascular coagulopathy (DIC)
- Thrombotic thrombocytopenic purpura (TTP)
- Replacement of isolated factor deficiencies (II, V, VII, IX, X, XI) when specific component therapy is unavailable
- Antithrombin III (AT-III) deficiency, when heparin is needed therapeutically (functions by accelerating the action of AT-III by 3000-fold)

- Infants with protein-losing enteropathy
- Contraindicated for augmentation of plasma volume or albumin concentration

Pharmacodynamics

- Donor WB is centrifuged and top plasma fluid layer is separated and frozen within 8 h (−18 to −30° C); rapid freezing helps prevent inactivation of labile coagulation factors V and VIII
- Plasmapheresis allows for a single donor (reducing recipient exposure to infection, HLA antibodies); extracorporeal therapy that involves removal of WB, plasma removal via a cell separator, and return of nonplasma components.
- After thawing, FFP contains near normal levels of many plasma proteins (procoagulant and inhibitory components of the coagulation cascades, acute phase proteins, immunoglobulins and albumin), fats, carbohydrates, and minerals in circulation
- Devoid of red cells, leukocytes, and platelets; does not carry risk of CMV (lacks leukocytes)

Pharmacokinetics

- One unit = 250 mL (~220 mL plasma, ~30 mL anticoagulant)
- Should be ABO compatible whenever possible (reference remains blood Type). In emergencies, Type AB (universal) is preferred (no antibodies in plasma to Type A, B, or AB blood)
- Should be transfused within 24 hours of thawing
- Not as viscous as pRBCs, does not need to be diluted with crystalloid

Adult Dosing

- 1 unit of plasma increases most factors ~2.5%; 4 plasma units ~ 10%
- A 10% increase in factor levels is typically necessary to make a significant change in coagulation status. However this will vary depending on patient's size and clotting factor levels.
- 1 mL plasma=1 unit of coagulation factors; 1 plasma unit = 220 units (freezing, thawing reduces factor recovery)

Pediatric Dosing

- 10–15 mL/kg gives an ~15%–20% rise in factor levels

Adverse Events/Reactions

- TRALI; association with female donors; in Europe male donors are preferred for FFP
- Infection transmission (see pRBCs)
- Prion disease
- Fluid/circulatory overload (colloidal)
- Allergic reactions 1%–3% incidence

References

Stanworth SJ, Hyde CJ, Murphy MF. Evidence for indications of fresh frozen plasma. *Trans Clin Biol*. December 2007. Volume 14, issue 6. 551–556.

Fresh frozen plasma: indications and risks. Consensus Development Conference Reports NIH Consensus Development Program.

Platelets

Clinical Uses/Relevance to Anesthesiology

- Platelet count < 10 000/microliters can result in spontaneous bleeding; in actively bleeding patients, a level >50 000/microliters is recommended.
- Prophylaxis for invasive procedures. Lumbar puncture, endoscopy >20 000/microliters; liver biopsy, procedures with insignificant blood loss, vaginal delivery >50 000/microliters; CNS >100 000/microliters. Empiric and few structured studies
- 50 000–100 000/microliters should be based on risk of bleeding
- Platelet dysfunction and microvascular bleeding despite adequate platelet count (uremia, aplastic anemia, chemotherapy, irradiation, ITP, DIC)
- Increased R time, reduced MA on thromboelastogram
- Massive transfusion/"Damage Control Resuscitation." 1:1:1 transfusion of pRBC:FFP:platelets reduces the potential for thrombocytopenia that can occur from the initial loss, followed by dilution from component therapy (FFP, pRBC devoid of platelets).
- Autoimmune thrombocytopenia. Autoantibodies to platelets; spontaneous bleeding is uncommon. Transfusion indicated to control serious active bleeding (not prophylactically). Transfused platelets have very short survival; need to administer 2–3 times more.
- Damage from extracorporeal devices. In the absence of anatomic problems, platelets should be given even when counts are >50 000/microliter.

Pharmacodynamics

- Small, irregularly shaped cell fragments (no nucleus). Upon endothelial cell injury, subendothelial collagen, vWF, and tissue factor are exposed to and activate circulating platelets that they come in contact with. Clumping occurs and the coagulation cascade is activated and strengthens the clot
- Pooled platelets. Buffy coat or platelet rich plasma techniques. Whole blood (450 mL) is centrifuged in two stages "hard spin" and "soft spin" to separate plasma from cell components.
- Plasmapheresis. Extracorporeal method that collects WB, and then separates RBCs and plasma from platelets. The platelets are removed and the remaining components (pRBCs, plasma) are returned to the donor. Process takes ~90 minutes; constitutes ~ 80% of US supply

- Cross-matching not necessary; however incompatibility can reduce posttrans-fusion counts. Platelets possess ABO antigens on their surface, and RBCs are present in small amounts (<0.5 mL). When several units needed, increased numbers of incompatible ABO RBCs may cause hemolysis; ABO matching is prudent in these cases
- Rh antigens are not present on the platelet surface, however RBCs (<0.5 mL) contained in the concentrate may lead to Rh immunization. Should avoid in women in their childbearing years; if necessary, do not withhold, but consider Rh Ig to prevent alloimmunization
- Platelet function is temperature sensitive; <18° C damages microcanalicular structures and induces clustering of platelet receptors; the clustered recep-tors are easily recognized by macrophages, which rapidly remove the pre-viously "chilled" platelets from circulation. Thus, need to be maintained at higher temp than other transfusion products and *cannot* be frozen, refriger-ated, or infused through warmed tubing.

Pharmacokinetics

- Endogenously produced platelets survive ~9–10 days; transfused platelets ~1–7 days posttransfusion.
- "Platelet concentrate" is the term used for the platelets separated from 1 unit of WB. ~5 platelet concentrates = 1 jumbo pack, or ~ 3×10^{11} platelets
- Plateletpheresis donors donate a "single" or "double" unit in a sitting. 1 plateletpheresis unit = 3×10^{11} platelets (equivalent to 1 jumbo pack or 1 unit of platelet concentrate)
- Storage time ~5 days (short because cannot be cooled to slow metabolism, blunt incidence of infection). At day 5, intravascular recovery is ~51%.
- Lack of response maybe due to pt factors (HLA antibodies, splenomegaly, DIC, amphotericin administration, fever) or long storage time. Consider HLA matching, cross-matching, or "fresh platelets" (<48 h after collection)
- Stored in special plastic containers with volume-to-surface ratios that allow sufficient gas exchange between the internal volume and external ambient air (hypoxia is detrimental to survival). Continuously agitated to reduce bacterial growth
- "Swirling" is a visual effect from diffraction when platelets are manually resus-pended and held up to a strong light. Its presence indicates that the platelets are high-quality and discoid; can be easily performed at bedside. Old platelets lack "swirling" since their morphology changes from discoid to spherical, a shape that does not diffract light.

Adult Dosing

- 1×10^{11} platelets increase platelet counts ~ 10 000/μL in a 70 kg pt
- 1 unit of plateletpheresis contains ~ 3×10^{11} platelets (would increase counts ~ 30–60 000/μL

- 1 unit of pooled platelets (pooled from ~5–10 units WB) contains ~ 3×10^{11} (would increase counts ~30–60 000/μL)
- Frequent transfusions of a lower dose of platelets may reduce total amount of platelets needed ($1/2$–1 jumbo pack or 1 plateletpheresis unit). Conversely, transfusion of larger doses extends the time between transfusion and may be more convenient for patient management (2 jumbo packs or 2 plateletpheresis units q 2–3 days)

Pediatric Dosing

- Roughly 1 platelet concentrate (derived from 1 unit of WB) per 10 kg
- Consider ordering specific amounts to reduce waste (eg, 20–25 mL); "volume reduce" by removing plasma to decrease volume load (however, results in loss of 15%–55% of platelets; alternatively, a smaller dose may be appropriate).
- May consider washing or removing plasma and resuspending with saline if donor ABO Type is incompatible with recipient or not available (reduces plasma antibodies and donor RBCs).

Adverse Events/Reactions

- Leukocytes increase risk of untoward complications; washing can reduce incidence
- Storage at higher temperatures increases risk of bacterial growth (~1:3000 units). Infection usually introduced by the needle entering the vein through skin that is ineffectively disinfected; rarely by donor bacteremia, or occult colon cancer. High mortality, particularly in immunocompromised patients with cancer or blood disorders.
- Febrile transfusion reactions. Secondary to leukocytes and soluble cytokines. May be avoided by transfusing leukocyte-reduced platelets.
- Rh alloimmunization.
- Acute Hemolytic Reactions. Type A and B antibodies in the plasma portion may react against recipient's red cells when large numbers of ABO-incompatible units are given
- GVHD
- TRALI. To reduce incidence, store in additive solutions instead of plasma
- Blood borne pathogens including HIV, HBV, HCV, CMV

References

McCullough J. Overview of platelet transfusion. *Semin Hematol.* 2010;47(3):235–242.

Stronek DF, Rebulla P. Platelet transfusions. *Lancet.* 2007; 370(9585):427–438.

Cryoprecipitate

Clinical Uses/Relevance to Anesthesiology

- Congenital fibrinogen deficiency, von Willebrand's disease, and Congenital Factor XIII deficiency for prevention (perioperative and peripartum) and treatment of bleeding
- Factor VIII, Factor XIII, and vWF deficiency should be managed with virally inactivated human-derived products or recombinant products if possible
- Massive transfusion with microvascular bleeding and fibrinogen <80–100 mg/dL (or if cannot be measured in a timely fashion); hemorrhage post cardiac surgery
- Treatment of hemorrhage secondary to thrombolytic therapy
- Management of bleeding due to snake venom
- Iatrogenic premature rupture of amniotic membranes
- Amniotic fluid embolism
- Uremia; prevention and treatment of bleeding
- Topical use as in fibrin glue (virally inactivated human-derived fibrin sealant products preferred)
- Fibronectin deficiency after major surgery, trauma, burns, and sepsis; deficiency impairs the reticuloendothelial system from clearing particulate debris in the circulation resulting in the accumulation of fibrin microaggregates, collagenous debris, and immune complexes

Pharmacodynamics

- Factor VIII (150 units/unit), von Willebrand factor (150 units/unit), fibrinogen (~350 mg/unit), fibronectin, factor XIII, and platelet microparticles.
- Fibrinogen is converted to fibrin by thrombin. Factor VIII and vWF mediate adhesion of circulating platelets to exposed subendothelium, and stabilizes coagulation factor VII in the plasma
- Factor XIII promotes clot stability by forming covalent bonds between fibrin monomers and by cross-linking alpha-2 antiplasmin, fibrinogen, fibronectin, collagen and other proteins to enhance the mechanical strength of the fibrin clot and protect the clot from proteolytic degradation
- Platelet microparticles can play active roles in thrombosis, inflammation, and vascular reactivity

Pharmacokinetics

- Prepared by thawing 1 unit of FFP at 1–6°C. The supernatant (rich in Factor VIII and XIII, vWF, fibrinogen, fibronectin, and platelet microparticles) is removed and refrozen within 1 h of thawing (<-18°C)
- Factor VIII is increased when the donor has higher baseline levels or exercises 5 minutes on a bicycle before donation; mixture is continuously mixed during

collection; time is minimized from donation to freezing of FFP; storage time is limited

- 1 unit cryoprecipitate = 0.25 g fibrinogen (10 units = 125 mL cryoprecipitate = 2.5 g fibrinogen). 1 unit FFP = 0.5 mg fibrinogen (5 units FFP = 1250 mL FFP = 2.5 g fibrinogen). Benefit is that can accomplish same dose with less volume
- Shelf life of 12 months
- ABO compatibility not required, due to the small volume of plasma transfused
- If pooled (10 units), needs to be used within 4 h; cannot be refrozen; use within 3 h after thawing
- Elimination half-time of 12 h
- Administer through a 180–260 μm standard blood tubing; consider mixing with 10–15 mL of NS to ensure complete removal of all material from each bag

Adult Dosing

- 1 unit cryoprecipitate increase fibrinogen by 5–8 mg/dL (>100 mg/dL is hemostatic). Effect can be monitored by fibrinogen level assay and clinical response
- Factor VIII and vWF when specific factor concentrates are unavailable: 1 unit = 150 units. ~ 6–12 units.

Pediatric Dosing

- 1 unit per 10 kg can increase fibrinogen ~60–100 mg/dL
- May consider ABO compatibility in neonates

Adverse Events/Reactions

- Viral transmission, risk is potentially higher given that adult dose of the product is 8–16 units.
- Rare reports of acute hemolytic transfusion reaction, nonhemolytic febrile and allergic reactions, or thrombosis
- Human derived fibrinogen is a potential alternative, however, adverse events include anaphylactic reaction, deep vein thrombosis

Reference

Callum JL, Karkouti K, Lin Y. Cryoprecipitate: the current state of knowledge. *Transfus Med Rev.* 2009; 23(3):177–188.

Clinical Case Scenario #1

Transfusion Requirements in Critical Care (TRICC) Trial randomized patients in the ICU to one of two transfusion groups: liberal transfusion (transfusion when Hg levels < 10 g/dL with a goal of 10–12 g/dL) or restricted transfusion

(transfusion when Hg < 7 g/dL with a goal of 7–9 g/dL). Hospital mortality was lower in the restrictive group, and 30-day mortality was lower among patients <55 y.o. or with APACHe II scores of 20 or less. In sicker or older patients, outcome parameters did not differ between the 2 groups.

Clinical Case Scenario #2

How would the following interventions affect oxygen-carrying capacity in a patient with a Hg of 10 g/dL, FIO_2 0.5, O_2 saturation 95%, paO_2 88 mmHg? O_2 content = [Hg * 1.39 *O_2 saturation] + [paO_2 * 0.003]. Currently, O_2 content = [10*1.39*0.95] + [88 * 0.003] = 13.46 mL of O_2/dL blood.# 1: Transfusion of 2 units of pRBCs. Assuming an increase in Hg of 2 g/dL, [12*1.39*0.95] + [88*0.003] = 16.11 mL of O_2/dL#2: Increasing FIO_2 to 1.0, which also results in increased paO_2 280 and O_2 saturation to 100%. [10 * 1.39 * 1] + [280 * 0.003] = 14.74#3: Implementing inotropic agents (milrinone or dobutamine) to increase contractility from 2.5 L/min to 4.8 L/min. Oxygen delivery (mLs O_2/min) = cardiac output (L/min) * (blood O_2-carrying capacity). At CO of 2.5 L/min, O_2 delivery = 2.5 * 13.46 = 33.65 mLs O_2/min. At CO of 4.8 L/min, O_2 delivery = 4.8 * 13.46=64.61 mLs O_2/min.Therefore, treatment of ischemia would include the simultaneous interventions of optimizing cardiac output, Hg level, and FIO_2/O_2 saturation. Note: increasing CO will result in increased myocardial O_2 consumption.

Clinical Case Scenario #3

Estimated blood volume can be calculated as follows: EBV = weight (kg) * average blood volume. Premature neonates = 95 mL/kg, full-term neonates = 85 mL/kg, infants = 80 mL/kg, adult men 75 mL/kg, adult women 65 mL/kg.

Calculates the following:

Premature neonate 1.5 kg: 1.5 kg * 95 mL/kg = 142.5 mL

Full term neonate 3.5 kg: 3.5 kg * 85 mL/kg = 297.5 mL

Infant 10 kg: 10 kg * 80 mL/kg = 800 mL

Male adult: 100 kg: 100 kg * 75 mL/kg = 7500 mL

Female adult 100 kg: 100 kg * 65 mL/kg = 6500 mL; Note: consider IBW in obese adults for calculation

Clinical Case Scenario #4

Allowable blood loss (ABL) can be calculated as follows:

ABL = [EBV * (H_i – H_t)]/H_i

Calculate the total body volume in an adult female who is 60 kg. Calculate the ABL if her starting Hct is 45%, to reach a Hct of 30%.

60 kg + 65 mL/kg= 3900 mL total blood volume. 3900 * [45–30]/45 = 1300 mL

Calculate the ABL of an 8 kg infant with a starting Hct of 38% before reaching 26%. Total blood volume: 8kg * 80 = 640 mL; 640 * [38–26]/38 = 202 mL.

Chapter 18

Electrolytes

Chapter 18.1

Sodium/Potassium/Calcium/ Phosphate

Tygh Wycoff, MD and John G. Augoustides, MD

Clinical Uses/Relevance to Anesthesiology

- Most abundant cation in the ECF
- Essential for the generation of action potentials in neurologic and cardiac tissue
- Primary determinant of ICF and ECF osmolality and consequent water balance
- Na^+/K^+ ATPase embedded in the cell membrane is responsible for maintaining electrochemical potentials
- Isotonic saline used to treat hyponatremia; hypertonic saline for severe hyponatremia
- Present in all crystalloids (except D5W) and to suspend colloids

Pharmacodynamics

- Normal plasma [Na^+] is 135–145 mEq/L
- Hyponatremia: < 135 mEq/L. Symptoms depend on the rate and amount of ↓; may include loss of appetite, nausea, vomiting, cramps, weakness, AMS, coma, and seizures. Causes are multifactorial; first step in diagnosis is determining the plasma osmolality. If low plasma osmolality (hypotonic hyponatremia), the second step is to determine total body sodium/extracellular fluid [ECF] volume. High, low, or normal ECF may be determined by assessing the urine osmolality, volume, and Na^+ along with clinical correlation. In hypotonic hyponatremia with normal or ↑ ECF, treatment involves water restriction and diuretics to remove total body water. In hypotonic hyponatremia with ↓ ECF volume, administration of isotonic saline is the primary therapy. The Na^+ dose required to correct a deficit can be calculated with the following equation:

$$Dose\ (mEq) = \{kg \times (140\text{-plasma }[Na^+])\} \times 0.6$$

- Slow correction to avoid central pontine myelinolysis. In symptomatic patients, serum Na^+ should be raised by 1–2 mEq/L/h and in asymptomatic patients, by

0.8 mEq/L/h (not to exceed 8 mEq/L over the first 24 h). Common causes of perioperative hyponatremia include TURP syndrome, SIADH (related to sympathetic activation, pulmonary or intracranial disorders), vomiting, diuretic use

- Hypernatremia: >145 mEq/L. Symptoms include AMS, weakness, neuromuscular irritability, focal neurological deficits, coma, and seizures. Diagnosis begins with an assessment of ECF volume. If the ECF is normal or ↓, assess urine osmolality, Na$^+$, and volume. Perioperative causes are often due to primary Na$^+$ gain or water deficit (water loss from the kidney, nonrenal or insensible losses through the skin, respiratory tract, or GI tract). Treatment involves stopping ongoing water losses and correcting the water deficit. The total body water deficit can be calculated from the following equation:
- Water Deficit (L) = {(plasma [Na$^+$] – 140)/140} x total body water (L)
- Central DI can be treated with intranasal DDAVP, while nephrogenic DI is treated with a low salt diet, diuretics, and NSAIDS. As in hyponatremia, the serum [Na$^+$] should be corrected slowly to avoid potential neurological complications. Plasma [Na$^+$] should be lowered by 0.5 mEq/L/h (not > than 12 mEq/L over the first 12 h).
- Hypernatremia ↑ the MAC of inhaled anesthetics, perhaps due to ↑ excitability of neuronal membranes

Pharmacokinetics

- Consumption of Na$^+$ far exceeds requirements in most healthy individuals; thus the kidney's primary function in Na$^+$ balance is excretion
- After filtration at the glomerulus, Na$^+$ reabsorption occurs in the PCT, loop of Henle, and DCT.
- Na$^+$ reabsorption is primarily controlled by the renin-angiotensin-aldosterone system (RAAS), ADH, and atrial natriuretic peptide (ANP)

Potassium

Clinical Uses/Relevance to Anesthesiology

- Major intracellular cation
- Membrane potential is maintained by the Na$^+$-K$^+$-ATPase pump that actively transports Na$^+$ extracellularly, and K$^+$ intracellularly in a 3:2 ratio
- Important for the generation and propagation of action potentials in cardiac and nervous systems
- Hypokalemia may result from medications, or other pathological states
- Hyperkalemia may result in deadly cardiac arrhythmias

Pharmacodynamics

- Normal plasma [K$^+$] is 3.5–5.0 mEq/L, with 1%–2% of total body K$^+$ extracellularly and the remainder located intracellularly. Therefore, small serum abnormalities may indicate large total body deficits or surpluses (assuming ICF and ECF compartment equilibrium)

- Hypokalemia: <3.5 mEq/L. Symptoms include fatigue, myalgias, and muscular weakness. Early EKG changes reflect prolonged ventricular repolarization (flattening or inversion of T waves resulting in U waves, which may progress to widening of the QRS complex and ventricular arrhythmias). Causes include ↓ intake, intracellular shifting, or ↑ excretion. Catecholamines (epinephrine, isoproterenol, terbutaline, and ritrodrine) shift serum K^+ intracellularly. Anesthesiologists should be aware of those patients receiving these drugs as tocolytics, bronchodilators, or as agents for cardiovascular support. Treatment includes correcting underlying etiology and replacing the K^+ deficit. PO doses are typically administered in 20 mEq doses BID-TID. IV infusion rates should not exceed 10 mEq/h (if concentration is >2.5 mEq/L); 40 mEq/h (if concentration <2.5 mEq/L); 1 mEq IV bolus, repeated as needed, if T wave flattening or U waves. Rapid IV K^+ infusion mandates continuous EKG monitoring. Outcome studies do not suggest ↑ perioperative morbidity or mortality for K^+ > or = 2.6 mEq/L.
- Hyperkalemia >5.0 mEq/L. Symptoms may include skeletal muscle weakness and SOB, cardiac toxicity from rapid ventricular repolarization (early EKG changes include peaked T waves, prolongation of the PR interval; may progress to widening of the QRS complex, and potentially VF and asystole). Causes include transcellular shifts: acidosis related to reperfusion of vascular beds that were previously ischemic (tourniquets, cross-clamping), medications, hypoventilation; ↓ renal excretion. Falsely ↑ serum $[K^+]$ (pseudohyperkalemia) may occur when intracellular K^+ leaks from hemolyzed cells following venipuncture. Treatment depends on the severity. Severe hyperkalemia (K^+ > 7.0 mEq/L, or EKG changes) is life-threatening emergency and requires urgent treatment. Cell membrane stabilization: 10 mL of 10% calcium gluconate over 2–3 min. Intracellular shifting: IV insulin (10–20 unit push) coadministered with 25–50 g of dextrose, IV bicarbonate (1 ampule), and IV or inhaled β-2 agonists. Removal: loop diuretics, cation exchange resins (sodium polystyrene sulfonate), dialysis (renal failure, or failure of other first-line therapies).

Pharmacokinetics

- After filtration at the glomerulus, 90% is reabsorbed in the PCT or collecting duct.
- Major site of K^+ *regulation* is the DCT where secretion is regulated by high urinary flow rates, hyperkalemia, and aldosterone

Cautions/Adverse Reactions

- Rapid peripheral IV infusion may cause intense pain on injection and local phlebitis.

Calcium

Clinical Uses/Relevance to Anesthesiology

• Essential for bone formation and neuromuscular function
• Critical for cardiac pacemaker activity and generation of the cardiac action potential
• Regulatory role in neurotransmitter and hormone activity, BP, enzymatic reactions
• Hyperkalemia treatment
• Hypotension treatment
• Magnesium toxicity in preeclampsia or eclampsia

Pharmacodynamics

• Normal ionized $[Ca^{++}]$: 1.1–1.4 mmol/L (4.5–5.6 mg/dL); normal total $[Ca^{++}]$: 2.2–2.6 mmol/L (9–10.5 mg/dL)
• Exists in the body in 3 states: bound to albumin, ionized (physiologically active form), and unionized and chelated with phosphate, sulfate, and citrate
• Extracellular ionized Ca^{++} can be measured directly. If unionized concentration is measured, should be interpreted with consideration of the plasma albumin (abnormally low plasma albumin results in falsely low unionized serum Ca^{++} levels). A commonly used formula is as follows:

$$\text{Corrected Ca++ (mg/dL)} = \text{Measured total Ca++ (mg/dL)} + 0.8(4.0 - \text{serum albumin level [g/dL]})$$

• Bone serves as an acid-base buffer. As a result, an ↑ in H+ in the body will bind to bone, displacing the Ca^{++} cation into the blood stream.
• Hypocalcemia: <1.1 mmol/L (4.5 mg/dL), or a total $[Ca^{++}]$ < 2.2 mmol/L (9 mg/dL). Symptoms of AMS, tetany, laryngospasm, hypotension; EKG changes include prolongation of the QT interval and heart block. Causes include hereditary or acquired hypoparathyroidism, poor vitamin D intake, alkalosis, ARF, acute hyperventilation, rapid infusion of blood preserved with citrate, Mg^{++} abnormalities. Acute treatment: Calcium gluconate 2 grams IV followed by infusion of 6 g in 500 ml D5W over 4–6 h. Long-term management involves correction of the underlying disorder and oral calcium and vitamin D supplementation.
• Hypercalcemia: >1.4 mmol/L (5.6 mg/dL) or a total $[Ca^{++}]$ > 2.6 mmol/L (10.5 mg/dL). Symptoms include GI effects (nausea, anorexia), CNS changes (stupor, ↓ mental status), and renal effects (polyuria, renal calculi, renal failure). EKG changes include shortened PR and QT intervals and widening of the QRS complex. May be caused by hyperparathyroidism, malignancy, acidosis (renal disease often results in slow "leeching" of bone, and osteoporosis or weakening), or thiazide diuretic therapy. Acute treatment involves diuretics (to excrete),

and IV fluid hydration (to dilute) serum Ca^{++}. Bone resorption can be inhibited with the use of pamidronate, plicamycin, and calcitonin. Glucocorticoids lower serum Ca^{++} levels through several mechanisms and are particularly effective in hypercalcemia associated with malignancy

- IV preparations: calcium gluconate has less tissue necrosis than calcium chloride if extravasated. Both are supplied as 100 mg/mL.
- PO preparations: calcium acetate or carbonate preferred with CRF. Provides a source of Ca^{++} and able to sequester phosphate in the intestine by forming insoluble phosphates that are excreted focally. Calcium carbonate may partially correct metabolic acidosis as well

Pharmacokinetics

- Excreted in the feces, urine, sweat glands. In the kidneys, ionized Ca^{++} is filtered by the glomerulus and then reabsorbed in the PCT, TAL, and the DCT
- Low Ca^{++} levels stimulate PTH release (causes Ca^{++} reabsorption in the kidney, GI tract, and bone)
- Poorly absorbed in the GI tract

Phosphorous

Role of Electrolyte in Body

- Stores and releases energy through high-energy bonds such as those in ATP and creatine phosphate
- Essential component of second-messenger systems such as cAMP
- Major component of nucleic acids, cell membranes, and phospholipids
- Promotes release of oxygen from hemoglobin as part of 2,3-diphosphoglycerate

Pharmacodynamics

- Normal serum phosphorus levels: 2.7–4.5 mg/dL
- Hypophosphatemia: <2.7 mg/dL. Symptoms include weakness, respiratory failure, confusion, stupor, seizures, and erythrocyte and leukocyte dysfunction. Caused by ↓ GI uptake, ↑ renal excretion, or transcellular shifts. In the perioperative setting, may result from acute respiratory alkalosis, malabsorption, refeeding after malnutrition, and alcohol abuse. Severe symptomatic hypophosphatemia should be treated with IV phosphate replacement, available as either sodium phosphate or potassium phosphate (15 mmol/250 ml D5W). An infusion of 0.08–0.16 mmol/kg should be administered over 6 h. Phosphate levels should be checked after initial infusion and repeat doses can be given if serum phosphate concentrations remain below 1.5 mg/dL. Mild asymptomatic hypophosphatemia can be treated with oral supplementation, available as Neutra-Phos (250 mg elemental phosphorus, 7 mEq sodium, and 7 mEq

potassium per capsule) or Neutra-Phos K (250 mg elemental phosphorus and 14 mEq potassium per capsule).

- Hyperphosphatemia >4.5 mg/dL. Symptoms are related to hypocalcemia and include ectopic calcification in skin and soft tissue, blood vessels, cornea, and kidneys. Can be caused by tissue damage or cell death (rhabdomyolysis or tumor lysis syndrome), renal failure, acidosis, and hypoparathyroidism. May result in severe hypocalcemia from ↓ calcitriol production, which leads to ↓ absorption of Ca^{++} in the GI tract. Additionally, phosphate can precipitate with Ca^{++} in the serum (further ↓ Ca^{++} levels). Ectopic calcification can occur as a result of phosphate-calcium precipitates. Treatment involves ↓ dietary phosphate intake and administration of oral phosphate binders such as calcium carbonate, aluminum hydroxide, and sevelamer. The goal of therapy is to maintain serum phosphorus levels between 4.5 and 6.0 mg/dL and the calcium-phosphorus product < 60.

Pharmacokinetics

- Largely unregulated absorption occurs through the duodenum and jejunum
- Approximately 90% of phosphate in the body is stored in bone
- Excreted in the GI tract and in the urine. Once in the kidneys, phosphate is filtered by the glomerulus and reabsorbed in the PCT by passive cotransport with Na^+
- PTH inhibits phosphate reabsorption in the kidney and promotes excretion in the GI tract

Clinical Case Scenario #1

A 76-year-old man undergoing transurethral resection of the prostate under spinal anesthesia becomes progressively confused and obtunded one hour into the procedure. An emergency serum chemistry panel shows a sodium concentration of 119 mEq/L.

Background: The patient has hyponatremia, likely from TURP syndrome.

Pathophysiology: The absorption of irrigating fluids, typically glycine, from the venous plexuses in the prostate leads to water overload and a hypotonic hyponatremia.

Treatment: The procedure should be stopped as soon as possible. A loop diuretic such as furosemide can be used to decrease extracellular fluid volume. Administer normal saline to correct serum sodium at a rate of 0.6–1 mEq/h. Hypertonic saline may be used in severe cases of hyponatremia with neurologic symptoms.

Clinical Case Scenario #2

A 47-year-old woman is admitted to the ward following an uneventful total thyroidectomy. The following morning she develops numbness and tingling in her hands bilaterally. Morning labs show an ionized calcium level of 0.74 mmol/L.

Background: The patient has hypocalcemia from inadvertent resection of parathyroid glands during her thyroidectomy.

Pathophysiology: The parathyroid glands, by secreting PTH, control calcium homeostasis. Normally, blood flow to the four glands is preserved during a thyroidectomy. If the parathyroid glands are removed or the blood supply is disrupted, hypocalcemia from an unintentional parathyroidectomy may result.

Treatment: Acutely, calcium gluconate should be administered intravenously. Once calcium levels have stabilized, oral calcium and vitamin D supplementation should be instituted.

References

1. Kaye AD, Kucera IJ. Intravascular fluid and electrolyte physiology. In: Miller RD, ed., *Miller's Anesthesia.* 6th ed. Philadelphia, PA: Elsevier; 2005: 1763–1798.

2. Prough DS, Wolf SW, Funston JS, et al. Acid-base, fluids, and electrolytes, In: Barash PG, Cullen BF, Stoelting RK, eds., *Clinical Anesthesia.* 5th ed. Philadelphia, PA: Lippincott Williams & Wilkins; 2006: 175–207.

3. Singer G. Fluid and electrolyte management. In: Ahya SN, Flood K, Pranjothi S, eds., *The Washington Manual of Therapeutics.* 30th ed. Philadelphia, PA: Lippincott Williams & Wilkins; 2001: 43–75.

4. Ives HE. Diuretic agents. In: Katzung BG, ed., *Basic & Clinical Pharmacology.* 9th ed. New York: McGraw-Hill; 2004: 241–258.

5. Singer GG, Brenner BM. Fluid and electrolyte disturbances. In: Fauci AS, Braunwald E, Kasper DL, et al., eds., *Harrison's Principles of Internal Medicine.* 17th ed. http://accessmedicine.com/content.aspx?aID=2868132.

6. Oh M, Carrol H. Disorders of sodium metabolism: hypernatremia and hyponatremia. *Crit Care Med.* 1992;20:94.

7. Tanifuji Y, Eger EI. Brain sodium, potassium, and osmolarity: effects on anesthetic requirement. *Anesth Analg.* 1978;57:404.

8. Halperin ML, Kamel KS. Potassium. *Lancet.* 1998;352:158.

9. Soni N. Electrolytes solutions and colloids. In: Evers AS, Maze, M, eds., *Anesthetic Pharmacology: Physiological Principles and Clinical Practice.* Philadelphia, PA: Elsevier; 2004: 751–762.

10. Micromedex. www.micromedex.com. Last accessed September 30, 2010.

11. Gennari FJ. Hypokalemia. *N Engl J Med.* 1998;339:451.

12. Kuvin JT. Electrocardiographic changes of hyperkalemia. *N Engl J Med.* 1998;338:662.

13. Ariyan CE, Sosa JA. Assessment and management of patients with abnormal calcium. *Crit Care Med.* 2004;32:S146.

14. Weisinger JR, Bellorini-Font E. Magnesium and phosphorus. *Lancet.* 1998;352:391.

15. Peppers MP, Geheb M, Desai T. Hypophosphatemia and hyperphosphatemia. *Crit Care Clin.* 2001;7:201.

Chapter 18.2

Sodium Bicarbonate

Nina Singh-Radcliff, MD

Clinical Uses/Relevance to Anesthesiology

- Treatment of hyperkalemia
- Alkaline diuresis hastens secretion of drugs (salicylates and TCAs) and may protect kidneys in rhabdomyolysis, hemolysis, and transfusion reactions
- Potentially renoprotective against contrast induced nephropathy (CIN) in patients with impaired renal function
- Alkalinization of local anesthetics
- Controversial efficacy in metabolic acidosis. Usually reserved for pH <7.1
- Plasma-expanding properties; maybe useful in HD shock.
- Rapid antacid action in stomach when taken PO

Pharmacodynamics

- Hyperkalemia. By reducing extracellular pH, provides a driving force/gradient for H^+ ion to flow out of the cell via the H^+/K^+ membrane exchanger to maintain homeostasis; results in K^+ *shifting* intracellularly (from intravascular and extracellular compartments). Does not reduce total body K^+
- Alkalinizes urine. Bicarbonate is filtered by the glomerulus as well as secreted into the tubules to maintain pH homeostasis. When acidic drugs bind to HCO_3^- in the renal tubules, drugs become charged and are unable to be reabsorbed into the bloodstream, allowing excretion via the urine (TCAs, salicylates, cocaine, amphetamines, quinine).
- Rhabdomyolysis and hemolysis can cause myoglobinuria and ARF. Urine alkalinization may reduce crystallization of myoglobin and uric acid within renal tubules (which can cause sludging, reduced GFR) and myoglobin's conversion to ferrihemate (nephrotoxic and occurs with pH <5.6). Rhabdomyolysis is also associated with acidemia (lactic acidosis from ischemia and uremia) and hyperkalemia (from lysis of cells), for which NaHCO3 can be helpful
- Alkalinizes local anesthetics. Uncharged LA can cross lipid bilayer of cell and access intracellular sodium receptor. Decreases time to onset and Cm as well as increases pH and reduces sting/pain with SQ injection.

- Acidemic states reduce inotropy and responsiveness to catecholamines and vasopressors. Non-gap acidosis results from loss/dilution of HCO_3^- (dilution with NaCl [>2 L], loss during diarrhea, renal tubular acidosis, hyperalimentation, acetazolamide tx, ureteroenteric fistula). Tx includes correction of primary cause, and $NaHCO_3$. Gap acidosis results from unmeasured cations or titratable acids (produced during DKA, alcohol abuse, toxins, anaerobic metabolism [lactic acidosis], and when not cleared during uremia). Tx includes correction of underlying cause; $NaHCO_3$ is controversial. $Na^+ + HCO_3^- + H^+ \longleftrightarrow H_2O + CO_2$ via carbonic anhydrase. Requires adequate ventilation to excrete CO_2 to prevent respiratory acidosis.

Pharmacokinetics

- 100 mEq of $NaHCO_3$ produces 2.24 L of CO_2; equivalent to 10 minutes of CO_2 production.
- Rapid bolus can cause transient fall in MAP, rise in ICP; can be alleviated by slow IV infusion.
- Excess $NaHCO_3$ can increase the nonionized fraction of basic drugs (opioids, local anesthetics); results in increased ability to cross lipid membranes to site of action and hence activity
- Antacid is highly soluble in stomach, short in duration. Increased urine pH, however, may last >24 hours and affect renal elimination of drugs.

Side Effects/Adverse Reactions

- Additives may be incompatible (norepinephrine and dobutamine)
- Hypernatremia (1 ampule contains 44.6–50 mEq Na^+); Na^+ retaining states (CHF, pulmonary edema, cirrhosis) can be exacerbated. Can reduce renin/aldosterone production.
- Hyperosmolality (1 ampule contains 90–100 mOsm)—can cause AMS
- Hypercapnia (1 ampule can produce ~1.12 L of CO_2, equivalent to 5 minutes of CO_2 production)—can cause increased ICP, AMS
- Hypokalemia—arrhythmias, exacerbate effects of digoxin
- Chronic alkalinization of gastric fluid can increase susceptibility to various acid sensitive bacilli; urine alkalinization may predispose individual to UTIs or urolithiasis.
- Urinary alkalinization may decrease levels of lithium, tetracyclines, chlorpropamide, methotrexate, and salicylates; increase levels of amphetamines pseudoephedrine, flecainide, mecamylamine, ephedrine, quinidine, and quinine
- Other physiologic effects: left shift in oxy-Hg curve, accelerated lactate production, CSF acidosis.

Dosages/Preparation

- 7.5% solution contains 0.9 mEq/mL of Na^+ and HCO_3^-, 44.6 mEq/ampule, 2 mOsm/mL.
- 8.4% solution contains 1 mEq/mL of Na^+ and HCO_3^-, 50 mEq/ampule 1.79 mOsm/mL.

- 4.2% suggested for <3 months (hyperosmolarity can cause IVH)
- Hyperkalemia – 1 ampule over 5 minutes (44.6–50 mEq).
- Metabolic acidosis – [0.3 x kg x {desired HCO_3 _ measured HCO_3}] = bicarbonate dose in mEq (0.3 assumes a 30% treatable body compartment [~21 L]). Administer half of calculated dose over 30 min to allow for time for equilibration into the extracellular compartment, and maneuvers to treat increased CO_2 production. Reassess ABG to guide management (pH, HCO_3^-, BE).
- Protection against CIN (unlabeled use)—154 mEq/L of NaHCO3 in D5W, with an initial infusion of 3 ml/kg/h one hour prior to contrast bolus, 1ml/kg/h for 6 h post procedure.
- Local anesthetics: typically 1 cc $NaHCO_3$: 10 cc lidocaine.
- 1 ampule $NaHCO_3$ is added to 1 L of 0.45 NS or D5W and infused at 200–400 mL/h IV for myoglobinuria 20–60 mEq/h); titrate urine pH >6
- Perform ABG, [K+] prior to initiation of NaHCO3 therapy, if possible.

Clinical Case Scenario

A 48-year-old male, 80 kg, is undergoing a right nephrectomy for tumor. After 1400 mL of EBL, the pt was given 2500 mL of crystalloid, and an ABG was ordered and revealed a pH of 7.14, pCO_2 39, pO_2 458, HCO_3^- 16, BE -13.2, Hct 7.3. The pt is requiring increasing doses of phenylephrine and ephedrine.

Background: The pt presents with severe metabolic acidosis likely from hypovolemia and anemia.

Pathophysiology: The metabolic acidosis is likely a gap acidosis due to lactic acid from anaerobic metabolism due to hypovolemia and anemia.

Treatment: Correct underlying disorder by administering fluids and pRBCs. Temporize with vasopressors until underlying cause is corrected. Reassess volume status and consider attaining repeat ABG to guide further treatment.

Alternative: Consider $NaHCO_3$ Calculate HCO_3^- deficit. Dose (mEq)= 0.3 x 80 kg x (24–16) = 192 mEq. Administer half of deficit (96 mEq), and repeat ABG. Continue treating underlying disorder

References

1. Proudfood AT, Krenzelok EP, Vale JA. Position paper on urine alkalinization. *J Toxicol Clin Toxicol.* 2004;42(1):1–26.
2. Bagley WH, Yang H, Shah KH. Rhabdomyolysis. *Intern Emerg Med.* 2007;2(3):210–218.
3. Tamura A, Goto Y, Miyamoto K, Naono S, Kawano Y, Kotuku M, Watanabe T, Kadota J. Efficacy of single-bolus administration of sodium bicarbonate to prevent contrast-induced nephropathy in patients with mild renal insufficiency undergoing an elective coronary procedure. *Am J Cardiol.* 2009;104(7):921–925.
4. Forsythe SM, Schmidt GA. Sodium bicarbonate for the treatment of lactic acidosis. *Chest.* 2000;17(1):260–267.

Chapter 19

Diuretics

Tygh Wycoff, MD and John G. Augoustides, MD

Normal Renal Tubule/Nephron Function

- Renal Corpuscle (comprised of glomerulus and Bowman's capsule). In the cortex, afferent arterioles form glomerular capillaries; they are compact and are also permeable to water, electrolytes, and metabolites of drugs and toxins (not proteins). These substances are "driven" out, or "filtered," from the capillaries by hydrostatic forces (charge and size also influence movement) into the surrounding Bowman's capsule to form "filtrate," or urine. Efferent arterioles, located distal to the renal corpuscle, regulate the filtration fraction by dilating or constricting. GFR is used to measure renal function; it is the rate (volume/time) at which blood is filtered through *all* glomeruli.

- Proximal Convoluted Tubule (PCT). Receives filtrate from the Bowman's capsule and delivers it to the Loop of Henle. The luminal surface contains microvilli that $\uparrow$ the surface area for reabsorption ("brush border"). The PCT is responsible for ~70% of Na^+ (via a Na^+/K^+ ATPase antiporter) as well as significant water, urea, organic acid, H^+, HCO_3^-, and phosphate (PTH dependent) reabsorption.

- Loop of Henle. As the PCT enters the hyperosmotic medulla, it becomes narrower, and forms the Loop of Henle, which will reenter the cortex as the thick ascending limb (TAL) and traverse back near the glomerulus. Electrolytes are actively transported out of the lumen to create a concentration gradient in the renal medulla

- Thick Ascending Limb (TAL). The Loop of Henle reenters the cortex as the TAL. It is water impermeable, but Na^+, K^+, and Cl^- cross via the Na-K-2Cl symporter (~25% Na^+ reabsorbed here). Additionally, K^+ transport creates a positive electrochemical gradient within the lumen (provides the driving force for divalent cations, Ca^{++}, Mg^{++}, to flow out of the lumen to be reabsorbed).

- Distal Convoluted Tubule (DCT). From the TAL, urine enters the DCT, where aldosterone affects $[Na^+]$ and $[K^+]$, PTH affects $[Ca^{++}]$, and pH homeostasis occurs. Vasopressin receptors are located here as well

- Collecting Duct. Receives filtrate from the DCT and delivers it to the ureters. Final nephron segment where fluid and electrolyte balance take place (~5% of Na$^+$ reabsorption; 5%-25% of water reabsorption depending on fluid status). ADH is secreted by the posterior pituitary in response to osmolality, volume status, and abnormal states such as SIADH. ADH $\uparrow$ water permeability in the collecting ducts (water flows down an osmotic gradient into the hyperosmotic renal medulla created by the countercurrent multiplier in the Loop of Henle). Aldosterone, a mineralocorticoid secreted by the adrenal cortex, is responsible for Na$^+$, K$^+$ regulation.

Mannitol

Clinical Use/Relevance to Anesthesiology

- $\downarrow$ ICP and IOP
- Renal protection for renal transplant surgery. When given prior to revascularization of a new renal graft, may result in $\downarrow$ incidence of acute kidney injury
- $\downarrow$ anuria or oliguria from large pigment loads to the kidney (eg, hemolysis or rhabdomyolysis)
- May provide renal protection (acute kidney injury) following CPB; controversial
- May provide renoprotection during aortic cross-clamping for AAA and thoracoabdominal aortic aneurysms; controversial
- Improved delivery of medications across blood-brain-barrier (BBB)
- Irrigating solution in TURPs ($\downarrow$ hemolytic effects of water)
- Cystic fibrosis; $\downarrow$ viscosity of mucus (clinical trials)

Pharmacodynamics

- Exogenous drug lacking appreciable metabolic, agonist, or antagonist effect. Osmotic and free radical scavenging properties are harnessed for therapeutic purposes.
- Acute $\downarrow$ of ICP by generation of osmotic gradient across an intact BBB. Draws intracellular water from brain parenchyma into the vasculature, which is then excreted by the kidneys. If BBB is disrupted, mannitol may enter the brain and paradoxically $\uparrow$ brain osmolality and ICP.
- Additionally, assists with transport of drugs across the BBB (high molarity injected into the intracarotid artery). Shrinks the BBB endothelial cells (water flows into vasculature; down osmotic gradient), stretching the tight junctions between them, and thereby creating "gaps" within 5 mins, and up to 30 mins after injection. During this time, drugs that are injected into the carotid artery can more easily diffuse through these gaps and enter into the brain (chemotherapeutic, Alzheimers)

- After filtration by the glomerulus, does not get reabsorbed or secreted into the bloodstream and will draw water into the descending limb of the Loop of Henle and the proximal collecting tubule (osmotically)
- Also ↑ urine volume and flow rate (rhabdomyolysis, excretion of toxins, uricemia) and ↓ Na^+ reabsorption time in the descending limb and collecting duct. "Opposes" the action of ADH in the collecting tubule; antagonizes effect, not receptor binding.
- Improves blood flow during ischemia. ↓ renal endothelial cell swelling, thereby ↑ the vessel diameter. May also have free radical scavenging properties.
- Currently being looked at for the treatment of CF and bronchiectasis. When orally inhaled as a dry powder, osmotically draws water into the lungs, thereby thinning the thick, viscous mucus seen in CF. May facilitate coughing the expectorant during physiotherapy

Pharmacokinetics

- Available as 5%, 10%, 15%, 20%, and 25% IV solutions
- No metabolism. Filtered by the glomerulus within 30–60 min
- ICP reduction: Onset 10–15 min; Duration: ~ 2 h (doses > 2 g/kg can prolong the duration, but do not further ↓ ICP). If dose is repeated, titrate to keep serum osmolality <320 mOsm/L
- ARF + oliguria: 0.25–2 g/kg infusions over 2–6 h
- Pediatric ICP/IOP reduction: 1–2 g/kg.

Cautions/Adverse Reactions

- Vascular smooth muscle dilation may cause transient hypotension; immediate
- Rapid expansion of the intravascular compartment via osmotic gradient drawing water from ECF and ICF compartments. Acute heart failure decompensation and florid pulmonary edema can occur.
- Hyponatremia from initial fluid shifts into vasculature (dilution). Hypernatremia may eventually result from potent water diuresis in excess of natriuresis
- Dehydration from excessive use of osmotic diuretics without water replacement
- Rebound intracranial hypertension may occur from a rapid ↓ in serum osmolality or accumulation in neurons and glia
- Hypokalemia from urinary excretion. During craniotomy, concurrent hyperventilation and intracellular K^+ shifting may compound effects.

Urea

- Use as an osmotic diuretic has fallen out of favor due to its ability to enter brain parenchyma and potentially increase ICP; also metabolized. Most common current use is topically on the skin for atopic dermatitis, psoriasis, and eczema.

- Available as 30% IV solution in D5W or D10W. ICP/IOP reduction: 0.5–1.5 g/kg administered as a slow IV infusion.
- Pediatric ICP dosing: 500–1500 mg/kg administered as slow IV infusion.

Loop Diuretics (Furosemide, Bumetanide, Torsemide)

Clinical Use/Relevance to Anesthesiology

- Chronic HTN; ↓ intravascular volume
- CHF; improves systemic and pulmonary edema.
- Edema ↓ in chronic kidney disease
- Promotes rapid diuresis. Ascites, cadaveric renal transplant (↓ injury to the new graft)
- Prevents anuria or oliguria from large pigment loads to the kidney (eg, hemolysis or rhabdomyolysis)
- Hypercalcemia, hyperkalemia, certain toxins; facilitates excretion renally
- ↓ ICP and IOP
- Hypercalcemia treatment

Pharmacodynamics

- Secreted into the renal tubule from the vasculature at the proximal tubule; competitive antagonist at the Cl^- binding site of luminal Na-K-Cl symporters in the TAL. Prevents Na^+ and Cl^- reabsorption, ↑ UOP, and ↓ blood volume.
- Effective diuretic because the TAL has a high Na^+ reabsorptive capacity (~25% of filtered Na^+ load) and distal segments cannot completely reabsorb the ↑ Na^+ load delivered to them.
- Divalent cations, Mg^{++}, Ca^{++}, also are prevented from being reabsorbed. Their reabsorption is dependent on the positive electrical potential that is generated in the tubule by K^+ via the Na-K-Cl symporter.
- Countercurrent exchange is impaired; Na^+, Cl^-, Mg^{++}, Ca^{++} reabsorption is prevented, further reducing the nephron's ability to concentrate urine
- Weakly inhibit carbonic anhydrase in the proximal tubule
- Effective in CHF to ↓ fluid overload. The body initially compensates to a ↓ CO, which results in ↓ renal blood flow, by retaining Na^+ and water via the renin-angiotensin system in order to ↑ cardiac filling pressures. However, this compensatory response becomes maladaptive when the pulmonary vasculature becomes congested or when cardiac function becomes impaired from poor oxygenation and ↑ right ventricular afterload
- Independent from their diuretic activity, vasodilatory effects also ↑ flow in several vascular beds including the lungs

Cautions/Adverse Reactions

- Electrolyte disturbances: hyponatremia, hypochloremia, hypokalemia, hypomagnesemia, hypocalcemia
- Dehydration
- Metabolic alkalosis.
- Concurrent renal disease or NSAIDS may ↓ loop diuretic efficacy
- Dose-related hearing loss; typically reversible. ↑ in pts with impaired renal function, or taking ototoxic drugs (aminoglycosides)
- Hyperuricemia may result from volume depletion and cause gouty attack in susceptible patients

Furosemide

Pharmacodynamics

- Coadministered with mannitol to ↓ ICP. Mannitol establishes an osmotic gradient across the BBB and ↑ intravascular volume; furosemide is capable of rapidly excreting the volume load.
- Inhibits compensatory volume-restoring mechanisms by blocking Cl⁻ channels in the cell membranes of neurons and glia

Pharmacokinetics

- IV onset: 5–20 min; PO onset: 40 min, bioavailability 60%
- Duration: PO 6 h
- Elimination 1 h (9 h ESRD).

Dose

- IV: available in 10 mg/mL solution
- PO: available in 20 mg, 40 mg, 80 mg tablets. PO is equivalent to ½ IV dosing (eg, 40 mg PO equal to 20 mg IV)
- ↓ICP: 0.5–1 mg/kg IV bolus; coadministration of mannitol may ↓ dosage for both drugs
- CHF/pulmonary edema: 20–40 mg IV BID; titrate by ↑ 20 mg/dose
- Hyponatremia from TURP, irrigation absorption: 10–20 mg IV initial dose (higher depending on severity), titrate to effect (volume status, electrolytes)
- Renal Transplant: 20–40 mg IV
- Hypercalcemia 20–40 mg; must be coadministered with IV fluids to avoid dehydration
- Hyperkalemia: 10–20 mg IV
- Pediatric dosing: CHF/pulmonary edema 1 mg/kg/dose q8–24 h

CHAPTER 19 Diuretics

Side Effects

- Neuromuscular blockade. ↑ intensity and duration. Likely a result of ↓ Ach production caused by an inhibition of ATP breakdown
- Tolerance with chronic use; likely from compensatory hypertrophy of distal tubule and collecting duct

Bumetanide

- More potent and complete absorption as well as ↓ individual bioavailability compared to furosemide. May be more effective in patients with renal insufficiency
- In 2008 NFL players suspended for steroid use were utilizing bumetanide to lower concentration of filtered substances in urine (attempted to hide). Also has been found to be an undisclosed ingredient in weight loss supplements.
- Renally metabolized. 97% protein binding
- IV: Available in 0.25 mg/mL solution. Onset 5 mins; half-life 60–90 minutes
- PO: Available 0.5 mg, 1 mg, 2 mg tablets. Onset 40 mins, duration 4 h
- CHF/edema: 0.5–1 mg q 2–3 hours, max 10mg/day
- Pediatric: not FDA-approved in children <18 years of age

Torsemide

- More prolonged effect, with less K⁺ loss and ototoxicity than furosemide.
- IV: available in 10 mg/mL solution. Onset: 5 min; half-life 2.2–3.8 h. Duration 4 h. Usual dose: 20 mg IV QD, double dose during titration up to max of 200mg/day.
- PO: available as 5 mg, 10 mg, 20 mg, 100 mg tablets. Bioavailability 85%; onset 40 min
- Safety and efficacy has not been established in children

Thiazide Diuretics (Hydrochlorothiazide)

Clinical Use/Relevance to Anesthesiology

- Chronic HTN; often 1st-line.
- Edema in CHF, ascites
- Nephrolithiasis from hypercalciuria; ↓ formation
- Nephrogenic DI; ↓ urine dilution in DCT and alleviates natriuresis
- Cheap, commonly utilized in developing world

Pharmacodynamics

- Secreted into the PCT from the bloodstream. Selectively inhibits Na-K-Cl transporters in the DCT and hinders Na⁺, Cl⁻ reabsorption (results in natriuresis, ↑ UOP, ↓ blood volume)
- Kaliuresis. Enhanced Na⁺/K⁺ exchange occurs in the distal tubule and collecting duct due to the high [Na⁺] in the tubule
- Calcium reabsorption is enhanced via the Na⁺/Ca⁺⁺ exchanger along the basolateral membrane of distal convoluted tubule epithelial cells. ↓ formation of

calcium-containing renal stones, ↑ total body Ca^{++} and bone mineral density, which may ↓ development of osteoporosis

- Renal prostaglandin synthesis is necessary for function and may be inhibited by concomitant use of NSAIDS.
- ↓ Hypertension-related morbidity and mortality is not well understood. Furthermore, the vasodilatory effect which persists after diuretic effect wears away is believed to be due to renal autoregulation, inhibition of carbonic anhydrase, or desensitization of vascular smooth muscles to Ca^{++}

Pharmacokinetics

- Rapidly absorbed from the gastrointestinal tract

Cautions/Adverse Reactions

- With prolonged administration, can cause a hypochloremic, hypokalemic metabolic alkalosis
- Hyperuricemia from competitive inhibition of uric acid secretion in the PCT and may precipitate attacks of gout in susceptible patients
- Hyperlipidemia; 5%-15% ↑ in low-density lipoproteins may occur
- Hyperglycemia; impaired insulin release and poor tissue utilization may be seen in diabetics or patients with impaired glucose tolerance
- Hyponatremia from ↑ ADH release and increased fluid intake can occur
- Hypokalemia with prolonged administration, or concomitant steroid use

Dose

- PO: available in 12.5 mg, 25 mg, 50 mg, and 100 mg tablets.
- HTN: 12.5–25 mg/day, titrate to maximum of 100 mg/day
- Edema: 50–100mg/day QD to BID
- Pediatric: 1–2 mg/kg

Potassium-Sparing Diuretics (Spironolactone, Triamterene, Amiloride)

Clinical Use/Relevance to Anesthesiology

- Hyperaldosteronism. Improvement in signs/symptoms from primary adrenal hypersecretion, ectopic ACTH production
- Edema from CHF, nephritic syndrome (secondary hyperaldosteronism)
- Ascites from hepatic cirrhosis
- Chronic HTN; intravascular volume depletion

Pharmacodynamics

- Weak diuretics

- ↓ production or function of Na⁺/K⁺ and Na⁺/H⁺ ion transporters
- Dependent on production of renal prostaglandins, similar to loop and thiazide diuretics. Efficacy of these drugs may be ↓ by patients taking NSAIDS

Cautions/Adverse Reactions

- Life-threatening hyperkalemia. ↑ risk in pts with renal disease, comcomitant use of K⁺-increasing drugs (beta-blockers, NSAIDS, ACE-inhibitors).
- Hyperchloremic metabolic acidosis may result from the inhibition of H⁺ secretion in the collecting tubules

Spironolactone

- Synthetic steroid; competitive aldosterone antagonist and blocks *production* of Na+/K+ and Na+/H+ cotransporters
- PO: available in 25 mg, 50 mg, or 100 mg tablets. Onset of action: several days. half-life ~ 1.4 h, effect may last for 2–3 days (result of mRNA-induced synthesis of Na⁺/K⁺ channels and Na⁺/H⁺ cotransporters)
- Edema (CHF, nephritic syndrome, hepatic cirrhosis): 25–200 mg QD-BID.
- Hyperaldosteronism: 100–400 mg QD. During surgery for adrenal adenomas, intraoperative hemodynamics may be better controlled when blood pressure and electrolytes are managed preoperatively with spironolactone
- Neonates: 0.5–1 mg/kg q8 h; pediatrics: 1–3 mg/kg q6–24 h
- Adverse effects: endocrine abnormalities such as gynecomastia, impotence, hirsutism, and benign prostatic hypertrophy

Triamterene

- Blocks Na⁺/K⁺ and Na⁺/H⁺ cotransporters
- PO: available in 50 mg, 100 mg tablets. GI absorption. half-life 3–5 h
- Edema (CHF, nephritic syndrome, cirrhosis): 100–150 mg PO BID
- Chronic HTN: 50–100mg PO QD-BID
- Pediatrics: 1–2 mg/kg PO BID; 1–4 mg/kg PO BID
- May cause megaloblastic anemia in pts with liver cirrhosis

Amiloride

- Blocks Na⁺/K⁺ and Na⁺/H⁺ contransporters
- PO: available 5 mg tablets. half-life 6–9 h
- Edema (CHF, nephrotic syndrome, hepatic cirrhosis): 5–20 mg QD
- Chronic HTN: 5–20 mg QD
- May cause glucose intolerance in diabetics
- Not FDA-approved in children

Carbonic Anydrase Inhibitors (Acetazolamide)

Clinical Use/Relevance to Anesthesiology

- Urine alkalinization/alkaline diuresis. Promotes clearance of certain drugs and harmful substances (myoglobin)
- ↓ IOP by reducing aqueous humor formation. Topical administration results in profound clinical effects without systemic side effects
- Metabolic alkalosis from bicarbonate depletion (diarrhea, overdiuresis). Useful when volume replacement may be contraindicated (CHF)
- Acute hyperphosphatemia
- Acute mountain sickness; improved signs and symptoms by ↓ CSF formation and pH

Pharmacodynamics

- Secreted from the bloodstream the PCT and inhibits carbonic anhydrase (carbonic acid cannot be converted to bicarbonate). Carbonic acid is charged and does not get reabsorbed.
- Aqueous humor and CSF quantity and pH reduction. Prevents ciliary body and choroidal plexus secretion of bicarbonate.
- Efficacy as a diuretic is ↓ after a few days of administration due to total-body sodium bicarbonate depletion and compensatory NaCl reabsorption in the nephron

Pharmacokinetics

- PO: rapid GI absorption; onset 30 min, peak 1–4 h, duration of action 12 h
- IV: onset 15 min
- half-life 4–8 h

Doses/Formulations

- PO: available in 125 mg, 250 mg, and 500 mg tablets
- IV: available in 500 mg powder that is typically dissolved in 10–50 mL NS or D5W.
- Glaucoma: 250–1000 mg/day divided into 2–4 doses
- Acute mountain sickness: 500–1000 mg/day divided into 2–4 doses
- Hyperphosphatemia: 500 mg q6 h
- Pediatric: acute mountain sickness 500–1000 mg QD, glaucoma 1–3 mg/kg q6–8 h, or 5–10 mg/kg q6 h

Cautions/Adverse Reactions

- Hypochloremic metabolic acidosis results from ↑ sodium bicarbonate excretion and necessitates frequent monitoring

- Nephrolithiasis may occur because of ↑ phosphate and calcium excretion
- Hypokalemia can result from bicarbonate-induced K^+ secretion into the collecting tubule
- In animal models, has been found to antagonize the effects of aniticholinesterases

Clinical Case Scenario #1

A 67 year-old female presents for resection of a right frontal lobe tumor after admission with nausea, vomiting, and slurred speech. Prior to coming to the OR, the neurosurgeon places a subarachnoid "bolt" that measures an ICP of 23 mm Hg.

Background: The patient has an increased ICP due to mass effect from the tumor.

Pathophysiology: Under normal conditions, the cranium is a fixed space that contains brain parenchyma, blood, and cerebrospinal fluid. When any one of these components is abnormally increased, pressure increases on other areas of the brain. If untreated, this may lead to brain herniation resulting in respiratory and/or cardiac arrest.

Treatment: ICP can be lowered by various methods including hyperventilation and the administration of steroids. Additionally, osmotic diuretics such as mannitol can reduce ICP by establishing an osmotic gradient that forces water from neurons and glia into the cerebral vasculature for excretion by the kidneys.

Clinical Case Scenario #2

A 39-year-old woman presents for laparoscopic resection of an adrenal adenoma. Her signs and symptoms include hypertension, weakness, and polyuria.

Background: The patient likely has an adrenal adenoma resulting in mineralocorticoid excess (Conn's syndrome). Primary aldosteronism generally occurs from a unilateral adenoma, although 25%-40% of patients are found to have bilateral adrenal hyperplasia.

Pathophysiology: Aldosterone, the major mineralocorticoid in humans, is secreted from cells in the adrenal cortex. The hormone causes sodium reabsorption and potassium excretion in the distal collecting tubules of the kidneys.

Treatment: Prior to resection, intravascular fluid volume and electrolytes should be restored to within normal limits. Spironolactone, an aldosterone antagonist, is effective in correcting sodium and potassium abnormalities, but can take 1–2 weeks to work completely. Furthermore, correction of serum potassium does not necessarily imply restoration of total-body deficits, which may range from 40 mEq to 400 mEq.

References

1. Cottrell JE, Robustelli A, Post K, et al. Furosemide- and mannitol-induced changes in intracranial pressure and serum osmolality and electrolytes. *Anesthesiology.* 1977;47:28.

2. Van Valenberg PLJ, Hoitsma AJ, Tiggeler RGWL, et al. Mannitol as an indispensable constituent of an intraoperative hydration protocol for the prevention of acute renal failure after renal cadaveric transplantation. *Transplantation.* 1987;44:784–788.

3. Ron D, Taitelman U, Michaelson M, et al. Prevention of acute renal failure in traumatic rhabdomyolysis. *Arch Intern Med.* 1984;144:277.

4. Ives HE. Diuretic agents. In: Katzung BG, ed., *Basic & Clinical Pharmacology.* 9th ed. New York: McGraw-Hill; 2004: 241–258.

5. Garwood S, Monk TG. Diuretics. In: Evers AS, Maze, M, eds., *Anesthetic Pharmacology: Physiological Principles and Clinical Practice.* Philadelphia, PA: Elsevier; 2004: 733–750.

6. Bendo AA, Kass IS, Hartung J, et al. Anesthesia for neurosurgery. In: Barash PG, Cullen BF, Stoelting RK, eds., *Clinical Anesthesia.* 5th ed. Philadelphia, PA: Lippincott Williams & Wilkins; 2006: 746–789.

7. Micromedex. www.micromedex.com. Last accessed September 30, 2010.

8. Gerber JG. Role of prostaglandins in the hemodynamic and tubular effects of furosemide. *Fed Proc.* 1983;42:1707–1710.

9. Kaye AD, Kucera IJ. Intravascular fluid and electrolyte physiology. In: Miller RD, ed., *Miller's Anesthesia.* 6th ed. Philadelphia, PA: Elsevier; 2005: 1763–1798.

10. Prough DS, Wolf SW, Funston JS, et al. Acid-base, fluids, and electrolytes, In: Barash PG, Cullen BF, Stoelting RK, eds., *Clinical Anesthesia.* 5th ed. Philadelphia, PA: Lippincott Williams & Wilkins; 2006: 175–207.

11. Kaissling B, Stanton BA. Adaptation of distal tubule and collecting duct to increased sodium delivery. I. Ultrastructure. *Am J Physiol.* 1985;248:F374-F381.

Antiarrhythmics

Chapter 20.1

Antiarrhythmics

Gaurav Malhotra, MD

- Prevent onset and progression to dangerous and possibly fatal arrhythmias as well as restoration of rhythm to normal sinus rhythm. Atrial fibrillation, atrial flutter, ventricular tachycardia, and ventricular fibrillation are commonly caused by heart disease (myocardial infarction, coronary artery disease and valvular disorders), cardiomyopathy, chronic medical illnesses (hypertension, diabetes, and hyperthyroidism), alcohol and drug abuse, excessive caffeine, and medications.

Pharmacodynamics

- Direct or indirect alteration to ion conductance, and hence action potentials across the cardiac myocyte.
- Classified into five main classes based primarily on which ion channels and currents they affect during the cardiac action potential
- **Class I** drugs affect Sodium (Na^+) channel; Phase 0
- **Class II** drugs are sympatholytic drugs that bind to beta-adrenoceptors and block binding of catecholamines such as epinephrine and norepinephrine
- **Class III** drugs affect Potassium (K^+) influx; Phase 1, 3
- **Class IV** drugs block calcium channel receptors and prevent the influx of Ca^{2+} into the cell; Phase 2
- **Class V** drugs work through miscellaneous mechanisms

Class I

- Block Na^+ channels and inhibit phase 0 depolarization. Lengthen both the action potential duration and the effective refractory period. Further classified into three subgroups (IA, IB, IC) based on their mechanism, duration of action, and affect on the Na^+ channel.

Class IA

- Inhibit fast Na^+ channels (Phase 0 depolarization), thereby slowing conduction. Also have moderate K+ channel blocking activity (slows rate of repolarization, prolongs action potential duration).

Quinidine

Clinical Uses

- Atrial fibrillation, atrial flutter to restore normal sinus rhythm.
- Life-threatening ventricular arrhythmias such as sustained ventricular tachycardia.
- Severe cases of *Plasmodium falciparum* malaria.

Pharmacodynamics

- Blocks the fast inward Na^+ current (delays phase 0 depolarization).
- Na^+ channel blockade is greater at increased heart rates, reduced at lower heart rates.

Pharmacokinetics

- Vd 2–3 L/kg; increased in cirrhosis, reduced in CHF
- Adults: 80%-90% of the drug is bound to plasma proteins; newborns: 50%-70% binding. Protein binding is decreased in cirrhosis, acute myocardial infarction, or cyanotic congenital heart disease.
- Metabolized hepatically via cytochrome P450 IIIA4 (mostly inactive compounds). Renally cleared.
- Elimination half-life 6–8 hours in adults, 3–4 hours in pediatric patients.

Side Effects

- Proarrhythmic effect that can be fatal, especially in patients with structural heart disease
- Prolongs the QT interval, which can lead to increased ventricular automaticity and polymorphic ventricular tachycardias, including Torsades de Pointes.
- Thrombocytopenia, granulomatous hepatitis, myasthenia gravis, and cinchonism (blurred vision, tinnitus, headache, psychosis) with drug toxicity. Patient occasionally can also have dizziness, dry mouth, urinary retention, nausea, and diarrhea.
- Inhibits cytochrome P450 2D6; can increase serum levels of lidocaine, beta blockers, opioids, and antidepressants.

Procainamide

Clinical Uses

- Supraventricular and ventricular arrhythmias; prevention and treatment
- Wolf-Parkinson-White syndrome treatment; lengthens the refractory period of the accessory pathway.

Pharmacodynamics

- Inhibits inward Na^+ current of fast Na^+ channels; also blocks outward K^+ current. This results in decreased myocardial excitability and increases the effective refractory period of the atria (and to a lesser extent the bundle of His-Purkinje system and ventricles of the heart).
- N-acetyl-procainamide (NAPA), a metabolite of procainamide has K^+ current blocking activity and thus prolongs cell repolarization.

Pharmacokinetics

- Vd is 2 L/kg for both adults and children; decreases in CHF, shock.
- 15%-20% plasma protein binding.
- Primarily metabolism hepatically to an active metabolite N-acetyl procainamide (NAPA).
- Excretion of drug and metabolite NAPA is primarily via the urine, with minimal fecal excretion.
- Elimination half-life is 2.5–4.5 hours in adults, 1.7 hours in children (NAPA elimination half-life ~2 times procainamide).

Side Effects

- Potentially fatal blood dyscrasias such as pancytopenia and agranulocytosis during the first three months of therapy, which requires regular CBC monitoring.
- Proarrhythmic effect in 3%-12% of patients, most commonly causing Torsades de Pointes.
- Chronic use can lead to development of a positive antinuclear antibody test in 50% of patients and may cause a drug induced lupus-like syndrome in 20%-30% of patients.
- Nonspecific systemic side effects such as nausea, vomiting, anorexia, headache, dizziness, insomnia, hallucinations, fever, rash, and myalgias.

Disopyramide

Clinical Uses

- Atrial and ventricular arrhythmias (suppression and prevention).
- Hypertrophic obstructive cardiomyopathy; medical management to suppress dangerous arrhythmias (lacks proarrhythmic risks).

Pharmacodynamics

- Decreases myocardial excitability and conduction velocity.
- Anticholinergic activity.
- Negative inotropic effects with up to 10% reduction of cardiac output, which can cause a reflexive increase in systemic vascular resistance.

Pharmacokinetics

- Vd is 1–2 L/kg.
- After PO intake, it is rapidly absorbed and reaches peak plasma levels usually within 2 hours.

- Metabolized to inactive metabolites in the liver by the CYP3A4 enzyme.
- Excreted primarily in the urine (40%-60%), with some fecal excretion (10%-15%).
- Mean elimination half-life of 6.7 hours.

Side Effects

- Anticholinergic side effects such as dry mouth (32%), urinary hesitancy (14%) and constipation (11%).
- Negative inotropic effects that causes a decrease in cardiac output and contractility, potentially leading to overt heart failure usually within the first three weeks of therapy.
- Rarely can cause hypoglycemia by increasing plasma insulin levels.
- Prolongs QT and can have proarrhythmic effects. If a preexisting 2nd or 3rd degree AV block is present, use of disopyramide can lead to complete heart block.

Class IB

- Blocks Na^+ channels (Phase 0), preventing inflow of Na^+ ions into the cardiac myocyte; shortens action potential and reduced refractoriness. Strong Na^+ channel blockers when the channel is in the inactivated state (during cell depolarization) and weak blockers when the channel is at rest (minimal effect at slower heart rates; more effective at faster heart rates such as tachyarrhythmias).

Lidocaine

- See "Local Anesthetics" chapter.

Tocainide

Clinical Uses

- Life-threatening ventricular arrhythmias.
- Trigeminal neuralgia, neuropathic pain (ameliorates pain).

Pharmacodynamics

- Primary analog of lidocaine.
- Suppresses automaticity of conduction tissue in the heart by blocking Na^+ channels and thus increasing the electrical stimulation threshold of the ventricle and His-Purkinje system.

Pharmacokinetics

- Vd is 2.5–3.5 L/kg.
- Does not undergo 1st-pass metabolism, unlike lidocaine.
- 2 enantiomers with the R isomer 4 times more potent than the S isomer.
- 10%–20% plasma protein binding.

- 30%-50% of the drug excreted unchanged by the kidneys. Remainder under-goes hepatic glucuronidation prior to renal excretion.
- Elimination half-life of 11 hours.

Side Effects

- Dizziness, loss of appetite, nausea/vomiting, tremor, and paresthesias.
- Blood dyscrasias such as agranulocytosis, bone marrow depression, leuko-penia, neutropenia, aplastic/hypoplastic anemia, thrombocytopenia, and se-quelae such as septicemia and septic shock have been reported.
- Interstitial pneumonitis within a few months of therapy (symptoms include exertional dyspnea, cough or wheezing, with bilateral infiltrates on chest x-ray). In most cases, symptoms remit after the medicine is discontinued.

Mexiletine

Clinical Uses

- Life-threatening ventricular arrhythmias.
- Refractory and chronic neuropathic pain; adheres to peripheral nerves and reduces pain signals carried to the central nervous system and brain.
- Diabetic neuropathy (experimental).
- Myotonia congenital (Thomsen disease) and myotonic dystrophy (Steinert's disease) muscle stiffness.

Pharmacodynamics

- Blocks Na^+ channels in the cardiac myocyte, decreasing the action potential duration by shortening the repolarization phase.

Pharmacokinetics

- Vd is 5–7 L/kg.
- Oral medication with minimal 1st-pass effect and is well absorbed.
- Peak plasma levels 2–3 hours.
- Plasma protein binding 50%-60%.
- Hepatically metabolized and renally excreted, with 10%-15% excreted as unchanged drug.

Side Effects

- Nausea, vomiting, lightheadedness, dizziness, tremor, numbness, and changes in sleeping habits.
- Truncal erythem and facial edema.
- Hypersensitivity syndrome, which is usually noted in Japanese males and pres-ents with fever, rash, eosinophilia, and elevated LFTs.
- Potent CYP1A2 inhibitor.
- Proarrhythmic effect; also a depressant effect on sinus node function and can cause sinus bradycardia or prolonged sinus node recovery time in patients.

Class IC

- Blocks open Na⁺ channels (depress the phase 0 depolarization) and slows conduction without having an effect on action potential duration. Dissociate slowly from the Na⁺ channels during diastole; thus have an increased effect at faster heart rates.

Flecainide

Clinical Uses

- Atrial fibrillation and supraventricular tachycardias such as AV nodal reentrant tachycardia and Wolff-Parkinson-White syndrome; suppression and treatment.
- Ventricular arrhythmias without acute ischemic injury.

Pharmacodynamics

- Inhibits Na⁺ channels and prolongs depolarization by slowing conduction at the AV node, His-Purkinje system, and the cardiac myocyte.
- At faster heart rates, has a greater effect on Na⁺ channels, and hence more effective in the treatment of tachyarrhythmias.

Pharmacokinetics

- Vd is 5–13 L/kg.
- PO form with minimal first pass metabolism and 85%-90% bioavailability.
- Rapid absorption with peak plasma concentration reached within 1.5–3 hours.
- Plasma proteing binding 40%-50%.
- Metabolized hepatically; excreted primarily by the kidneys (10%-50% as unchanged drug).
- Average elimination half-life of 20 hours; increased in heart failure or renal dysfunction.

Side Effects

- Proarrhythmic effect.
- Cardiac arrest, mortality in pts with structural heart disease such as recent history of MI, LVD (Cardiac Arrhythmia Suppression Trial (CAST). *N Engl J Med.* 1989;321:406–412)
- Profound bradycardia in pts with prior sinus node disease; due to its affect on the the AV node.
- Negative inotropic effect that can decrease ventricular EF, worsen heart failure.
- Nausea, vomiting, loss of appetite, dizzyness, headache, or blurry vision.

Propafenone

Clinical Uses

- Paroxysmal atrial fibrillation, atrial flutter, and other supraventricular arrhythmia treatment.
- Life-threatening ventricular arrhythmias.

Pharmacodynamics

- Blocks fast Na⁺ current channels and prolongs phase 0 depolarization of the cardiac myocyte.
- Exhibits some beta-blocking properties.

Pharmacokinetics

- Vd is 2–5 L/kg.
- PO medication, well absorbed; peak levels in 3.5 hours.
- Significant 1st-pass metabolism with a bioavailability of 3.4%-10.6%.
- Plasma protein binding 85%-90%.
- Metabolized primarily by the liver. 2 different metabolism groups: extensive metabolizer group, which comprises of 90% of the population, has an elimination half-life of 2–10 hours and the poor metabolizer group, which comprises 10% of the population, and an elimination half-life of 10–32 hours.

Side Effects

- Negative inotropic effects, especially in patients with reduced LV function.
- Proarrhythmic activity.
- Increases the PR and QRS intervals, leading to bundle branch block or increased level AV blockade.
- Dizziness, blurry vision, nausea, and loss of appetite.
- Lupus-like reaction and agranulocytosis.

Class II

- Competitively binds to beta-adrenoceptors, inhibiting binding of endogenous catecholamines; reduces sympathetic activity in the cardiac myocyte. Beta-blockers slow the automaticity of the sinus node and other cardiac pacemaker cells and increase the refractory period of the atrioventricular node, therefore acting as an antiarrhythmic for supraventricular tachycardias. These drugs usually block the β1 receptors in the heart and β2 receptors in the lungs, skeletal muscle, heart and blood vessels. See "Beta-Blockers."

Class III

- Blocks potassium channels and prolongs action potential duration, repolarization, and refractory period of the cardiac myocyte (Phase 1 and 3). They preferably bind to fast channels and therefore are more effective against reentrant tachycardia by selectively blocking the reentrant circuit.

Amiodarone

Clinical Uses

- Ventricular tachycardia.
- Ventricular fibrillation refractory to defibrillation; second-line after epinephrine.
- Atrial fibrillation/flutter and other supraventricular tachycardias.

Pharmacodynamics

- Possesses characteristics of all 4 classes. Inhibits sodium channels at rapid pacing frequencies (Class I); suppresses AV node via sympatholytic activity (Class II); blocks potassium channels, which prolongs the cardiac action potential (Class III); negative inotropy by blocking L-type calcium channels (Class IV).
- Negative inotropic effect results in peripheral vasodilation; opposite effects typically balance out but can occasionally result in hypotension.

Pharmacokinetics

- Available IV and PO. IV doses are given as a load, followed by a continuous infusion or intermittent doses. Oral absorption can be slow with onset of action within 2 to 3 weeks.
- Vd is 66 L/kg.
- 96% plasma protein binding.
- Metabolized hepatically via cytochrome CYP 2C8 and 3A4 to inactive metabolites.
- Long elimination half-life of 40–55 days.
- Excreted renally and focally; not dialyzable.

Dose

- Cardiac arrest: 300 mg IV rapid bolus (diluted in 20–30 mL NS or D5W).
- Arrhythmias (3 phase sequence): 150 mg IV over 10 minutes, followed by 360 mg IV over 6 hours, and then 450 mg/18 hours maintenance.

Side Effects

- Pulmonary toxicity and side effects: chronic interstitial pneumonitis (most common), acute respiratory distress syndrome (ARDS), penumonia, and lung nodules. Signs and symptoms include dyspnea, a productive cough, pleuritic chest pain, fever, and weight loss.
- Hyper or hypothyroidism. Significantly increases the iodine load, which can result in decreased T3 production.
- Neurological side effects include tremors, peripheral neuropathy, paresthesias, ataxia, and photosensitivity.
- Cardiac: bradycardia, heart failure, shock, or asystole. Proarrhythmic effect in 2%–3% of patients (usually Torsades de Pointes, occasionally ventricular fibrillation). Hypotension and bradycardia appear to be related to rate of infusion.

- Gastrointestinal side effects: nausea, vomiting, diarrhea, and anorexia. Elevation of aminotransferase (25% incidence). Symptomatic hepatitis (less than 3%; possible risk of progressing to cirrhosis or hepatic failure).
- Corneal microdeposits are commonly noted in patients. Risk of optic neuropathy and blindness after long-term use of this medication.
- Peripheral vein phlebitis (central line preferable); adsorbed into polyvinyl chloride bags and tubing.

Ibutilide

Clinical Uses
- Rapid conversion of atrial fibrillation and atrial flutter to sinus rhythm.
- Not approved for ventricular arrhythmias.

Pharmacodynamics
- Increases the action potential duration by activating the slow inward Na^+ current and thus increasing atrial and ventricular refractoriness.
- Blocks the inward potassium channels during phase 3, however its interaction with the potassium channels is complex and not completely understood.

Pharmacokinetics:
- IV formulation; onset of action within 90 minutes.
- Vd is 11 L/kg.
- 40% plasma protein binding.
- Metabolized hepatically by oxidation.
- Elimination half-life 6 hours. Excreted primarily by the kidneys, with 19% excreted in feces.

Side Effects
- Headache and nausea most commonly seen.
- Cardiac: Proarrhythmic side effects (Torsade de Pointes or other ventricular arrhythmias). Hypotension (2%), sinus bradycardia (1.2%), supraventricular tachycardia (2.7%), atrioventricular (1.5%), or bundle branch block (1.9%).

Dofetilide

Clinical Uses
- Supraventricular tachycardia and atrial fibrillation/flutter; treatment and prevention of recurrence after conversion to sinus rhythm.
- Life-threatening ventricular arrhythmias; prevention.
- Arrhythmias in postmyocardial infarction with LV dysfunction and in CHF.

Pharmacodynamics
- Selectively blocks the delayed rectifier outward potassium current in myocardial cells and therefore increases their refractory time.

Pharmacokinetics

- PO formulation; bioavailability of >90%.
- Vd is 3 L/kg.
- Peak plasma concentration within 2–3 hours and a steady state plasma level in 2–3 days.
- Plasma protein binding is 60%-70%.
- Elimination half-life of 10 hours and is metabolized in the liver by the CYP3A4 enzyme.
- Renal filtration and active tubular secretion; 80% is excreted in original form, with 20% metabolized to inactive metabolite that is renally cleared. Dose adjustment should be made based on CrCl.

Side Effects

- Cardiac: Torsades de Pointes; due to the increase in QT and QTc. Dose-related, variable: 0.3%-10.5% ventricular tachycardia or supraventricular tachycardia.
- Headache, chest pain, dizziness, nausea, diarrhea and insomnia are possible side effects.

Bretylium

Clinical Uses

- Ventricular tachycardia and ventricular fibrillation; treatment and prevention.

Pharmacodynamics

- Blocks inward flow of potassium current during phase 3 of the cardiac cell depolarization.
- Decreases the sympathetic outflow by blocking the release of noradrenaline from peripheral nerve terminals.

Pharmacokinetics

- IV: VF suppression within 2 minutes; VT suppression 20 min-2 hours.
- Elimination half-life ~ 7.8 hours
- Renally excreted as original compound. 70%-80% excreted within the first 24 hours.

Side Effects

- Postural hypotension (50%); may be associated with vertigo, lightheadedness, and syncope.
- Bradycardia, increased premature ventricular contractions, transient hypertension, and chest pain can be seen.
- Nausea and vomiting (3%). Diarrhea, abdominal pain, flushing and macular rash.

Sotalol

Clinical Uses

- Ventricular tachycardia, ventricular fibrillation; treatment and prevention of recurrence.
- Atrial fibrillation, atrial flutter; maintenance of sinus rhythm.
- Fetal supraventricular tachycardia.

Pharmacodynamics

- Sotalol is a recemic mixture of L and D isomers.
- The D-isomer blocks the inward flow of potassium current (phase 3) in the cardiac cells thereby prolonging repolarization.
- The L-isomer has beta-blocker activity and decreases atrioventricular conduction and slows sinus rate by around 25%.

Pharmacokinetics

- PO form: bioavailability of 90%-100%.
- Onset: 1–2 hours, with duration of 8–16 hours.
- Reaches peak plasma concentration in 2.5–4 hours and steady state level in 2–3 days.
- Vd is 1.2–2.4 L/kg.
- No plasma protein binding.
- Elimination half-life of 12 hours.
- Undergoes no metabolism and is excreted by the kidneys as unchanged drug.

Side Effects

- Cardiac: ventricular arrhythmias (particularly Torsades de Pointes from QT prolongation), bradycardia, bradyarrhythmias. May aggravate heart failure in patients with decreased ventricular function.
- Fatigue, dyspnea, dizziness, and anxiety are also seen.

Class IV

- Binds to L-type calcium channels on the cardiac myocyte, SA and AV nodes, and vascular smooth muscle; inhibits inflow of calcium ions into the cell. Results in a decreased HR, conduction velocity within the heart, and inotropy; as well as increased refractory period of the AV node. These properties make them good antiarrhythmic drugs, especially against supraventricular tachycardia. See Calcium Channel blockers.

Class V

- Consists of miscellaneous drugs.

Adenosine

Clinical Uses

- Supraventricular tachycardia, especially reentrant arrhythmias that use the AV node; treatment.
- Pharmacological stress during nuclear stress tests.

Pharmacodynamics

- Endogenously produced purine nucleoside that acts at adenosine receptor subtypes (A1, A2A, A2B, A3) that are G protein coupled.
- A1 receptor binding inhibits L-type calcium channels in cardiac tissue, decreasing conduction through the SA and AV nodes.
- A2 receptors binding results in vascular smooth muscle relaxation (dilation).
- Anti-inflammatory properties at A2A receptors.
- Inhibits release of norepinephrine by binding to adenosine receptors on sympathetic nerve terminals.

Pharmacokinetics

- Very rapid onset of action.
- Very brief duration of action with an elimination half-life of 10 seconds.
- Metabolized in blood and tissue to inosine, which is broken down into hypoxanthine and uric acid and excreted renally. Can also be salvaged to adenosine monophosphate.

Dose

- SVT treatment or diagnosis: 6 mg IV fast bolus; if no effect, 12 mg IV fast bolus 1–2 minutes after first dose; an additional 12 mg IV fast bolus 1–2 minutes (6–12–12).
- Stress test: 0.14 mg/kg/min for 5–6 minutes.

Side Effects

- Facial flushing, palpitations, chest pain, and hypotension are most common.
- Cardiac: can produce a transient 1st, 2nd, or 3rd degree AV block. More common when adenosine used as an infusion during cardiac stress tests. Can cause ventricular fibrillation when used in patients with Wolff-Parkinson-White.
- Respiratory: can cause dyspnea, chest tightness, hyperventilation, and bronchoconstriction in asthmatics if administered by inhalation.
- Can also cause headache, dizziness, blurry vision, numbness, diaphoresis, and metallic taste.

Digoxin

Clinical Uses

- Rate control for atrial fibrillation, atrial flutter, or rapid ventricular rates (reentrant).
- Mild-moderate heart failure.

Pharmacodynamics

- Binds to the α subunit of the Na^+/K^+ ATPase channel in cardiac myocytes, decreasing its function. This results in increased intracellular sodium (concentration gradient), which increase the influx of calcium ions via a sodium-calcium exchange pump.
- The increased intracellular calcium within the cardiac cells will lead to increased storage in the sarcoplasmic reticulum. The result is an increase in calcium released with each action potential and hence an increase in contractility.
- Can directly suppress AV node by increasing vagal activity.

Pharmacokinetics:

- Onset of action 5–60 min (IV administration) or 1–2 hours (oral administration).
- Vd is 6–7 L/kg, decreased in renal failure and increased in hyperthyroidism.
- Duration of action: 3–4 days.
- 25% plasma protein binding.
- Metabolized in the stomach and by the liver.
- Renally excreted with 50%-70% as unchanged drug.
- Elimination half-life of 36–48 hours in normal adults.

Side Effects

- Cardiac: premature ventricular contractions, paroxysmal atrial tachycardia with AV block, AV dissociation, bigeminy, ventricular tachycardia, and fibrillation.
- Gastrointestinal: nausea, vomiting, diarrhea, loss of appetite and abdominal pain.
- Neurological: dizziness, headache, confusion, visual disturbances, hallucination, depression, and weakness.

Clinical Case Scenario

78-year-old with history of IDDM, HTN, CAD s/p CABG 3 years ago presents for a femoral-popliteal bypass. Intraoperative anesthetic uneventful and patient brought to the PACU with stable vital signs and on 4L NC oxygen. Within 30 minutes of being in PACU, patient noticed to be in ventricular tachycardia and unresponsive.

Airway secured with endotracheal intubation and CPR started. Chest compressions performed while defibrillator and code medications accessed.

Defibrillator used as quickly as possible, initially at 200 Joules.

If ventricular fibrillation or ventricular tachycardia persists 1 mg IV epinephrine given. Can be redosed q3–5 minutes

Subsequent defibrillator shocks at 360 Joules.

If VFib/VTach persists, can give one time dose of 40 U IV vasopressin.

If VFib/Vtach refractory to shocks and epinephrine or vasopressin, amiodarone 300 mg IV push can be given. Amiodarone may be repeated once at
150 mg IV in 3–5 minutes. Maximum cumulative dose is 2.2 g IV/24 hours.
  Lidocaine may also be used at 1.0–1.5 mg/kg IV q3–5 minutes with a maximum dose of 3 mg/kg.

References

1. From the Centers for Disease Control and Prevention. Availability and use of parenteral quinidine gluconate for sever or complicated malaria *JAMA*. 2001;285(6):730.

2. Sherrid MV, Barac I, McKenna WJ, Elliott PM, Dickie S, Chojnowska L, Casey S, Maron
BJ. Multicenter study of the efficacy and safety of disopyramide in obstructive hypertrophic cardiomyopathy. *J Am Coll Cardiol*. 2005;45(8):1251–1258.

3. Di Bianco R, Gottdiener JS, Singh SN, Fletcher RD. A review of the effects of disopyramide phosphate on left ventricular function and the peripheral circulation. *Angiology*.
1987;38(2 Pt 2):174–183.

4. Fenster PE, Nolan PE. Antiarrhythmic drugs. In: Bressler R, Katz MD, eds., *Geriatric
Pharmacology*. New York: McGraw-Hill; 1993: 6:105–149.

5. Feinberg L, Travis WD, Ferrans V, Sato N, Bernton HF. Pulmonary fibrosis
associated with tocainide: report of a case with literature review. *Am Rev Respir Dis*.
1990;141(2):505–508.

6. Burton ME. *Applied Pharmacokinetics & Pharmacodynamics: Principles of Therapeutic
Drug Monitoring*. 4th ed. Philadelphia: Lippincott Williams & Wilkins; 2006.

7. Podrid PJ, Lampert S, Graboys TB, Blatt CM, Lown B. Aggravation of arrhythmia by
antiarrhythmic drugs: incidence and predictors. *Am J Cardiol*. 1987;59(11):38E-44E.

8. Murray, KT . Ibutilide. *Circulation*. 1998;97(5):493–497.

9. Stambler BS, Wood MA, Ellenbogen KA, Perry KT, Wakefield LK, VanderLugt JT.
Ibutilide Repeat Dose Study Investigators. Efficacy and safety of repeated intravenous doses of ibutilide for rapid conversion of atrial flutter or fibrillation. *Circulation*.
1996;94(7):1613–1621.

10. Abi-Mansour P, Carberry PA, McCowan RJ, Henthorn RW, Dunn GH, Perry KT. Study
Investigators. Conversion efficacy and safety of repeated doses of ibutilide in patients
with atrial flutter and atrial fibrillation. *Am Heart J*. 1998;136(4 Pt 1):632–642.

11. Torp-Pedersen C, ller M, M⊠ Bloch-Thomsen PE, et al. Danish Investigations of
Arrhythmia and Mortality on Dofetilide Study Group. Dofetilide in patients with congestive heart failure and left ventricular dysfunction. *N Engl J Med*. 1999;341(12):857–865.

12. Roden DM. Usefulness of sotalol for life-threatening ventricular arrhythmias. *Am J
Cardiol*. 1993;72:51A.

13. Mason, JW . A comparison of seven antiarrhythmic drugs in patients with ventricular
tachyarrhythmias. Electrophysiological study versus Electrocardiographic Monitoring
Investigators. *N Engl J Med*. 1993;329:452.

14. McMahon WS, Holzgrefe HH, Walker JD, et al. Cellular basis for improved left ventricular pump function after digoxin in experimental left ventricular failure. *J Am Coll
Cardiol*. 1996;28:495.

15. Gheorghiade M, Van Veldhuisen DJ, Colucci WS. Contemporary use of digoxin in the
management of cardiovascular disorders. *Circulation*. 2006;113:2556.

Antihyperglycemic Agents

Chapter 21.1

Insulin

Elizabeth Valentine, MD and Nina Singh-Radcliff, MD

Role in the Practice of Anesthesiology/Relevance to Anesthesiology

- Perioperative normoglycemic management for insulin resistance, hyperglycemia, or DM; hyperglycemia may be associated with ↑ morbidity and mortality in critically ill and some subsets of surgical patients (studies to define optimal glucose control have conflicting results; currently, practice varies based on the patient, the surgery, and hospital and clinician resources)
- Perioperative normoglycemia may ↓ impaired wound healing, infection, dehydration, and worsened neurologic injuries in ischemic insults; ↓ hyperviscosity and thrombogenesis (particularly in patients with DM)
- Diabetic ketoacidosis (DKA); prevention and treatment
- Hyperglycemic hyperosmolar syndrome (HHS); prevention and treatment
- Long-term, to prevent microvascular (neuropathy, nephropathy, retinopathy) and macrovascular (CAD, PVD, HTN, CHF, and autonomic neuropathy) complications
- Hyperkalemia treatment

Pharmacodynamics

- Primary endogenous hormone responsible for controlling uptake and utilization of nutrients. Insulin binds to an alpha subunit on the insulin receptor (comprised of 2 alpha and 2 beta subunits) embedded in the plasma membrane. A complex feedback system regulates insulin release. Receptor agonism results in a conformation change that induces autophosphorylation of tyrosine residues present in the beta subunit. These residues proceed in a complex signaling cascade to stimulate intracellular uptake and storage of glucose amino acids, and fatty acids while inhibiting breakdown of glycogen, protein, and fat; functions as a "rest-and-digest" hormone.
- Exogenous insulin binds to insulin receptors on cell membranes to stimulate glucose intake and storage, prevent nutrient breakdown, and shift K+ intracellularly

Pharmacokinetics

- A number of insulin preparations are available with differing time to peak and duration of action; clinically, they are divided into *rapid-*, *intermediate-*, and *long-acting*

- Under stable metabolic conditions, these agents are typically used in combination; usually a short-acting insulin in combination with an intermediate- or long-acting preparation given in divided doses throughout the day. Some motivated patients may have a continuous infusion pump.

- For patients on home insulin therapy, it may be prudent to adjust their preoperative regimen to prevent hypoglycemia while NPO. A common strategy is to take one-half to two-thirds of an intermediate or long-acting agent on the evening prior to surgery and omit any scheduled insulin dose on the morning of surgery. Blood sugar should be checked preoperatively and monitored closely intraoperatively. Dextrose-containing IVF should be readily available

- In patients with continuous insulin infusion pump it is up to the discretion of the clinician whether to provide a continuous baseline infusion via patient's pump or to deactivate it perioperatively. Some advocate deactivation to prevent unintended hypoglycemic episodes, or improved control during changing metabolic demands seen perioperatively, instead utilizing intermittent boluses, continuous infusion, short-acting preparations. Key is titration to desired goal, monitor blood sugars, and effect of therapy

Side Effects/Adverse Reactions

- Hypoglycemia. Most common adverse reaction; increased likelihood with tighter glucose control. Autonomic symptoms of hypoglycemia (eg, sweating, palpitations, difficulty concentration, irritability) are masked by general anesthesia. Serial blood glucose should be monitored closely when administering insulin in the OR and should be considered for all diabetic patients.

- Allergy. Rare; usually due to added components (eg, protamine in NPH) or minor contaminants. May range from local sensitivity to severe, life-threatening systemic reactions. Treatment involves discontinuation of triggering agent, intravenous fluids, antihistamines (H1- and H2-blockers), glucocorticoids, and epinephrine.

- Hypokalemia. Insulin administration drives potassium intracellularly. Thus, while administration of insulin does not change total body potassium concentration, it does change the extra- to intracellular concentrations (hence, its use to treat hyperkalemia).

- Hypophosphatemia

- Hypomagnesemia

- Tight glucose control outcomes. Controversial, as some studies suggest tight glucose control (blood glucose [BG] 80–110) compared to conventional treatment (blood glucose < 180–200) have reduced morbidity and or/mortality, others suggest increased mortality with no differences in major morbidity. Meta-analyses of randomized controlled trials have had similarly conflicting results.

Oral Antihyperglycemic Agents

Sulfonylureas

Clinical Uses

- Insulin resistant diabetes mellitus; oral, long acting antihyperglycemic
- Acute stroke, traumatic brain injury, spinal cord injury (clinical trials underway; IV formulation)

Pharmacodynamics

- Insulin secretagogue. Stimulates the release of insulin from pancreatic β cells via ATP-dependent potassium channel; ineffective in the absence of functioning beta cells (separate binding site than meglitinides). Binding inhibits potassium flow through the channel extracellularly, resulting in the membrane potential becoming positive and the opening of voltage-gated calcium channels. Increased intracellular calcium results in pro(insulin) filled vesicles binding to the cell membrane and releasing its contents into the bloodstream
- Extrapancreatic effects may occur with long-term use: enhanced peripheral sensitivity to insulin, reduced basal hepatic glucose production and hepatic clearance of insulin.
- Mild diuresis via enhanced free water clearance.
- Antiarrhythmic effect

Pharmacokinetics

- Metabolized by the liver, excreted by the kidney. Cautious use in either hepatic or renal insufficiency.
- Highly protein bound.

Side Effects/Adverse Reactions

- Hypoglycemic episodes. Perioperative implications since long-acting and pts are NPO prior to surgery. Increased risk in renal or hepatic insufficiency (reduced clearance). Patients should be instructed to hold sulfonylureas on the day of surgery.
- Nausea and vomiting, agranulocytosis, aplastic and hemolytic anemias, dermatologic sensitivities, generalized hyperreactivity, flushing, hyponatremia, and cholestatic jaundice.
- Increased vascular tone, decreased tolerance to ischemic injury mediated by an inhibition of ischemic preconditioning have been reported. ATP-dependent potassium channels may play a central role in the phenomenon of ischemic preconditioning; blocking the channel may result in deleterious effects.
- **Glyburide (Micronase, Diabeta, Glycron, Glynase).** Often first-line therapy for DM. Potent. Long-term use may have extrapancreatic effects. May be used in combination with metformin. Hypoglycemia in 20%-30% of users. Minimally removed by hemodialysis

- **Glipizide (Glucotrol).** Does not alter glucagon secretion. Increased insulin binding in erythrocytes after long-term use
- **Tolbutamide (Orinase, Tol-tab).** Onset 30–60 minutes, peak 3–5 hours. Shortest duration of action.
- **Glimepiride (Amaryl).**
- **Acetohexamide (Dymelor).**

Meglitinides

Clinical Uses

- Insulin resistant diabetes mellitus; oral, long-acting antihyperglycemic

Pharmacodynamics

- Insulin secretagogue. Stimulates release of insulin from pancreatic B cells via ATP-dependent potassium channels in pancreatic β cells (separate binding site than sulfonylureas). Binding inhibits potassium flow through the channel extracellularly, resulting in the membrane potential becoming positive and the opening of voltage-gated calcium channels. Increased intracellular calcium results in pro(insulin) filled vesicles binding to the cell membrane and releasing its contents into the bloodstream

Pharmacokinetics

- Metabolism is primarily hepatic with renal excretion.
- Rapidly absorbed by GI tract and peak blood levels obtained within 1 hour of administration, allowing for multiple preprandial dosing (sulfonylureas with 1–2 daily doses)

Side Effects and Adverse Reactions

- Hypoglycemia.
- Weight gain.
- **Repaglinide (Prandin)**: Small amount of renal metabolism. Use cautiously in patients with hepatic or renal insufficiency.
- **Nateglinide (Starlix):** derived from D-phenylalanine. Promotes a more rapid but less sustained release of insulin; most useful in reducing postprandial hyperglycemia. May have fewer instances of hypoglycemia than either repaglinide or sulfonylureas.

Biguanides (Metformin)

Clinical Uses

- Insulin resistant diabetes mellitus; oral, long-acting antihyperglycemic. Metformin is the only drug of its class currently in use. May be utilized with other oral antihyperglycemic agents
- Malaria therapy
- Polycystic ovarian disease

Pharmacodynamics

- Decreases hepatic gluconeogenesis and sensitizes peripheral tissue to insulin.
- Does not affect the secretion of other hormones such as glucagon, somatostatin, cortisol, or growth hormone.
- Modest effects on lipid metabolism, including decreasing triglycerides and LDL cholesterol, increasing HDL cholesterol, and promoting weight loss; may improve endothelial function
- Reduces microvascular and macrovascular disease; less weight gain than other oral agents
- Decreased plasminogen activator inhibitor 1 and enhanced fibrinolysis

Pharmacokinetics

- Absorbed by small intestine and excreted unchanged in urine. Not protein bound.

Side Effects/Adverse Reactions

- Lactic acidosis. Potentially fatal complication. Discontinue preoperatively, and hold for a minimum of 48 hours postoperatively, or until renal function is shown to be normal. Contraindicated in patients with renal impairment, hepatic disease, lactic acidosis from other sources, heart failure requiring treatment, and chronic hypoxic lung disease.
- Nausea and vomiting, bloating, abdominal pain, anorexia, and metallic taste.

Thiazolidinediones

Clinical Uses

- Insulin resistant diabetes mellitus; long-acting, oral antihyperglycemic
- Polycystic ovarian disease
- Nonalcoholic steatohepatitis
- Psoriasis
- Autism
- Breast cancer

Pharmacology

- Insulin sensitizing agents. Selective agonist for nuclear peroxisome proliferator-activated receptor (PPAR®), found in adipose tissue, skeletal myocytes, hepatocytes, and vascular endothelium. Activation results in the transcription of genes responsible for carbohydrate and lipid metabolism.
- Also increase expression of genes that encode proteins that enhance adipogenesis in the subcutaneous tissue. Results in the redistribution of fat stores from the muscle and visceral adipose tissue
- May lower hepatic glucose production. Requires insulin for action.
- Favorable effects on markers of atherosclerosis (inhibit plasminogen activator inhibitor 1, C-reactive protein, TNF-a, IL-6, nitric oxide). May inhibit infarct

size, attenuate postinfarct left ventricular remodeling and failure. However, no improvement in morbidity or mortality seen.

Pharmacokinetics
- Extensive hepatic metabolism; highly protein bound

Side Effects/Adverse Reactions
- Rare cases of hepatotoxicity; contraindicated if evidence of hepatic dysfunction or elevated LFTs.
- Edema, weight gain, and plasma volume expansion; use cautiously in NYHA Class I-II patients; contraindicated in Class III-IV.
- Slow onset, requiring up to 12 weeks to reach maximum effect
- **Rosiglitazone (Avandia):** Recent evidence of significantly increased risk of myocardial infarction and a near-significant increased risk of death from cardiovascular events for rosiglitazone-containing drugs compared to other drugs. This has led to a black box warning from the FDA and the requirement that the drug be limited only to patients who cannot control their diabetes with other drugs or for patients already taking the drug who demonstrate improvement and acknowledge the associated risks.
- **Pioglitazone (Actos):** Does not appear to carry increased cardiovascular risk of rosiglitazone. May increase risk of bladder cancer

Alpha Glucosidase Inhibitors
Clinical Uses
- Insulin resistant diabetes mellitus, oral antihyperglycemic
- Insulin deficient diabetes mellitus

Pharmacology
- Inhibits alpha glucosidase enzyme in intestinal brush border, thus inhibiting carbohydrate absorption.

Pharmacokinetics
- Poorly absorbed from gastrointestinal tract; should be administered at the start of meal.

Side Effects and Adverse Reactions
- Abdominal bloating, flatulence, diarrhea. Because carbohydrates do not get absorbed from the GI lumen, they will eventually pass into the colon. Digestion by bacteria results in these untoward side-effects.
- **Acarbose (Precose).** Well absorbed. Blocks pancreatic alpha-amylase, which is responsible for hydrolyzing complex starches to oligosaccharides within the small intestine
- **Miglitol (Glyset).** Poorly absorbed

Glucagon-like Peptide Analogs
Clinical Uses
- Insulin resistant diabetes mellitus

Pharmacology

- Augments glucose-dependent insulin secretion, reduces glucagon production, slows gastric emptying, and decreases appetite.

Pharmacokinetics

- Glucagon-like peptide is rapidly inactivated by depeptidylpeptidase IV enzyme; therefore, analogs must be resistant to this enzyme.

Side Effects

- Nausea, weight loss, hypoglycemia if administered with insulin secretagogues, acute pancreatitis
- **Exendin (Byetta):** derived from salivary gland of Gila monster. Must be given as twice daily injection.
- **Liraglutide (Victoza):** Phase I Trials of oral variant currently underway

Clinical Case Scenario

A 58-year-old, 90-kg male presents to preoperative clinic prior to a planned cholecystectomy. His past medical history is significant for long-standing Type 2 diabetes mellitus, controlled with metformin and glyburide. What should you tell him in regard to his medication management perioperatively?

Background: In 2007, there were an estimated 23.6 million people in the United States with diabetes, or approximately 7.8% of the population. Type 2 diabetes mellitus accounts for 90% of cases of diabetes worldwide. Thus, it is one of the most common comorbidities encountered by anesthesiologists.

Preoperative Counseling: Patients should discontinue metformin 48 hours prior to any surgery or prior to administration of intravenous contrast due to concerns for lactic acidosis, a rare but potentially fatal side effect of metformin administration. It should be held at least forty-eight hours postoperatively and until normal renal function is demonstrated. Any sulfonylurea should also be discontinued on the morning of surgery, as it may precipitate a hypoglycemic episode in a patient kept nil per os for surgery. Blood glucose should be checked preoperatively and coverage provided with insulin if necessary.

Perioperative Concerns: Blood glucose should be monitored serially both intra- and postoperatively to prevent diabetic ketoacidosis (DKA) or hyperglycemic hyperosmotic syndrome (HHS). Additionally, these patients are at increased risk of cardiovascular disease and silent ischemia, diabetic autonomic neuropathy leading to intraoperative hemodynamic instability, gastroparesis leading to increased aspiration risk, and renal insufficiency. Diabetics are also at risk for difficult airway status secondary to limited atlantoaxial joint mobility and temporomandibular joint mobility due to glycosylation of proteins and abnormal cross-linking of collagen.

References

1. Van den Berghe G, Wouters P, Weekers F, et al. Intensive insulin therapy in critically ill patients. *N Engl J Med.* 2001;345:1359–1367.

2. Van den Berghe G, Wilmer A, Hermans G, et al. Intensive insulin therapy in the medical ICU. *N Engl J Med.* 2006;354:449–461.

3. Van den Berghe G, Wilmer A, Milants I, et al. Intensive insulin therapy in mixed medical/surgical intensive care units: benefit versus harm. *Diabetes.* 2006;55:3151–3159.

4. The NICE-SUGAR Study Investigators. Intensive versus conventional glucose control in critically ill patients. *N Engl J Med.* 2009;360:1283–1297.

5. Green DM, O'Phelan KH, Bassin SL, Chang CW, Stern ST, Asai SM. Intensive versus conventional insulin therapy in critically ill neurologic patients. *Neurocrit Care.* 2010: Published online first August 2010.

6. Wiener RS, Wiener DC, Larson RJ. Benefits and risks of tight glucose control in critically ill adults: a meta-analysis. *JAMA.* 2008;300:933–944.

7. Langley J, Adams G. Insulin-based regimens decrease mortality rates in critically ill patients: a systematic review. *Diabetes Metab Res Rev.* 2007;23:184–192.

8. Davis Stephen N. Chapter 60. Insulin, oral hypoglycemic agents, and the pharmacology of the endocrine pancreas. In: Brunton LL, Lazo JS, Parker KL, eds., *Goodman & Gilman's The Pharmacological Basis of Therapeutics.* 11th ed. http://www.accessmedicine.com/content.aspx?aID=958974.

9. Wall RT III. Chapter 16. Endocrine disease. In: Hines RL, Marschall KE, eds., *Stoelting's Anesthesia and Co-Existing Disease.* 5th ed. Philadelphia: Churchill-Livingstone; 2008.

10. National Diabetes Information Clearinghouse. http://diabetes.niddk.nih.gov/dm/pubs/statistics Accessed November 21, 2010.

11. Woodcock J, Sharfstein JM, Hamburg M. Regulatory action on rosiglitazone by the U.S. Food and Drug Administration. *N Engl J Med.* 2010:363:1489–1491.

12. Nissen SE, Wolski K. Effect of rosiglitazone on the risk of myocardial infarction and death from cardiovascular causes. *N Engl J Med.* 2007;356:2457–2471.

13. Riveline JP, et al. Sulfonylureas and cardiovascular effects: From experimental data to clinical use. Available data in humans and clinical applications. *Diabetes Metab.* 2003;29. 207–222.

Chapter 22

Mood Stabilizers and Antidepressants

Chapter 22.1

Monoamine Oxidase Inhibitors (MAOIs)

Gregory Moy, MD and Nabil Elkassabany, MD

Clinical Uses/Relevance to Anesthesiology

- Depression; popularity has ↓ with the introduction of newer and safer drugs. Still used in atypical or refractory depression
- Potentially serious drug interactions, however anesthesia can be safely conducted
- Adverse reactions with sympathetic stimulants, serotoninergic drugs, and meperidine have been reported
- Exaggerated response to vasopressors, especially indirect-acting agents

Pharmacodynamics

- Blocks monoamine oxidase (MAO) from deaminating and inactivating amine neurotransmitters (dopamine, serotonin, norepinephrine, epinephrine); results in ↑ levels in the cytoplasm of nerve terminals
- Two isoenzymes, MAO-A and MAO-B; selective and nonselective inhibitors; irreversible and reversible inhibitors

Pharmacokinetics

- Absorbed from GI tract, except transdermal preparation of selegiline
- Reversible inhibitors with half-lives of 1–3 h
- Irreversible inhibitors of MAO may have effects that persist as long as 2 weeks
- Metabolized by the liver and excreted in the urine

Side Effects/Adverse Reactions

- Exaggerated response to vasopressors, especially indirect-acting agents (direct-acting agents in small doses should be used)
- Sympathetic stimulation; avoid drugs that enhance sympathetic activity (ketamine, pancuronium, epinephrine in local anesthetics)
- Hypertensive crisis following ingestion of tyramine-containing foods
- Serotonin toxicity can occur when coadministered with meperidine or other serotonin-potentiating drug. Mild symptoms (tachycardia, diaphoresis,

Table 22.1.1 Dosages/Preparation

Phenelzine (Nardil)	30–60	oral	NE, 5-HT, DA	11.6
Tranylcypromine (Parnate)	20–30	oral	NE, 5-HT, DA	2.5
Selegiline (Eldepryl)	10	oral, patch	DA, ?NE, ?5-HT	9

myoclonus, fever) to severe symptoms (autonomic instability, coma, seizure). When switching antidepressants, drug's half-life must be considered.

- Orthostatic hypotension, seizures, urinary retention, agitation, tremor, paresthesias, jaundice, muscle spasms are the most common side effects

Clinical Case Scenario

A 47-year-old female is in the PACU after a lumpectomy for breast cancer. Her temperature is 97.4°F, and she is shivering. The nurse asks if the patient can receive meperidine to treat the shivering. The patient has a history of atypical depression, for which she has been taking phenelzine. The PACU anesthesia staff decided to place a warming blanket and to avoid giving meperidine.

The synthetic opioid meperidine may be used for the treatment of postoperative shivering. The use of meperidine with MAOIs in this patient would not be recommended because meperidine blocks the neuronal uptake of serotonin, causing the potential for serotonin syndrome.

Serotonin syndrome is a potentially lethal, though uncommon, adverse drug reaction that can occur when multiple serotonergic drugs are given or with overdose of a single agent. The excess serotonergic activity may present with mild symptoms (tachycardia, fever, diaphoresis, myoclonus) to severe symptoms (autonomic instability, coma, seizure).

References

1. Brunton L, Lazo J, Parker K, eds. *Goodman and Gilman's The Pharmacological Basis of Therapeutics*. 11th ed. New York: McGraw-Hill; 2006.
2. Morgan G, Mikhail M, Murray M. *Clinical Anesthesiology*. 4th ed. New York: Lange; 2006.
3. Huyse F, Touw D, van Schijndel R, de Lange J, Sleats J. Psychotropic drugs and the perioperative period: a proposal for a guideline in elective surgery. *Psychosomatics*. 2006;47:8–22.
4. Yao F. *Yao & Artusio's Anesthesiology: Problem-Oriented Patient Management*. 5th ed. Philadelphia: Lippincott Williams & Wilkins; 2003.

Chapter 22.2

Selective Serotonin Reuptake Inhibitors (SSRIs)

Gregory Moy, MD and Nabil Elkassabany, MD

Role in the Practice of Anesthesiology/Relevance to Anesthesiology

- Depression; first-line agents (less adverse effects: little or no anticholinergic activity or affect on cardiac conduction)
- Obsessive-compulsive, panic, and eating disorder treatment
- Chronic pain; component of multimodal therapy
- May be continued perioperatively; long half-life gives some leeway in the event of a missed dose
- May ↑ intraoperative bleeding

Pharmacodynamics

- Selectively inhibits the reuptake of serotonin (5-HT) at presynaptic nerve membrane
- Serotonin functions as a neurotransmitter between nerve cells; released by presynaptic cell, crosses synapse, binds to postsynaptic receptor, and elicits a signaling cascade. The receptor action is terminated by reuptake into the presynaptic cell by monoamine transporters.
- Major depression is believed to be due to low levels of serotonin. Thus, by ↓ monoamine transporter reuptake, SSRIs ↑ serotonin levels in the synapse.

Pharmacokinetics

- Well absorbed after PO intake
- Variable pharmacokinetic behavior; but generally long half-lives. Fluvoxamine has a half-life of 18 h; fluoxetine has half-life of 50 h (active metabolite up to 240 h)
- Hepatic metabolization by cytochrome P450 enzyme system; SSRIs also inhibit P450. Renal excretion of metabolites

Side Effects/Adverse Reactions

- Nausea/vomiting, headache, sexual dysfunction, agitation, and insomnia
- Cytochrome P450 inhibition; potentiates effects of several drugs including antipsychotics, TCAs, benzodiazepines, carbamazepine, antibiotics

- Serotonin toxicity when combined with MAOIs or other serotonin-potentiating agents. Mild symptoms (tachycardia, diaphoresis, myoclonus, fever) to severe symptoms (autonomic instability, coma, seizure). When switching antidepressants, drug's half-life must be considered.
- Decrease platelet aggregation and combined with NSAIDs could ↑ surgical blood loss

Dosages/Preparation

- Oral preparations
- Citalopram (Celexa) 20–40 mg; escitalopram (Lexapro) 20–40 mg; fluoxetine (Prozac) 20–40 mg; fluvoxamine (Luvox) 100–200 mg; paroxetine (Paxil) 20–40 mg; sertraline (Zoloft) 100–150 mg

Clinical Case Scenario

A 41-year-old female who is having cosmetic surgery in 4 weeks presents for preoperative consultation. She is healthy with only a history of depression, for which she has been taking sertraline. She states that she has been reliant on this medication for many years and asks if she should continue to take this medication before her surgery. At the end of the consultation, she is told that she does not need to discontinue taking sertaline before her surgery.

Knowledge of drug interactions is crucial in the perioperative management of patients with psychiatric disorders. Discontinuation of SSRIs has the risk of withdrawal symptoms, including nausea, dizziness, and anxiety. However, there are no serious interactions with commonly used anesthetic agents. They are generally considered safe to continue perioperatively.

Guidelines do not exist for the perioperative use of psychotropic drugs. The literature suggests that the risks are related to the type of psychiatric disorder, the specific psychotropic drug, the patient physical status, and other drugs used. One must evaluate the perioperative risks of continuing or discontinuing these medications, considering the potential anesthetic interactions and the patient's psychiatric dependence on the drug. Consultation with the patient's psychiatrist may be useful.

References

1. Brunton L, Lazo J, Parker K, eds. *Goodman and Gilman's The Pharmacological Basis of Therapeutics.* 11th ed. New York: McGraw-Hill; 2006.

2. Morgan G, Mikhail M, Murray M, eds. *Clinical Anesthesiology.* 4th ed. New York: Lange; 2006.

3. Huyse F, Touw D, van Schijndel R, de Lange J, Sleats J. Psychotropic drugs and the perioperative period: a proposal for a guideline in elective surgery. *Psychosomatics.* 2006;47:8–22.

4. De Baerdemaeker L, Audenaert K, Peremans K. Anaesthesia for patients with mood disorders. *Curr Opin Anaesthesiol.* 2005;18:333–338.

Chapter 22.3

Tricyclic Antidepressants (TCAs)

Gregory Moy, MD and Nabil Elkassabany, MD

Clinical Uses/Relevance to Anesthesiology

- Depression treatment
- Neuropathic pain; postherpetic neuralgia and diabetic neuropathy
- Chronic pain syndromes at lower doses than antidepressants
- May ↑ anesthetic requirements due to enhanced brain catecholamine activity
- Potential interactions with sympathetic stimulating drugs, serotonergics, and meperidine; however, anesthesia can be safely conducted

Pharmacodynamics

- Inhibits norepinephrine (NE) and serotonin reuptake transporters; thereby ↑ synaptic levels.
- Norepinephrine and serotonin function as neurotransmitters between nerve cells; they are released by presynaptic cells, cross the synapse, bind to postsynaptic receptor, and elicit a signaling cascade. The receptor action is terminated by reuptake into the presynaptic cell by monamine transporters.
- Major depression is believed to be due to low levels of serotonin and norepinephrine.
- Secondary amines (desipramine, nortriptyline) are relatively selective for NE effects, while tertiary amines (amitriptyline, clomipramine, doxepin, imipramine) also affect serotonin
- Antagonizes alpha-1 adrenergic, histamine, muscarinic ACh, and NMDA receptors; inhibits Na^+ channel and L-type calcium channels

Pharmacokinetics

- Well absorbed after PO administration
- Hepatic metabolism—primarily by cytochrome P450 enzymes; metabolites are excreted via the kidney
- The tertiary amines have active metabolites with longer half-lives (see Table 22.3.1)

Table 22.3.1 Dosages/Preparation

	Usual Doses (mg/day)	Amine Effects	Half-Life in Hours, Parent (Metabolite)
Amitriptyline (Elavil)	100–200	NE, 5-HT	16 (30)
Clomipramine (Anafranil)	100–200	NE, 5-HT	32 (70)
Doxepin (Adapin)	100–200	NE, 5-HT	16 (30)
Imipramine (Tofranil)	100–200	NE, 5-HT	12 (30)
Desipramine (Norpramin)	100–200	NE	30
Nortriptyline (Pamelor)	75–150	NE	30

Side Effects/Adverse Reactions

- Anticholinergic actions: dry mouth, blurred vision, constipation, and urinary retention; secondary amines have less anticholinergic effects. Can potentiate centrally acting anticholinergic agents (atropine and scopolamine) and ↑ likelihood of postoperative confusion and delirium
- Cardiac effects: depletion of myocardial catecholamines can potentiate anesthetic-induced myocardial depression (hypotension, impair contractility); tachycardia, T-wave flattening or inversion, prolongation of PR, QRS, and QT intervals (particularly with amitriptyline)
- Lower seizure threshold
- Orthostasis, sedation, weight gain, and sexual dysfunction
- Exaggerated response to indirect-acting vasopressors and sympathetic stimulation; avoid pancuronium, ketamine, meperidine, and epinephrine-containing local anesthetics
- Discontinuation or abrupt discontinuation can result in anxiety, insomnia, headache, and malaise
- Toxicity manifests as anticholinergic, cardiac, CNS, pulmonary, and GI effects; treated with alkaline diuresis and supportive measures

   Oral preparations for all TCA

Clinical Case Scenario

A 39-year-old male with history of car accident 2 years ago presents for pain management consultation for treatment of his chronic cervical neck pain. He has been prescribed increasing doses of opioids by his primary care physician. After obtaining further history and physical exam, there is a neuropathic component to his pain. The patient is prescribed amitriptyline starting at 25 mg at night.

TCAs are useful in the treatment of neuropathic pain. The increased levels of monoamines caused by the TCAs most likely also affect endogenous pain pathways. Other possible mechanisms include NMDA antagonism and sodium channel blockade.

They produce analgesia at lower doses than those typically needed for the treatment of depression. Initial doses of amitriptyline are 10 to 25 mg, depending on the age of the patient. The dose is increased every week until there is there is analgesia or until adverse effects develop. Some may experience relief with 10–25 mg, while others may require up to 150 mg daily. As sedation is common, they are typically dosed at nighttime.

References

1. Brunton L, Lazo J, Parker K, eds. *Goodman and Gilman's The Pharmacological Basis of Therapeutics*. 11th ed. New York: McGraw-Hill; 2006.

2. Huyse F, Touw D, van Schijndel R, de Lange J, Sleats J. Psychotropic drugs and the perioperative period: a proposal for a guideline in elective surgery. *Psychosomatics*. 2006;47:8–22.

3. Bryson H, Wilde M. Amitriptyline: a review of its pharmacological properties and therapeutic use in chronic pain states. *Drugs Aging*. 1996;8:459–476.

Chapter 22.4

Antipsychotics

Gregory Moy, MD and Nabil Elkassabany, MD

Clinical Uses/Relevance to Anesthesiology

- Schizophrenia, manic phase of bipolar illness, and acute idiopathic psychotic illnesses
- Potent antiemetics; prophylactic and therapeutic
- Postoperative delirium treatment
- Hiccups therapy
- Sedative and anxiolytic properties may ↓ anesthetic requirements
- Chronic therapy may be associated with abnormalities of the endocrine, immune, and cardiovascular systems
- Predispose for arrhythmias, perioperative hypotension, intraoperative core hypothermia, prolonged narcosis, and postoperative confusion

Pharmacodynamics

- Variable drug effects on neurotransmitters; all antipsychotics are dopamine receptor antagonists with the potential risk for extrapyramidal neurological effects
- Psychosis has been attributed to ↑ levels of dopamine in the mesolimbic centers of the brain; extrapyramidal neurological effects are attributed to ↑ levels of dopamine at the nigrostriatal and mesocortical pathways
- Newer generation are atypical antipsychotics; have significantly lower risk of extrapyramidal effects and potentially prominent antiserotonergic, antiadrenergic, and antihistaminic activity

Pharmacokinetics

- Most are highly lipophilic, protein-bound, and accumulate in vessel-rich tissues, such as the brain
- Metabolized hepatically by cytochrome P450, glucuronidation, sulfation, and other conjugation processes; excretion via urine and bile
- Variable half-lives (see Table 22.4.1)

Table 22.4.1 Dosages/Preparation

Drug	Class	Usual dose, in mg (Form)	Extrapyramidal Effects	Half-Life, in hours (Range)
Haloperidol (Haldol)	Butyrophenone	2–20 daily (O, L, I) 2–5 per dose IM	++++	24 (12–36)
Droperidol (Inapsine)	Butyrophenone	2.5–10 (I) for sedation 0.625–2.5 (I) for PONV	++	2
Chlorpromazine (Thorazine)	Phenothiazine	200–800 (O, L, I, S, SR) 25–50 per dose IM	++	24 (8–35)
Thioridazine (Mellaril)	Phenothiazine	150–600 (O, L)	+	24 (6–40)
Risperidone (Risperdal)	Atypical	2–8 (O, I)	++	20–24
Olanzapine (Zyprexa)	Atypical	5–10 (O, I)	+	30 (20–54)
Quetiapine (Seroquel)	Atypical	300–500 (O)	0	6
Clozapine (Clozaril)	Atypical	150–450 (O)	0	12 (4–66)
Aripiprazole (Abilify)	Atypical	10–15 (O)	0	75

*Dosage forms indicated as follows: I, injection; L, oral liquid; O, oral solid; S, suppository; SR, oral sustained-release

Side Effects/Adverse Reactions

- Cardiovascular effects: orthostatic hypotension, depression of cardiac repolarization, prolongation of QT intervals, flattening of T-waves, depression of ST segments, and prolongation of PR interval
- Extrapyramidal motor system: acute dystonia, akathasia, parkinsonism, neuroleptic malignant syndrome (NMS), perioral tremor, and tardive dyskinesia
- NMS (rare). Can occur hours to weeks after administration. It results from dopamine blockade in the basal ganglia and hypothalamus and impaired thermoregulation. Signs and symptoms include muscle rigidity, hyperthermia, rhabdomyolysis, autonomic instability, altered consciousness. Differential diagnosis under GA include MH (high $ETCO_2$) and serotonin toxicity (very high CPK). Treatment is with dantrolene or bromocriptine.
- Can worsen Parkinsonian symptoms
- Decreases seizure threshold (caution with ketamine); can also prolong postoperative hallucinations or delirium
- Atypical antipsychotics have less risk of extrapyramidal, but increased risk of hypotension and DM, seizure, weight gain, and hyperlipidemia.

Droperidol

- Clinically used for premedication, neuroleptanalgesia, antiarrhythmia (less commonly today), PONV, hiccups. Centrally acting competitive antagonist at dopamine, alpha, and GABA receptors. Neuroleptic activity reduces motor activity and provides sedative effects; effects at chemoreceptor trigger zone (CTZ) in CNS produce potent antiemetic effects. Delayed awakening limits intraoperative use to low doses. Avoid use if prolonged QT interval. May cause QT prolongation or Torsades de Pointes (black box warning). Can be administered PO, IM, and IV. Antiemetic response within 180 seconds after IV administration. Dosing: 0.3–0.625 mg IV q8–12 h.

Haloperidol

- Clinically used for the treatment of schizophrenia, hiccups, postoperative delirium, and persistent vomiting. It can also be used for premedication due to its sedative properties. Centrally acting competitive antagonist at dopamine, alpha, and GABA receptors. Neuroleptic effects reduce motor activity and provides sedative effects and indifference to environment; effects at CTZ in CNS produce potent antiemetic effects. Avoid use if prolonged QT interval. Increased mortality in elderly patients with dementia related psychosis (black box warning). Available in PO, IM, and IV forms. Dosing: PO 1–15 mg; IM 2–15 mg; IV 1–5 mg. Longer duration of action than droperidol.

Clinical Case Scenario

A 72-year-old female is in the PACU after a laparoscopic cholecystectomy. She is confused and is attempting to pull out her IV access.

Postoperative delirium is not uncommon in the elderly. Initial consideration must be given to find and treat any organic cause of the confusion, recognizing that delirium in the elderly may be the presenting signal for conditions such as MI or sepsis. When organic causes are ruled out, prompt treatment can be instituted with the use of antipsychotics.

Haloperidol is a first-line agent because there are several ways to administer the drug and few adverse effects when given in low doses and short duration. There are no significant hypotensive or autonomic effects. One to 5 mg IM or IV may be given for prompt control.

References

1. Brunton L, Lazo J, Parker K, eds. *Goodman and Gilman's The Pharmacological Basis of Therapeutics.* 11th ed. New York: McGraw-Hill; 2006.

2. Kudoh A. Perioperative management for chronic schizophrenic patients. *Anesth Analg.* 2005;101:1867–1872.

3. Parikh S, Chung F. Postoperative delirium in the elderly. *Anesth Analg.* 1995;80:1223–1232.

4. Morgan G, Mikhail M, Murray M. *Clinical Anesthesiology.* 4th ed. New York: Lange; 2006.

Chapter 22.5

Lithium

Gregory Moy, MD and Nabil Elkassabany, MD

Clinical Uses/Relevance to Anesthesiology

- Acute mania, bipolar disease (mania); mood stabilizing drug
- Chronic pain adjunct to multimodal therapy
- Perioperative risks must be weighed against risks of discontinuing drug; long elimination half-life
- Lithium levels may need to be performed to determine if within therapeutic range; preoperative clinical assessment of cardiac, thyroid, and renal function is advised
- Hypothermia can occur if coadministered with diazepam; prolongs effects of neuromuscular blocking drugs

Pharmacodynamics

- Precise mechanism of action is unknown
- Possibly alters CNS cation distribution and metabolism of biogenic monoamines

Pharmacokinetics

- Absorbed through the GI tract
- Max plasma concentration reached after 2 to 4 h
- Elimination half-life 20–24 h
- Primarily renally excreted (95%); renal reabsorption and excretion in the tubules parallels that of sodium. Salt restriction and thiazide diuretics results in retention and toxicity. Furthermore, increased sodium intake, osmotic diuretics, and acetazolamide increase renal excretion; possibly requiring larger dose

Side Effects/Adverse Reactions

- Nausea, diarrhea, drowsiness, polyuria, weight gain, fine hand tremor, headache
- Narrow therapeutic window; effective dose 0.6–1.2 mEq/L and toxicity with doses >1.5 mEq/L; requires regular testing of serum concentration

- Acute intoxication: Vomiting, profuse diarrhea, tremor, confusion, hyperreflexia, ataxia, coma, convulsions, and seizure. Severe cases are treated with hemodialysis; mild toxicity is treated with supportive measures (sodium and fluid repletion). Toxic effects can be potentiated by drugs that reduce lithium excretion or increase reabsorption, such as NSAIDs, ACE-inhibitors, thiazide diuretics, and metronidazole
- Cardiac effects: although relatively well tolerated, there have been reports of sinus dysfunction, T-wave flattening, ventricular arrhythmia, and myocarditis
- Potentiation of depolarizing and nondepolarizing neuromuscular blocking drugs
- Acquired nephrogenic diabetes insipidus with long-term use
- Benign thyroid enlargement; rarely hypothyroidism
- Significant risk of delirium if given with electroconvulsive therapy

Dosages/Preparation

- Available as tablets, capsules, liquids; also slow-release preparations
- Outpatients: 900–1500 mg PO QD; manic inpatients: 1200–2400 mg PO QD

Clinical Case Scenario

A 27-year-old male sustained multiple gunshot wounds to his extremities and was intubated in the trauma bay with etomidate and rocuronium. He arrives to the OR for exploration of his injuries. The patient remains hemodynamically stable throughout the case. Extubation is considered at the end of the procedure, however he does not appear to be making any respiratory effort. The differential diagnosis for his lack of respiratory drive includes concurrent head injury, drug and/or alcohol intoxication prior to injury, overuse of opioids and sedating medications perioperatively, and continued neuromuscular blockade.

More medical history is obtained from the patient's family during the procedure, and it is discovered that he has bipolar disorder and has been maintained on lithium. His train-of-four is tested, and he does not have any twitches.

Lithium has interactions with several different classes of medications. The patient was emergently intubated with the nondepolarizing muscle relaxant, rocuronium, without knowledge of this medical history. His prolonged duration of neuromuscular blockade can be explained by his chronic use of lithium.

References

1. Brunton L, Lazo J, Parker K. *Goodman and Gilman's The Pharmacological Basis of Therapeutics.* 11th ed. New York: McGraw-Hill; 2006.

2. Huyse F, Touw D, van Schijndel R, de Lange J, Sleats J. Psychotropic drugs and the perioperative period: a proposal for a guideline in elective surgery. *Psychosomatics.* 2006;47:8–22.

3. De Baerdemaeker L, Audenaert K, Peremans K. Anaesthesia for patients with mood disorders. *Curr Opin Anaesthesiol.* 2005;18:333–338.

Antibiotics and Antivirals

Chapter 23.1

Antibiotics

Nina Singh-Radcliff, MD and Kris E. Radcliff, MD

Clinical Uses/Relevance to Anesthesiology

- Patients currently on antibiotic regimen, should be continued intraoperatively
- Prophylactic administration to reduce surgical site infections (SSIs) in clean-contaminated, contaminated, and dirty procedures (in addition to aseptic technique). SSIs occur when local innoculum is sufficient to overcome host defenses and establish growth.
- Prophylaxis for clean procedures should be considered with the following risk factors: DM, chronic steroids; obesity; extremes of age; multiple (>3) preoperative comorbidities; malnutrition; recent surgery; ASA Class 3, 4, or 5; massive transfusion; insertion of prosthetic devices; electrocautery; injection with epinephrine; wound drains; hair removal with razor; previous radiation of site.
- Administration should occur prior to procedure, <30 minutes before incision, not >1 hour. In situations of obesity, (women >80 kg, men >100 kg) the dose should be increased
- Readministration should be done 1–2.5 half-lives of the antibiotic for the duration of the procedure to ensure adequate levels. If EBL >1500 mL, the antibiotic should be redosed regardless of when the last dose was previously given. Antimicrobial activity is not dependent on increasing concentration, however, it is critical that a minimum inhibitory serum concentration is maintained (time dependent)
- Prophylaxis does not need to exceed operative period unless gross contamination occurs secondary to ruptured viscus or severe trauma.
- Antibiotic selection should target anticipated bacteria that could cause infection, achieve adequate local tissue levels, have minimal side effects, and be relatively inexpensive.
- S. *aureus* and S. *epidemidis* may cause infection in the majority of procedures not violating mucosa or a hollow viscus; 1st generation cephalosporins provide good coverage
- GI cases (endoscopies, colonoscopies) in pts with low gastric acidity, stasis or obstruction, UGI bleeding, advanced malignancy may have increased bacteria count/wound infection; *consider* antibiotics

- Surgical Care Improvement Project (SCIP). A national quality partnership of organizations focused on reducing the incidence of surgical complications. Approximately 1 million wound infections/year in the United States; increases average hospital stay by 1 week, additional $1.5 billion in health care costs annually. SCIP compliance has potential financial rewards; noncompliance may result in penalties.
- Bacterial endocarditis prophylaxis. New guidelines state prophylaxis is not indicated for dental, GI, or GU tract procedures unless high risk patients (prosthetic cardiac valve; previous endocarditis; cyanotic CHD that is unrepaired, including those with palliative shunts and conduits; completely repaired CHD with prosthetic material or device, either surgical or catheter intervention, for the first 6 months postprocedure; repaired CHD with residual defects at the site or adjacent to the site of a prosthetic patch or prosthetic device; cardiac transplantation recipients with cardiac valvular disease).

Pharmacodynamics

- Bactericidal antibiotics are lethal to bacteria by inhibiting cell wall synthesis. Bacteriostatic drugs limit growth and reproduction of bacteria without killing them (interferes with protein production, DNA replication, cellular metabolism)
- Beta-lactam rings are present in penicillins, cephalosporins, and carbapenems and bestow their therapeutic function; the side chains can confer traits such as resistance to enzymes that degrade penicillin, changes in half-life of the drug, mechanism of cell wall penetration, and side effects

Penicillins (Penicillin, Amoxicillin, Methicillin, Oxacillin, Ampicillin)

- Oldest class of antibiotics, bactericidal, beta-lactams.
- Inhibit the necessary cross-linking of the peptidoglycan cell wall structure; the beta-lactam ring mimics the substrate of transpeptidase enzyme resulting in weakening and lysing of the cell wall.
- Mammalian cells do not have cell walls, and thus, are not affected.
- Penicillinase is a bacterial enzyme that cleaves natural penicillins; methicillin and oxacillin are penicillinase-resistant.
- Ampicillin and amoxicillin are synthetic (aminopenicillins) and have an extended spectrum of action compared with natural penicillins.
- Hypersensitivity may be common, and cross-allergenicity with cephalosporins has been reported. 1%-4% of beta-lactam administration results in allergic reaction, however only 0.004%-0.15% of these reactions results in anaphylaxis.

Cephalosporins

- Bactericidal, beta-lactams, similar mechanism of action to penicillins (beta-lactam ring mimics transpeptidase enzyme substrate and disrupts synthesis of the peptidoglycan layer of bacterial walls).
- Effective against a broader spectrum of bacteria compared with penicillins; preferred agent for surgical prophylaxis.
- Subgrouped into 1st, 2nd, 3rd, and 4th generations; each generation has a broader spectrum of activity than the one before (1st generation predominantly active against Gm (+) bacteria, successive generations have increased activity against Gm (–).
- 3rd generation cephalosporins can cross the BBB and may be used to treat meningitis and encephalitis. Cefoxitin is highly active against anaerobic bacteria, which offers utility in treatment of abdominal infections.
- Can cause diarrhea, nausea, rash, pain, or inflammation at the injection site. Penicillin allergy cross-sensitivity is ~2%-7%; penicillin anaphylaxis cross-reactivity is as high as 50%.

Macrolides (Erythromycin, Clarithromycin, Azithromycin)

- Bacteriostatic; inhibits protein synthesis by binding to a subunit of the bacterial ribosome.
- Efficacy against Gm (+), staphylococci, and streptococci. Most Gm (–) are resistant to macrolides.
- Erythromycin, a prototype of this class, has a spectrum and use similar to penicillin. Azithromycin and clarithromycin, have a high level of lung penetration and thus are effective in pulmonary infections. Clarithromycin has been widely used to treat H. pylori, the cause of stomach ulcers.
- Erythromycin may aggravate the weakness of patients with myasthenia gravis. Azithromycin may rarely cause angioedema, anaphylaxis, and dermatologic reactions (Stevens-Johnson syndrome, toxic epidermal necrolysis).

Lincosamides (Clindamycin and Lincomycin)

- Bacteriostatic; inhibits protein synthesis by binding to the 50S subunit of bacterial RNA.
- Effective against anaerobes, as well as serious staphylococcus, pneumococcus, and streptococcal infections in penicillin-allergic patients.
- Clindamycin has restricted range, resistance is common; needs to be infused over 10–20 minutes.

Quinolones/Fluoroquinolones (Ciprofloxacin, Levofloxacin, Ofloxacin).

- Synthetic bactericidal drug; inhibits bacterial DNA gyrase and hence supercoiling of DNA
- Effective against Gm (+) cocci.
- Quinolones have high renal clearance (passive and active excretion) and are useful in UTIs, pyelonephritis, bacterial prostatitis. Fluoroquinolones are broad-spectrum, do not have a beta-lactam ring, and are well distributed into bone tissue.
- Serious adverse effects include CNS and tendon toxicity, QT prolongation, convulsions, Torsades de Pointes; and increased incidence of C. difficile and MRSA infections.

Sulfonamides such as Co-trimoxazole and Trimethoprim.

- Bacteriostatic; folate synthesis inhibition (competitively inhibits enzyme DHPS, which catalyzes a key step in folate synthesis). Folate is a necessary component of nucleic acid synthesis; in its absence, cells are unable to divide.
- Broad range against Gm (+) and Gm (−) bacteria; used primarily in UTIs and nocardia infections. When used in combination with trimethoprim, blocks two distinct steps in folic acid metabolism, preventing emergence of resistant strains.
- Untoward reactions include porphyria, Stevens Johnson syndrome and toxic epidermal necrolysis (3% incidence; however up to 60% in pts with HIV).

Tetracyclines (Tetracycline, Doxycycline).

- Bacteriostatic; inhibits protein synthesis by binding to an RNA subunit. Chemical structure with four rings
- Broad-spectrum, Gm (+) and Gm (−). Used in GU infections and prostatitis; may be used in URI, sinusitis, middle ear infections in patients with beta-lactam and macrolide allergies.
- Resistance is common, so culture and susceptibility testing are recommended. Do not use in children <8 y.o., and during periods of tooth development (may cause staining and impairment of bone and tooth structure); may exacerbate systemic lupus erythematosus and myasthenia gravis; Fanconi syndrome may result from breakdown products that affect proximal tubular function in the nephrons of the kidney.

Aminoglycosides (Gentamicin, Tobramycin)

- Bacteriocidal; irreversibly binds to an RNA subunit and inhibits protein synthesis. When synergized with beta-lactams that inhibit cell wall synthesis, aminoglycosides have increased permeability.
- Gm (+) and Gm (–) bacteria, Pseudomonas auriginosa; not effective against anaerobes (oxygen is required for uptake of antibiotic) or intracellular bacteria.
- Causes renal toxicity and ototoxicity (need to have periodic testing of kidney function and hearing); resistance is common.

Glycopeptides (Vancomycin)

- Bacteriocidal against enterococci; bacteriostatic against Gm (+); narrow spectrum. Inhibits cell wall synthesis by interfering with the formation of peptidoglycan.
- First-line therapy in methicillin-resistant S. aureus (MRSA); coagulase-negative staphylococcus (cnS) from central lines, prostheses, and sternotomies; CNS shunt infection or endocarditis by MRSA; ampicillin-resistant enterococcal infections; prophylaxis for major surgical procedures involving prosthetic implants or devices at hospitals with a high rate of MRSA. Second-line therapy in patients with true beta-lactam allergy; for mild and moderate Gm (+) infections consider clindamycin.
- "Red man syndrome" is a common side effect caused by histamine release (flushing, tingling, pruritus, tachycardia, red rash on face, upper torso, back, and arms); can be reduced by slow rate of infusion, dilution, antihistamine prophylaxis. Nephrotoxicity, blood disorders (neutropenia and deafness are reversible once therapy is discontinued); necrosis or phlebitis; hypotension (30% drop). Not cleared by standard HD or PD, but removed by CVVH. Infuse vancomycin over 1 h (2 h for higher doses), entire dose must be administered prior to skin incision. <70 kg 1 g, 71–99 kg 1.25G, >100 kg 1.5 g. If pt on vancomycin, redose at 8 h; if <8 h give ½ dose.

References

1. Woods RK, Dellinger P. Current guidelines for antibiotic prophylaxis for surgical wounds. *Am Fam Physician*. 1998;57:2731–2740.

2. Classen DC, Evans RS, Pestotnik SL, Horn SD, Menlove RL, Burke JP. The timing of prophylactic administration of antibiotics and the risk of surgical-wound infection. *N Engl J Med*. 1992;326:281–286.

3. CDC Draft Guideline for the Prevention of Surgical Site Infection. *Fed Regist*. 1998;63:33167–33192.

4. Page CP, Bohnen JM, Fletcher JR, McManus AT, Solomkin JS, Wittmann DH. Antimicrobial prophylaxis for surgical wounds: guidelines for clinical care. *Arch Surg*. 1993;128:79–88.

Chapter 23.2

Antivirals

Meghan Lane-Fall, MD and Todd Miano, PharmD, BCPS

Antiretroviral Drugs/Treatment of Human Immunodeficiency Virus (HIV)

Clinical Uses/Relevance to Anesthesiology

- Human immunodeficiency virus (HIV), and some may inhibit hepatitis B virus
- Affects hepatic cytochromes and can increase or decrease clearance of perioperative medications
- Efforts should be made to restart perioperatively when possible.

367

Pharmacodynamics/Pharmacokinetics

- Several classes. Nucleoside/nucleotide reverse transcriptase inhibitors (NRTIs): lamivudine*, zidovudine, didanosine, tenofovir*. Nonnucleoside reverse transcriptase inhibitors (NNRTIs): efavirenz, delavirdine, nevirapine. Protease inhibitors (PIs): indinavir, ritonavir, atazanavir, saquinavir. Entry inhibitors: enfuvirtide. *Also exhibits activity against hepatitis B virus
- Clinically relevant effects on drug metabolism are fount with the NNRTIs and the PIs. Other classes of antiretrovirals have no discemable effect on the CYP P450 system
- NNRTIs—Delavirdine generally inhibits CYP3A4, leading to decreased clearance of CYP3A4 substrates. In contrast, nevirapine generally acts as an enzyme inducer. Efavirenz has a mixed profile depending on the specific enzyme.
- All members of the PI class have the potential to inhibit CYP P450 enzymes. The extent varies depending on the agent and enzyme involved. Some agents also act as enzyme inducers. Interactions with the PIs relevant to anesthesia involve significantly decreased clearance of midazolam and fentanyl due to inhibition of CYP3A4. Inhibitory effects are most potent with ritonavir. Ritonavir also prolongs the elimination of CYP3A4 substrates propafenone, amiodarone, ergot derivatives
- These classes of drugs exhibit variable pharmacokinetics

Side Effects/Adverse Reactions

- Nausea/vomiting, fatigue, malaise (most pronounced on initiation of therapy)
- Toxicities of NRTIs are likely related to mitochondrial DNA synthesis inhibition, and include peripheral neuropathy, anemia, and pancreatitis

- Elevations in hepatic transaminases are common with NNRTI therapy
- Lipodystrophy can occur with longstanding use of highly active antiretroviral therapy (HAART; use of more than one class of agents)
- Tenofovir can cause nephrotoxicity

Antiherpesvirus Drugs

Clinical Uses/Relevance to Anesthesiology

- Herpes simplex (HSV), varicella zoster (VZV), cytomegalovirus (CMV), Epstein-Barr (EBV), and human herpesvirus 8 (HHV-8)
- Acyclovir perioperative continuation should be considered due to short half-life
- Consider preoperative electrolyte panel; may result in electrolyte disturbances

Pharmacodynamics/Pharmacokinetics

- Guanosine analogs (acyclovir, valacyclovir, ganciclovir, valganciclovir) and miscellaneous (foscarnet*, cidofovir**, docosanol, trifluridine, fomivirsen); *Also exhibits activity against HIV; **Also active against adenovirus and HPV
- Acyclovir is an analogue of nucleoside 2'-deoxyguanosine; it is activated within the virus via phosphorylation. Incorporated into the DNA primer template and inhibits viral DNA polymerase, thereby hindering elongation of the viral DNA chain
- This class of drugs is predominantly renally excreted

Side Effects/Adverse Reactions

- Nephrotoxicity is a concern with the following agents, in order of risk; cidofivovir > foscarnet > acyclovir. This risk is increased by volume depletion and concomitant use of other nephrotoxic agents such as aminoglycosides and loop diuretics. Electrolyte disturbances (hypokalemia, hypomagnesemia, hypo- or hypercalcemia, hypo- or hyperphosphatemia) can also be seen and are most common with foscarnet and cidovovir.
- Intravenous acyclovir can cause neurotoxicity (seizure, mental status changes)

Other Antiviral Agents

Clinical Uses/Relevance to Anesthesiology

- Anti-influenza drugs (amantadine, rimantadine, oseltamavir, zanamivir) have no known important interactions in the perioperative period
- Ribavirin and interferon used in the treatment of hepatitis C have no known important interactions in the perioperative period

Pharmacodynamics

- Anti-influenza A (amantadine*, rimantadine); Anti-influenza A and B (neuraminidase inhibitors; oseltamivir, zanamivir); *Also used in the treatment of Parkinsonian symptoms

Side Effects/Adverse Reactions

- Amantadine may cause exacerbation of preexisting seizure disorder or psychiatric symptoms
- Interferon and ribavirin may cause myelosuppression

Dosages

- Variable

Clinical Case Scenario

A 28-year-old man presents for elective repair of an inguinal hernia. His medications include lamivudine and lopinavir/ritonavir for HIV-1 infection.

After ilioinguinal and genitofemoral peripheral nerve blocks, sedation and monitored anesthesia care is initiated with midazolam and fentanyl and the case proceeds uneventfully.

In the PACU, the patient remains sedated and does not meet criteria for discharge 2 hours postprocedure.

Background: Midazolam is metabolized by the CYP3A4 cytochrome pathway. Ritonavir is both a potent inhibitor and moderate inducer of CYP3A4, and prolongs the duration of action of drugs metabolized in this pathway.

Treatment: Drugs metabolized by CYP3A4 should be dosed with caution in patients taking ritonavir.

Alternative: Consider using anesthetic agents not metabolized by CYP3A4.

References

1. Hayden FG. Chapter 49. Antiviral agents (nonretroviral). In: Brunton LL, Lazo JS, Parker KL, eds., *Goodman & Gilman's The Pharmacological Basis of Therapeutics*. 11th ed. http://www.accessmedicine.com/content.aspx?aID=950476. Accessed December 15, 2010.

2. Flexner C. Chapter 50. Antiretroviral agents and treatment of HIV infection. Brunton LL, Lazo JS, Parker KL, eds., *Goodman & Gilman's The Pharmacological Basis of Therapeutics*. 11th ed. http://www.accessmedicine.com/content.aspx?aID=951131. Accessed December 15, 2010.

3. Safrin S. Chapter 49. Antiviral agents. In: Katzung BG, ed., *Basic & Clinical Pharmacology*. 11th ed. http://www.accessmedicine.com/content.aspx?aID=4521594. Accessed December 16, 2010.

4. von Moltke LL, Greenblatt DJ, Granda BW, et al. Inhibition of human cytochrome P450 isoforms by nonnucleoside reverse transcriptase inhibitors. *J Clin Pharmacol*. 2001;41:85–91.

5. Ma Q, Okusanya O, Smith P, et al. Pharmacokinetic drug interactions with non-nucleoside reverse transcriptase inhibitors. *Expert Opin Drug Metab Toxicol.* 2005;1:473–485. doi: 10.1517/17425255.1.3.473

6. Eagling VA, Back DJ, Barry MG. Differential inhibition of cytochrome P450 isoforms by the protease inhibitors, ritonavir, saquinavir and indinavir. *Br J Clin Pharmacol.* 1997;44:190–194. doi: 10.1046/j.1365–2125.1997.006

7. Olkkola KT, Palkama VJ, Neuvonen PJ. Ritonavir's role in reducing fentanyl clearance and prolonging its half-life. *Anesthesiology.* 1999;91:681–685.

Chapter 24

Statins: HMG-CoA Reductase Inhibitors

(Lovastatin, Pravastatin, Simvastatin, Atorvastatin, Fluvastatin)

Jason Choi, MD and John G. Augoustides, MD

Clinical Uses/Relevance to Anesthesiology

- Hyperlipidemia and hyperlipoproteinemia treatment; ↓ cholesterol synthesis. Widely shown to be effective in primary and secondary prevention of cardiovascular events in patients with or at high risk of CAD (hypertension, diabetes, tobacco history). Additionally, ↓ total mortality and thromboembolic events (eg, MI, stroke) in patients with and without atherosclerosis

- Acute coronary syndrome mortality reduction

- Pleiotropic effects: improved vascular endothelial function, stabilization of atheromatous plaques, immunomodulation, and protection against thrombosis have expanded their use in perioperative medicine

- Perioperative risk reduction in cardiothoracic and vascular procedures. Cardioprotective (stabilizes atheromatous plaques), neuroprotective (reduced risk of stroke), and nephroprotective (reduced risk of acute kidney injury) and are therefore recommended for all cardiovascular surgeries. Furthermore, postoperative discontinuation of statin therapy is associated with ↑ risk of cardiac morbidity and mortality.

- Potential therapeutic roles in sepsis, airway reactivity, and the prevention of venous thromboembolism

- In future investigations, indications for perioperative statin use are likely to be expanded and further delineated

Pharmacodynamics

- Competitively inhibits 3-hydroxy-3-methylglutaryl-coenzyme A (HMG-CoA) reductase in the liver. HMG-CoA reductase catalyzes the rate-limiting step in cholesterol biosynthesis (conversion of HMG-CoA to mevalonate).

- In a dose dependent manner, statins up-regulate LDL-receptors and ↓ release of lipoproteins resulting in ↑ clearance of LDL and VLDL. LDL and VLDL drawn out of circulation are used to produce bile salts that are eventually excreted and recycled
- Mechanism for pleiotropic effects have yet to be determined

Phamacokinetics

- Rapid GI absorption
- Metabolized by liver via CYP3A4 with extensive first-pass effect; also excreted unchanged via urine and feces
- Levels are ↑ when combined with drugs that inhibit CYP3A4 (eg, amiodarone, cyclosporine, grapefruit juice, verapamil, itraconazole, ketoconazole, erythromycin, clarithromycin, telithromycin, nefazodone, and HIV protease inhibitors)

Cautions/Adverse Reactions

- Myalgia/cramps; approximately 4%
- Elevation of transaminase; approximately 5%. Can reach up to 3 times the upper normal limit in 0.5%-2% of cases
- Hepatotoxicity (jaundice, elevated LFTs, hepatic tenderness) is less common
- Rhabdomyolysis leading to myoglobinuria and ARF is rare (0.08% of cases) but a severe side effect; signs and symptoms include muscle pain, tenderness, weakness, or brown urine. Risks are dose-dependent and more common when statins are combined with fibrate therapy or other moderate to strong CYP3A4 inhibitors.
- Contraindicated for active liver disease, unexplained transaminitis; use with caution in severe renal impairment (CrCl <10 ml/min)
- Caution in pregnancy and breast-feeding as cholesterol synthesis is essential to fetus

Key Statin Clinical Trials

4S (1994): Landmark trial showed improved survival with long-term statin therapy in patients with known cardiovascular disease (CVD) and hypercholesterolemia.

MIRACL (2001): Treatment of patients with acute coronary syndrome should include statin therapy irrespective of baseline LDL levels.

Heart Protection Study (2003): Statin therapy reduces the risk of cardiovascular events in patients with diabetes but no CVD or hypercholesterolemia.

ASTEROID (2006): Trial showed direct ultrasound evidence of plaque regression within coronary arteries with statin therapy alone.

JUPITER (2008): The first trial to show that statin use in patients without hypercholesterolemia or CVD resulted in lower rates of MI, stroke, and death.

DECREASE III (2009): For patients undergoing vascular surgery, perioperative statins decrease postoperative myocardial ischemia and are associated with reduction in death from cardiovascular causes.

Clinical Case Scenario

59-year-old male with history of diabetes, hyperlipidemia, tobacco use, and peripheral vascular disease is scheduled to undergo an elective right femoral-popliteal artery bypass graft for claudication. You speak with him the day prior to surgery and he asks which medications he should continue to take until surgery.

Discussion: In regard to statins, the patient should be advised to continue to take his statin up until surgery. Also, it should be restarted postoperatively as soon as possible. The beneficial pleiotropic effects of statins for patients undergoing cardiovascular surgery and possibly even noncardiac surgery have significant potential. A long-acting statin such as fluvastatin extended release may provide more benefit as its effect can extend into the postoperative period.

The risks and perioperative safety of statins have been well established. Myalgia and liver toxicity require the trending of creatine kinase and liver enzyme levels. The rarer but severe complication of rhabdomyolysis warrants prompt discontinuation of the statin and appropriate supportive care to prevent/ameliorate acute renal failure. Furthermore, concurrent fibrate therapy is known to increase the risk of rhabdomyolysis.

References

1. Evers AS, Maze M. *Anesthetic Pharmacology: Physiologic Principles and Clinical Practice.* Philadelphia: Churchill Livingstone; 2004.

2. National Institute for Health and Clinical Excellence (May 2008, reissued March 2010). Lipid modification: cardiovascular risk assessment and the modification of blood lipids for the primary and secondary prevention of cardiovascular disease; quick reference guide.

3. Paraskevas KI. Applications of statins in cardiothoracic surgery: more than just lipid-lowering. *Eur J Cardiothorac Surg.* 2008;33:947–948.

4. Singh N, Patel P, Wyckoff T, Augoustides J. Progress in perioperative medicine: focus on statins. *J Cardiothorac Vasc Anesth.* 2010;24:892–896.

5. Micromedex. www.micromedex.com. Last Accessed December 2, 2010.

Chapter 25

Vitamins/Herbals

Ellen Wang, MD

Clinical Uses

- Herbal medications are classified as dietary supplements (Dietary Supplement Health and Education Act of 1994), and thus exempt from the strict regulations of prescription drugs. The contents can vary widely, often due to poor manufacturing standards, and can contain varying amounts of the active ingredient as well as contaminants.
- Without direct questioning, pts do not often volunteer this information (~70%)
- Use is ↑; in the United States, up to 37% of adults use herbal medicines and spend more than $27 billion/year
- Anesthetic implications include bleeding, ↓ protein binding, electrolyte disturbances, organ toxicity, stroke, heart attack, transplant rejection, and death.
- The ASA recommends discontinuing all herbals 2–3 weeks before elective surgery.
- The ASRA states that herbals, by themselves, do not ↑ the risk of spinal hematoma in pts requiring neuraxial anesthesia.
- For pts undergoing major surgery with risk of significant blood loss, consider ruling out coagulation and bleeding issues.

Echinacea (Purple Coneflower Root)

Clinical Uses

- Stimulates immune system; prevention and treatment of viral, bacterial, and fungal infections, especially URIs
- Wounds and burns

Pharmacology

- Unknown
- Constituents cause immunostimulation through ↑ phagocytosis and nonspecific T-cell stimulation

Cautions/Adverse Reactions/Anesthetic Implications

- Allergic reactions, some reports of anaphylaxis
- Hepatotoxicity when coadministered with anabolic steroids, amiodarone, methotrexate, ketoconazole
- Organ rejection in transplant recipients; contraindicated in systemic and autoimmune disorders
- ↓ effectiveness of corticosteroids

Ephedra (*Ephedra sinica*) (Ma Huang)

Clinical Uses

- Weight loss
- Energy supplement
- Asthma, bronchitis

Pharmacology/Pharmacokinetics

- Ephedrine, the active compound, is a noncatecholamine, sympathomimetic agonist at α_1, β_1, and β_2 adrenergic receptors and indirectly releases endogenous norepinephrine
- Dose-dependent ↑ in BP and HR
- Elimination half-life of 5.2 h with 70%-80% excreted unchanged in urine

Cautions/Adverse Reactions

- Hepatotoxicity
- MI, stunned myocardium, fatal arrhythmias and strokes
- Tachyphylaxis with long-term use due to depletion of endogenous catecholamine stores
- Concomittant use with MAO-inhibitors may have life-threatening interactions
- Recommended discontinuation at least 24 h prior to surgery
- Perioperative HD instability due to depletion of endogenous catecholamine stores; use of direct-acting sympathomimetics may be necessary

Garlic (*Allium sativum*) (Ajo)

Clinical Uses

- ↓ atherosclerosis by ↓ BP and thrombus formation
- ↓ serum lipid and cholesterol levels

Pharmacology

- Active compounds: sulfur-containing compounds (allicin and its transformation products)

- In addition to inhibition of platelet aggregation, may irreversibly potentiate platelet inhibitors (prostacyclin, forskolin, indomethacin, and dypyridamole)

Cautions/Adverse Reactions/Anesthetic Implications

- Inhibits platelet aggregation
- Recommended discontinuation at least 7 days prior to surgery
- May ↑ postoperative surgical bleeding; bleeding time ↑ for 3 days after discontinuation. Case reports of bleeding during laparoscopic surgery as well as spontaneous epidural hematoma; potentiates warfarin
- May potentiate hypotension

Ginger (*Zingiber officinale*)

Clinical Uses

- Dyspepsia, colic
- Motion sickness, nausea/vomiting (symptoms of hyperemesis gravidarum)
- Vertigo

Pharmacology

- Alters platelet aggregation; potent inhibitor of thromboxane synthetase enzyme
- Mild sympathomimetic effect

Cautions/Adverse Reactions

- May ↑ perioperative bleeding and alter bleeding time; may potentiate warfarin

Ginseng (*Panax ginseng*) (American ginseng, Asian ginseng)

Clinical Uses

- Protection from stress and illness
- ↑ energy levels
- Antioxidant
- ↓ postprandial blood glucose levels

Pharmacology

- Active compounds: ginsenosides (including panaxynol)
- Incompletely understood given many heterogeneous and sometimes opposing effects of different ginsenosides
- May augment adrenal steroidogenesis
- Inhibits platelet aggregation, possibly irreversible
- Elimination half-life between 0.8–7.4 h

Cautions/Adverse Reactions

- Ginseng abuse syndrome with large doses: sleepiness, hypertonia, edema
- Prolongs PT, PTT
- Recommend discontinuation at least 7 days prior to surgery
- Perioperative HTN and intraoperative HD variability, hypoglycemia, worsens bleeding, and can prolong warfarin activity

Gingko (*Gingko biloba*) (Duck Foot Tree, Maidenhair Tree, Silver Apricot)

Clinical Uses

- Memory enhancement; improves or stabilizes cognitive functions in Alzheimer and non-Alzheimer dementia
- Circulatory stimulant; ↓ claudication in PVD, Raynaud's phenomena
- Age-related macular degeneration
- Erectile dysfunction
- Vertigo, tinnitus, and altitude sickness treatment

Pharmacology

- Active compounds: terpenoids and flavonoids, derived from the leaf of *Ginkgo biloba*
- Alters vasoregulation through modulation of nitric oxide
- Antioxidant properties
- Anti-inflammatory effects
- Modulates neurotransmitter and receptor activity
- Inhibits platelet activating factor
- Elimination half-life between 3–10 h

Cautions/Adverse Reactions

- Suggest avoiding gingko if taking NSAIDs (bleeding), anticonvulsant drugs (↓ effectiveness), and TCAs (potentiate seizure threshold-lowering action)
- Recommend discontinuation at least 36 h prior to surgery
- Cases of spontaneous bleeding and prolonged postoperatively bleeding

St. Johns Wort (*Hypericum perforatum*) (Amber, Goat Weed, Hardhay, Klamatheweed)

Clinical Uses

- Mild to moderate depression, short-term treatment (not effective in major depression)

Pharmacology

- Active compounds: hypericin and hyperforin
- Modulation of GABA neurotransmission
- Inhibits serotonin, norepinephrine, and dopamine reuptake by neurons
- ↑ cytochrome P_{450} metabolism, thereby ↓ effects of many commonly used medications (warfarin, midazolam, calcium channel blockers, NSAIDs)
- Elimination half-life is 43.1 h (hypericin) and 9.0 h (hyperforin)
- Peak plasma level is 6.0 h (hypericin) and 3.5 h (hyperforin)

Cautions/Adverse Reactions

- Central serotonin syndrome (tremors, hypertonicity, myoclonus, autonomic dysfunction, hyperthermia, hallucinations)
- Photosensitivity is possible
- Recommend discontinuation at least 5 days prior to surgery
- ↑ metabolism of some perioperative drugs (midazolam)
- May prolong the effects of GA
- Potential heart transplant rejection

Kava (*Piper methysticum*) (Awa, Intoxicating Pepper, Kawa)

Clinical Uses

- Anxiolysis (without amnesia) and sedation, useful in treatment of insomnia
- Antidepressant properties
- Anticonvulsive and neuroprotective effects

Pharmacology

- Active compounds: kavain and methysticin, derived from dried root of the pepper plant *Piper methysticum*
- Possibly binds to the alpha subunit of the GABA receptor, hyperpolarizing postsynaptic membranes, making neuronal cells resistant to activation (similar to benzodiazepine activity)
- Na^+ channel blockade, similar to local anesthetics; relaxes arterial vascular smooth muscle causing ↓ SVR; direct myocardial depressant; ↓ level of neuronal cellular excitability and may be neuroprotective
- Calcium-channel blockade; causes ↓ BP through peripheral arterial vasodilatation, ↓ HR via atrial and AV nodes, and may cause direct myocardial depression
- Cyclooxygenase inhibition, with potency similar to NSAIDs
- Reversible MAO-B inhibition (equipotent to amitriptyline)
- Elimination half-life is 9 h, unchanged metabolites excreted through urine and feces; peak plasma levels at 1.8 h.

Cautions/Adverse Reactions

- Heavy use produces a skin condition known as *kava dermopathy* (reversible scaly cutaneous eruptions)
- GA and sedative effects may be prolonged; may potentiate benzodiazepines, barbiturate, ethanol effects
- Renal and hepatic toxicity may occur (prohibited in the UK); ↓ RBF via inhibition of cyclooxygenase
- Inhibition of platelet aggregation
- Hypotension perioperatively
- Recommend discontinuation at least 24 h prior to surgery

Valerian (*Valeriana officinalis*) (All Heal, Garden Heliotrope, Vandal Root)

Clinical Uses/Indications

- Sedative, treatment of insomnia
- Found in virtually all herbal sleep aids

Pharmacology

- Active compounds: sesquiterpenes
- Modulation of GABA neurotransmission
- Pharmacokinetics have not been studied, though effects thought to be short-lived

Cautions/Adverse Reactions

- May potentiate the sedative effects of anesthetics
- Abrupt discontinuation may cause a benzodiazepine-like withdrawal

Feverfew (*Tanacetum parthenium*)

Clinical Uses/Indications

- Migraine headaches
- Fever reduction
- Arthritis
- Digestive problems

Pharmacology

- Active compound: parthenolide
- Inhibits serotonin release from aggregating platelets

- ↓ 86%-88% of prostaglandin production without inhibition of the cyclooxygenase enzyme
- May also have GABAergic effects

Cautions/Adverse Reactions

- Inhibits platelet activity; potentiates warfarin and other anticoagulants
- Withdrawal syndrome with abrupt discontinuation after long- term use; rebound headaches and muscle/joint pains
- Allergic reactions can occur
- GI upset; nausea, vomiting, pain, diarrhea
- Contraindicated in pregnancy

Vitamin E

Clinical Uses/Indications

- Protects cells against effects of free radicals (by-products of metabolism)
- ↓ cellular aging, ↓ the risk of certain kinds of cancer (eg, melanoma)
- Prevents abnormal clotting and ↓ the risk of ischemic and CAD
- Protects immune function
- ↓ risk of Alzheimer's disease

Pharmacology

- Fat-soluble antioxidant that stops production of reactive O_2 radicals formed during fat oxidation
- ↓ production of prostaglandins (thromboxane) that cause platelet clumping
- Acts as a cell membrane stabilizer by allowing for tighter packing of the membrane (more orderliness)

Cautions/Adverse Reactions

- Doses > 800 IU/day, interferes with vitamin K synthesis, causing warfarin-like effects
- Can increase bleeding
- Doses > 400 IU/day can worsen HTN particularly in hypertensives

Fish Oil (Omega-3 Fatty Acids)

Clinical Uses/Indications

- ↓ the risk of MI and CAD; ↓ LDL and ↑ HDL
- Antiaging, delays or ↓ tumor development in certain forms of cancer (eg, breast, colon, prostate)

- ↓ risk of developing age-related macular degeneration
- ↑ memory function, ↓ risk of developing Alzheimer's and dementia
- Depression, bipolar disorder, schizophrenia treatment
- ↓ inflammation, treatment of rheumatoid arthritis, ulcerative colitis, SLE
- Prenatal supplement to aid in fetal development of brain, retina, and nervous system

Pharmacology

- Most notable eicosapentaenoic acid (EPA) and decosahexaenoic acid (DHA)
- Competes with omega-6 family of polyunsaturated fatty acids for incorporation into cell membranes, displacing arachidonic acid from membranes, which diminishes production of arachidonic acid-derived mediators of inflammation and production of prothrombotic agent thromboxane A_2.
- Also modulates intracellular signaling pathways, indirectly modulating inflammatory response
- ↑ lifespan of cells by slowing deterioration of telomeres
- Antiplatelet activity

Cautions/Adverse Reactions

- Temporary diarrhea or greasy stools
- Perioperative bleeding
- Hypotension
- Recommend discontinuation 2–3 weeks prior to surgery

Clinical Case Scenario

A 68-year-old woman with a history of hypertension and osteoarthritis is scheduled for total hip replacement in 7 days. Her medications include atenolol, hydrochlorothiazide, and alendronate. She also reports taking gingko biloba, ginseng, and echinacea.

Background: The pt presents for a surgery with risk of blood loss.

Recommendations: Tell the patient to stop the herbals now and tell her to take only atenolol on the morning of surgery. Echinacea can cause immunosuppression. Gingko and ginseng can cause prolonged postoperative bleeding. Preoperative coagulation labs should be ordered.

Illicit Substances

Chapter 26.1

Cocaine

Nabil Elkassabany, MD

Role in the Practice of Anesthesiology/Relevance to Anesthesiology

- Used as a topical anesthetic for ENT procedures because of its vasconstrictive and local anesthetic properties. Recent studies suggest that safer alternatives for topical anesthesia with equal effectiveness are available.
- Used in combination with other local anesthetic (tetracaine-adrenaline-cocaine) TAC for repair of head and neck lacerations in the emergency department. Cocaine-free topical anesthetics are currently available and are equally effective, with the benefit of decreased risk and cost.
- One of the most frequently abused drugs. In 2008, almost 15 percent of Americans had tried cocaine, with 6 percent having tried it by their senior year of high school.
- Cocaine induced myocardial ischemia is a concern for the anesthesiologist in the perioperative period. It is still controversial whether to proceed with elective surgical cases in patients who test positive for cocaine preoperatively.

Pharmacodynamics

- Cocaine blocks norepinephrine reuptake in peripheral sympathetic nerve terminals, thereby increasing the norepinephrine concentration in the synaptic cleft. This blockage results in the sympathomimetic state associated with cocaine use.
- The euphoric effect of cocaine (the cocaine high) results from prolongation of dopamine's activity in the limbic system and the cerebral cortex.
- Blockage of the voltage gated sodium channel is responsible for the local anesthetic effect and may contribute to the arrhythmogenic properties of cocaine.

Pharmacokinetics

- Routes of administration include inhalation (smoking), oral, transmucosal, and intravenous.
- Peak effect is achieved within 1–3 minutes through inhalation (smoking)

- Cocaine is an ester local anesthetic that is metabolized by plasma esterases. Major metabolites are benzylecgonine, ecgonine methyl ester (EME), and nor-cocaine. Metabolites are water soluble and are excreted in urine.
- Serum half-life is 90 minutes. Metabolites can be detected in urine for 72 hours or longer.
- Urine drug screen tests for cocaine metabolites rather than the parent drug.
- Cocaine is an inhibitor of the enzyme cytochrome P450 2D6, pharmacokinetic interaction with other drugs is unlikely to be clinically relevant.

Additives/Adjuvants

- The deleterious effects of cocaine on myocardial oxygen supply and demand are exacerbated by concomitant cigarette smoking. This combination substantially increases the metabolic requirement of the heart for oxygen and simultaneously decreases the diameter of diseased coronary arterial segments.
- Concomitant use of cocaine and alcohol is common. Persons who abuse cocaine in temporal proximity to the ingestion of ethanol produce cocaethylene, a metabolite synthesized by hepatic-transesterification. Like cocaine, it blocks the reuptake of dopamine at the synaptic cleft, thereby possibly potentiating the systemic toxic effects of cocaine.

Side Effects/Adverse Reactions
- **Cardiovascular side effects:**
  - Mycordial ischemia: the mechanism of which include
  - Hypertension and tachycardia resulting from the sympathomimetic effect of cocaine.
  - Coronary vasoconstriction.
  - Induction of platelet activation.
  - Beta-blockers must be used cautiously for treatment in cocaine induced myocardial ischemia. Blocking B receptors can leave the alpha effect, coronary and other vascular beds vasoconstriction, unopposed. Short-acting B blockers and B blockers with mixed alpha and Beta effects have been used with success.
  - Arrhythmia: prolonged QT syndromes and ventricular fibrillation have been reported with acute cocaine toxicity.
  - Case reports of aortic dissection and rupture of aortic aneurysms.
- **Central nervous system side effect:** cerebrovascular strokes have been reported with acute cocaine toxicity.
- **Pulmonary side effects:** Acute lung injury has been reported after inhalation of cocaine. Ciliary function of the tracheobronchial tree is impaired with long-term smoking.
- **Interaction with anesthetic agents:** Ketamine. Pancuronium and other drugs that can cause tachycardia and hypertension are better avoided.

- Some authors suggested impaired metabolism of succinylcholine in acute cocaine toxicity as both drugs are metabolized via plasma esterases. Clinical studies refuted this claim.
- Minimum alveolar concentration (MAC) of inhaled agents is increased with cocaine toxicity.

References

1. De R, Uppal HS, Shehab ZP, Hilger AW, Wilson PS, Courteney-Harris R. Current practices of cocaine administration by UK otorhinolaryngologists. *J Laryngol Otol.* 2003;117(2):109–112.

2. Harper SJ, Jones NS. Cocaine: what role does it have in current ENT practice? A review of the current literature. *J Laryngol Otol.* 2006;120(10):808–811.

3. Bush S. Is cocaine needed in topical anaesthesia? *Emerg Med J.* 2002;19(5):418–422.

4. Eidelman A, Weiss JM, Enu IK, Lau J, Carr DB. Comparative efficacy and costs of various topical anesthetics for repair of dermal lacerations: a systematic review of randomized, controlled trials. *J Clin Anesth.* 2005;17(2):106–116.

5. Schilling CG, Bank DE, Borchert BA, Klatzko MD, Uden DL. Tetracaine, epinephrine (adrenalin), and cocaine (TAC) versus lidocaine, epinephrine, and tetracaine (LET) for anesthesia of lacerations in children. *Ann Emerg Med.* 1995;25(2):203–208.

6. *National Survey on Drug Use & Health* [Internet]. Rockville, MD: National Institute of Drug Abuse.

7. Hernandez M, Birnbach DJ, Van Zundert AA. Anesthetic management of the illicit-substance-using patient. *Curr Opin Anaesthesiol.* 2005;18(3):315–324.

8. Bhargava S, Arora RR. Cocaine and cardiovascular complications. *Am J Ther.* 2010;18:e95-e100.

9. Elkassabany NM. *Evidence Based Practice of Anesthesiology.* 2nd ed. Fleisher LA, ed. Philadelphia, PA: Elsevier; 2010.

10. Billman GE. Mechanisms responsible for the cardiotoxic effects of cocaine. *FASEB J.* 1990;4(8):2469–2475.

11. Jones RT. Pharmacokinetics of cocaine: considerations when assessing cocaine use by urinalysis. NIDA monograph. Rockville, MD: National Institute of Drug Abuse. 1997;175:221–234.

12. Du C, Tully M, Volkow ND, Schiffer WK, Yu M, Luo Z, Koretsky AP, Benveniste H. Differential effects of anesthetics on cocaine's pharmacokinetic and pharmacodynamic effects in brain. *Eur J Neurosci.* 2009;30(8):1565–1575.

13. Levine SR, Brust JC, Futrell N, Ho KL, Blake D, Millikan CH, Brass LM, Fayad P, Schultz LR, Selwa JF. Cerebrovascular complications of the use of the "crack" form of alkaloidal cocaine. *N Engl J Med.* 1990;323(11):699–704.

14. Fernandez Mere LA, Alvarez Blanco M. [Cardiac arrhythmia during general anesthesia in a former cocaine user]. *Rev Esp Anestesiol Reanim.* 2007;54(6):385–386.

15. Restrepo CS, Rojas CA, Martinez S, Riascos R, Marmol-Velez A, Carrillo J, Vargas D. Cardiovascular complications of cocaine: imaging findings. *Emerg Radiol.* 2009;16(1):11–19.

16. DuPont RL, Baumgartner WA. Drug testing by urine and hair analysis: complementary features and scientific issues. *Forensic Sci Int.* 1995;70(1–3):63–76.

17. Tyndale RF, Sunahara R, Inaba T, Kalow W, Gonzalez FJ, Niznik HB. Neuronal cytochrome P450IID1 (debrisoquine/sparteine-type): potent inhibition of activity by (-)-cocaine and nucleotide sequence identity to human hepatic P450 gene CYP2D6. *Mol Pharmacol.* 1991;40(1):63–68.

18. Moliterno DJ, Willard JE, Lange RA, Negus BH, Boehrer JD, Glamann DB, Landau C, Rossen JD, Winniford MD, Hillis LD. Coronary-artery vasoconstriction induced by cocaine, cigarette smoking, or both. *N Engl J Med.* 1994;330(7):454–459.

19. Farooq MU, Bhatt A, Patel M. Neurotoxic and cardiotoxic effects of cocaine and ethanol. *J Med Toxicol.* 2009;5(3):134–138.

20. Parker RB, Laizure SC. The effect of ethanol on oral cocaine pharmacokinetics reveals an unrecognized class of ethanol-mediated drug interactions. *Drug Metab Dispos.* 2010;38(2):317–322.

21. Brogan WC III, Lange RA, Glamann DB, Hillis LD. Recurrent coronary vasoconstriction caused by intranasal cocaine: possible role for metabolites. *Ann Intern Med.* 1992;116(7):556–561.

22. Benzaquen BS, Cohen V, Eisenberg MJ. Effects of cocaine on the coronary arteries. *Am Heart J.* 2001;142(3):402–410.

23. Heesch CM, Wilhelm CR, Ristich J, Adnane J, Bontempo FA, Wagner WR. Cocaine activates platelets and increases the formation of circulating platelet containing microaggregates in humans. *Heart.* 2000;83(6):688–695.

24. Damodaran S. Cocaine and beta-blockers: the paradigm. *Eur J Intern Med.* 2010;21(2):84–86.

25. Perera R, Kraebber A, Schwartz MJ. Prolonged QT interval and cocaine use. *J Electrocardiol.* 1997;30(4):337–339.

26. Yildirim AB, Basarici I, Kucuk M. Recurrent ventricular arrhythmias and myocardial infarctions associated with cocaine induced reversible coronary vasospasm. *Cardiol J.* 2010;17(5):512–517.

27. Daniel JC, Huynh TT, Zhou W, Kougias P, El Sayed HF, Huh J, Coselli JS, Lin PH, Lemaire SA. Acute aortic dissection associated with use of cocaine. *J Vasc Surg.* 2007;46(3):427–433.

28. Lalouschek W, Schnider P, Aull S, Uhl F, Zeiler K, Deecke L, Lesch OM. [Cocaine abuse—with special reference to cerebrovascular complications]. *Wien Klin Wochenschr.* 1995;107(17):516–521.

29. Levine SR, Brust JC, Futrell N, Brass LM, Blake D, Fayad P, Schultz LR, Millikan CH, Ho KL, Welch KM. A comparative study of the cerebrovascular complications of cocaine: alkaloidal versus hydrochloride—a review. *Neurology.* 1991;41(8):1173–1177.

30. Karila L, Lowenstein W, Coscas S, Benyamina A, Reynaud M. [Complications of cocaine addiction]. *Rev Prat.* 2009;59(6):825–829.

31. Forrester JM, Steele AW, Waldron JA, Parsons PE. Crack lung: an acute pulmonary syndrome with a spectrum of clinical and histopathologic findings. *Am Rev Respir Dis.* 1990;142(2):462–467.

32. Luft A, Mendes FF. Anesthesia in cocaine users.]. Rev Bras Anestesiol. 2007 Jun;57(3):307–14.

33. Skerman JH. The cocaine-using patient: perioperative concerns. *Middle East J Anesthesiol.* 2005;18(1):107–122.

34. Hoffman RS, Henry GC, Wax PM, Weisman RS, Howland MA, Goldfrank LR. Decreased plasma cholinesterase activity enhances cocaine toxicity in mice. *J Pharmacol Exp Ther.* 1992;263(2):698–702.

35. Jatlow P, Barash PG, Van Dyke C, Radding J, Byck R. Cocaine and succinylcholine sensitivity: a new caution. *Anesth Analg.* 1979;58(3):235–238.

36. Bernards CM, Kern C, Cullen BF. Chronic cocaine administration reversibly increases isoflurane minimum alveolar concentration in sheep. *Anesthesiology.* 1996;85(1):91–95.

37. Stoelting RK, Creasser CW, Martz RC. Effect of cocaine administration on halothane MAC in dogs. *Anesth Analg.* 1975;54(4):422–424.

Drugs of Abuse

William Gao and Nabil Elkassabany, MD

Methamphetamine

Anesthetic Implications

- Amphetamine-induced myocardial ischemia and other cardiovascular compli-cations are strong concerns in the perioperative period.
- Volatile anesthetics should be avoided in patients undergoing general anes-thesia if possible. Isoflurane potentiates vasoconstriction and increases the risk of arrhythmias, whereas halothane sensitizes the myocardium to the effects of catecholamines.
- With acute amphetamine exposure, patients may have higher anesthetic requirements, including increased MAC of inhaled anesthetics and decreased response to succinylcholine. Instances of shorter duration of action of thio-pental have also been seen.
- Regional anesthesia has the possibility of inducing hypertension from vasocon-striction, ephedrine-resistant hypotension, and altered pain perception.
- With chronic amphetamine use, patients may have markedly diminished anes-thetic requirements possibly secondary to chronic catecholamine depletion in the central nervous system.

Pharmacodynamics

- Methamphetamine is a potent CNS stimulant from the amphetamine family of synthetic drugs. It is the most commonly abused type of amphetamine.
- Inhibition and reversal of norepinephrine reuptake transporters at the presyn-aptic adrenergic nerve terminals causes increased levels of neurotransmitters at the synapse. This results in sympathomimetic activity by increasing stimu-lation of the postsynaptic adrenergic receptors. Similar action on dopamine reuptake transporters in the nucleus accumbens and ventral tegmental area results in activation of the reward pathway and euphoria.
- Physiological effects include vasoconstriction, increased blood pressure, increased heart rate, increased respiratory rate, and bronchodilation. Other

common effects include hyperthermia, increased muscle activity, decreased gastrointestinal motility, and dilation of the pupils.

Pharmacokinetics

- Methamphetamine is most commonly administered through intravenous injection, inhalation, ingestion, or insufflation.
- Predominant route of elimination is direct renal excretion of the unchanged form. A small amount is metabolized by the hepatic cytochrome P450 system, which converts it to amphetamine by N-demethylation or to hydroxymethamphetamine by hydroxylation before being excreted.
- The half-life of methamphetamine is about 9 to 12 hours. Although very similar to cocaine in mechanism and presentation, it is distinguishable by its significantly longer pharmacodynamic and pharmacokinetic half-life. It also allows for detection of methamphetamine in the blood about 40 to 48 hours after use.
- Under normal circumstances, it can be identified in urine up to 3 to 6 days after administration. Because it is a weak base, excretion may be enhanced when the urine is acidified, such as with ammonium chloride.

Presentation

- Symptoms: euphoria, increased energy and alertness, improved concentration and mental acuity, aggression, decreased appetite, palpitations, headache, and loss of visual acuity.
- Signs: hypertension, tachycardia, dyspnea, hyperthermia, diaphoresis, psychomotor agitation, and mydriasis.

Clinical Uses

- Only clinical use of methamphetamine approved by the FDA is under the trade name Desoxyn. It can be prescribed for the treatment of ADHD in children or exogenous obesity in persons older than 12 years old. Off-label uses include ADHD in adults, narcolepsy, and treatment-resistant depression.

Street Names

- Meth, ice, crank, chalk, crystal, fire, glass, go fast speed.

Clinical Case Scenario #1: Methamphetamine

A 22-year-old male is diagnosed in the emergency department with appendicitis and is immediately scheduled for an emergent appendectomy. On preoperative evaluation, he presents with tachycardia, hypertension, diaphoresis, and appears restless and agitated. On questioning, he admits to recent ingestion of methamphetamine several hours earlier. The surgery continues as scheduled due to it serious nature. Postoperatively the patient is found to have difficulty speaking and right-sided weakness. CT scan of the head reveals a left-sided hemorrhagic stroke.

Pathophysiology: The mechanism of amphetamine-induced strokes likely involves a number of factors. Acute hypertensive surges and cerebral vasoconstriction inhibit the blood supply and perfusion to the brain. Additionally, cerebral vasculitis, enhanced platelet aggregation, and cardioembolism can contribute to strokes. Underlying arteriovenous malformations (AVMs) and aneurysms increase the risk of hemorrhagic strokes.

Treatment: Management of amphetamine-induced strokes mostly follows that of other strokes due to limited development of medications specifically targeted for this purpose. Recent research has indicated dihydropyridine antagonists may show promise in preventing cerebral ischemia.

Cannabis

Anesthetic Implications

- Acute exposure can enhance the effect of anesthetic drugs on blood pressure and cardiac activity. At low or moderate doses, tachycardia and increased cardiac output usually predominate, and thus anesthetic drugs increasing heart rate, such as epinephrine, atropine, ketamine, and pancuronium, should be avoided. At higher doses, bradycardia and hypotension are prominent, which can cause myocardial depression in patients on potent inhalation agents for general anesthesia.

- Life-threatening arrhythmias are not typical with cannabis, but electrocardiogram changes including reversible ST-segment and T-wave abnormalities have been known to occur.

- The depressant action on the brain can be potentiated with barbiturates, benzodiazapines, opioids, and phenothiazines, resulting in profound CNS depression.

- Pulmonary complications are of significant concern because it is the most common route of exposure. Irritation of the respiratory airways may lead to laryngospasm or bronchospasm. Impaired airway epithelial function and damage to bronchial tissue may also cause decreased lung function.

Pharmacodynamics

- Cannabis refers to a variety of preparations of the hemp plant (*Cannabis sativa*). It contains many active compounds, but the main psychoactive component is the cannabinoid l-Δ^9-tetrahydrocannabinol (THC).

- Involves the activation of presynaptic cannabinoid 1 (CB1) receptors by THC. These G protein coupled receptors are prevalent throughout the brain and less so in the peripheral nervous system. When activated, neuromodulation occurs predominately through inhibition of cyclic adenosine monophosphate formation and changes in Ca^{2+} and K^+ transport across the neuronal membrane.

- Inhibition of glutamate and GABA release from the presynaptic nerve terminal has been of particular interest in explaining the effects of THC. Because glutamate and GABA are the main excitatory and inhibitory neurotransmitters of the central nervous system, interference with their release is likely a central cause of the respective depressant and stimulant effects of cannabis.
- Because GABAergic neurons inhibit dopamine neurons of the nucleus accumbens and ventral tegmental area, cannabis removes this inhibition and stimulates the dopaminergic activity of the reward pathway.
- Physiological effects include decreased blood pressure, increased heart rate, increased respiratory rate, and smoking-related issues. Other significant effects include increased cerebral blood flow, decreased gastrointestinal motility, delayed gastrointestinal disturbances, reduced intraocular pressure, conjunctival hyperemia, hypothermia, analgesia, muscle relaxation, and immune suppression.

Pharmacokinetics

- Marijuana is prepared from the dried flowering tops and leaves, and hashish is derived from dried cannabis resin and compressed leaves. Different parts of the hemp plant contain different concentrations of THC, thus the THC in marijuana typically ranges between 0.5% to 5% and between 2% to 20% in hashish. Both forms can be smoked or ingested, but smoking is most common.
- THC is rapidly distributed to the tissues and, due to its high lipophilicity, more prominently distributes to the brain and adipose tissue, which have higher lipid content. It accumulates in the adipose tissue before being released back into the circulation.
- Cannabinoids undergo hydroxylation and oxidation by the hepatic cytochrome P450 system. One of the predominant products is 11-hydroxy-THC, a potent compound which may be responsible for some of the physiological and psychological effects.
- The half-life of THC in occasional users is about 56 hours, while in chronic users it is about 28 hours. THC is hard to detect in the blood after 8 to 12 hours since it is rapidly distributed into the tissue.
- Metabolites can easily be detected in urine within 3 to 4 days of exposure, but excretion can occur for approximately 4 to 5 weeks in more chronic users.

Presentation

- Symptoms: euphoria, reduced anxiety, depersonalization, distortion of time and space, heightened sensory perception, misperceptions, hallucinations, lethargy and sedation, mental clouding, loss of concentration, disconnected thoughts, impaired decision-making, and impaired memory.
- Signs: hypotension, bradycardia, tachypnea, hypothermia, conjunctival hyperemia, muscle weakness and incoordination, tremulousness, dysarthria, and increased appetite.

Clinical Uses

- FDA has approved the use of the synthetic cannabinoids nabilone and dronabinol. Both can be prescribed in the treatment of nausea and vomiting from cancer chemotherapy when other conventional antiemetic treatments have failed. Dronabinol can additionally be prescribed to stimulate appetite in patients with anorexia or cachexia from AIDS or AIDS-related illnesses.
- Other less studied clinical uses include decreasing intraocular pressure in glaucoma, prevention of seizures in epilepsy, treatment of movement disorders such as multiple sclerosis and Parkinson's disease, analgesia in chronic pain syndromes, and bronchodilation in asthma.

Street Names

- Hashish: boom, gangster, hash, hash oil, hemp. Marijuana: blunt, dope, ganja, grass, herb, joint, bud, Mary Jane, pot, reefer, green, sinsemilla, skunk, weed.

Clinical Case Scenario #2: Cannabis

A 26-year-old female is diagnosed in the emergency department with a ruptured ectopic pregnancy. On preoperative evaluation, she is found to have tachycardia, hypertension, and conjunctival injection. On questioning, she admits to ingesting hashish a couple hours earlier. Because of the possible fatal complications of her condition, surgery continues as initially planned. Intraoperatively, the patient has prolonged episodes of tachycardia despite adequate fluid maintenance and exclusion of other immediate causes. No complications are noted postoperatively.

Pathophysiology: The mechanism of tachycardia in cannabis exposure likely involves sympathomimetic action on the heart, which stimulates cardiac activity. Complications such as myocardial ischemia and infarction are not common occurrences in comparison to cocaine or amphetamine use.

Treatment: Management of cannabis-induced tachycardia may include beta-blockers, but should be used cautiously due to the risk of unopposed alpha activity and resulting vasoconstriction.

Heroin

Anesthetic Implications

- Acute exposure affects inhalation anesthetics, producing a dose-dependent and concentration-dependent decrease in the minimal alveolar concentration and anesthetic requirements for these drugs.
- Chronic exposure can cause cross-tolerance to anesthetic drugs and other depressants most likely from chronic receptor stimulation. This can pose significant therapeutic and ethical challenges in postoperative pain management

due to decreased analgesic response and decreased pain threshold. Incomplete pain control is a significant incentive for opioid use.

- In recovering addicts, effective regional anesthesia, especially with nonsteroidal anti-inflammatory drugs, may preclude the need for opioids. It can also be administered safely in patients with recent heroin use, although hypotension should be anticipated.

- Opioid antagonists or agonist-antagonists, such as naloxone or buprenoprhine, should not be administered to opioid users due to the high risk of precipitating acute withdrawal.

Pharmacodynamics

- Heroin, also known as diacetylmorphine, is a central nervous system depressant synthesized from the opioid morphine, a derivate of the opium poppy (*Papaver somniferum*).

- After crossing the blood-brain-barrier, it is converted back to morphine, which acts as a potent agonist on the opioid receptors, specifically the mu (μ) subtype. These G protein coupled receptors stimulate voltage-gated Ca^{2+} channels on presynaptic nerve terminals to close, thus decreasing release of neurotransmitters such as glutamate, while K^+ channels are opened, which hyperpolarizes, inhibiting postsynaptic neurons. Because glutamate is an important excitatory amino acid, its combined action with postsynaptic inhibition is an overall central nervous system depressant.

- Mu receptors are found in high concentration in the nucleus accumbens and ventral tegmental area, the reward pathway. Activation decreases release of GABA from presynaptic nerve terminals, which normally inhibits postsynaptic dopaminergic neurons. Dopaminergic activity is thus increased and induces the euphoria and reward involved in reinforcement.

- Central effects of heroin use are respiratory depression, sedation, analgesia, stimulation of chemoreceptor trigger zone, suppression of the cough reflex, hypothermia, and pupil constriction. Peripheral effects include decreased blood pressure, decreased heart rate, decreased gastrointestinal motility, contraction of the biliary and urinary sphincters, and pruritis from histamine release.

Pharmacokinetics

- Heroine, like many other drugs of abuse, is most commonly administered through intravenous injection, inhalation, ingestion, or insufflation.

- In the tissues, it is rapidly deacetylated to the inactive 3-monoaceteylmorphine and the active 6-monoacetlymorphine (6-MAM), which is converted to morphine, the major mu receptor agonist of heroin. Morphine has a longer half-life of about 2 to 3 hours, which likely accounts for heroin's longer duration of action given its short half-life.

- It is metabolized mostly in the liver to morphine-3-glucuronide (M3G) and morphine-6-glucuronide (M6G) via glucuronidation and excreted in the urine along with 6-MAM.

- The half-life is approximately 2 to 5 minutes, making detection in the blood extremely difficult and rarely done outside of the research setting.
- Urine drug tests are designed to detect the heroin metabolites and are able to do so within 2 to 3 days of administration or even longer after prolonged exposure. The presence of 6-MAM specifically differentiates the use of heroin versus other opioids because it is a unique metabolite.

Presentation

- Symptoms: euphoria, reduced anxiety, relaxation, perception of heavy extremities, lethargy and sedation, alternating drowsy and alert states, mental clouding, detachment and disorientation, and delirium.
- Signs: hypotension, bradycardia, respiratory depression, hypothermia, miosis, decreased pain sensation, dry mouth, nausea and vomiting, constipation, urinary retention, and urticaria.

Clinical Uses

- There are currently no approved clinical uses of heroin, but numerous other drugs of the opioid class have widespread applications in medicine for their therapeutic benefits.
- Morphine, hydromorphone, oxycodone, and fentanyl are often given for analgesia in pathological or postoperative pain. Loperamide and diphenoxylate can be prescribed in cases of severe diarrhea not responsive to other treatments. Opioids such as codeine and hydrocodone are beneficial as antitussive agents for cough suppression.

Street Names

- Smack, brown sugar, hope, H junk, skag, white horse, China white, cheese (with OTC cold medicine and antihistamine).

Clinical Case Scenario #3: Heroin

A 42-year-old female is recovering from open reduction and internal fixation of a fibular fracture following a bicycle accident. In the postoperative period, the patient continues to complain of severe, constant pain at the sight of repair. Morphine had initially been prescribed for analgesia and provided adequate pain relief, but the patient is later switched to as-needed oral acetaminophen with hydrocodone. She now describes only minimal pain relief and requests stronger medications. Upon questioning, she is discovered to have a history of chronic heroin and opioid abuse for over a decade.

Pathophysiology: Opioid tolerance is not a rare occurrence with chronic heroin, or other opioid, abuse. This is most likely a result of chronic, repeated stimulation of the opioid receptors, which results in decreased effect and response to opioids.

> **Treatment:** Management of pain is a difficult task in patients with opioid tolerance. Postoperatively, intravenous patient-controlled analgesia (PCA) is often effective for patients who abuse opioids. When converting to oral formulations, a combination of long-acting and short-acting oral medications are most effective in providing pain relief. Additionally, methadone is also an option because it is an effective analgesic and less likely to be diverted. Relying only on as-needed medications is not optimal because it may not be given promptly and thus unable to provide adequate pain relief.

Phencyclidine

Anesthetic Implications

- Phencyclidine (PCP) potentiates adrenergic stimulation and sympathetic activity and thus the implications common to other stimulants are of concern.
- Phencyclidine may prolong the effects of succinylcholine through the inhibition of its metabolic pathway, the plasma cholinesterase enzyme. However, current research has shown that this interaction appears to have minimal clinical effect.

Pharmacodynamics

- Phencyclidine, also known as 1-(1-phenylcyclohexyl-piperidine), is a synthetic hallucinogenic drug first developed as an anesthetic agent but was later discontinued because of its intense dissociative side effects.
- Noncompetitive antagonism of glutamate at N-methyl-D-aspartic acid (NMDA) receptors interferes with Ca^{2+} channels and the transport of Ca^{2+} across the cell membrane, inhibiting neurotransmitter release. High affinity for sites in the cortex and limbic system are responsible for the diverse psychotic symptoms and cognitive deficits characteristic of its use.
- Interaction with opioid receptors produces the analgesia, lethargy, sedation, and coma for which it was initially used in anesthesia. Reuptake inhibition of monoamines, such as norepinephrine, results in sympathomimetic activity similar to that of stimulants. Complicated interactions with nicotinic and muscarinic receptors result in anticholinergic and cholinergic activity, which can have an array of physiological effects.

Pharmacokinetics

- PCP is most often smoked but must be mixed with a leafy material such as tobacco or cannabis. Ingestion and insufflation are also common, whereas intravenous injection is rarely done.
- It rapidly distributes to all the tissues because it is highly lipophilic. It most prominently distributes to the brain and the adipose tissue due to their high lipid content and can later be released when the adipose tissue is metabolized.

- PCP is hydroxylated by the hepatic cytochrome P450 system to several inactive compounds such as 4-phenyl-4-(1-piperidinyl)-cyclohexanol (PPC) and 1-(1-phenylcyclohexyl)-4-hydroxypiperidine (PCHP). These metabolites are excreted by the kidneys along with small amounts of unchanged drug.
- The half-life of PCP varies greatly with a range of about 7 hours to 5 days, although the usual average is about 20 to 21 hours. It can usually only be detected in the blood for 1 to 3 days following use since it is rapidly distributed from the blood into the tissues.
- It can be detected in urine up to 7 days after exposure and by 10 days most all has been metabolized and excreted. Because it is a weak base, excretion can be enhanced when the urine is acidified thus decreasing the window of detection.

Presentation

- Symptoms: euphoria, dissociation, detachment from the surroundings, disorientation, depersonalization, disordered thought, impaired concentration, perceptual distortions, belief of invulnerability, delusions, hallucinations, anxiety, agitation, combativeness and violence, psychosis, and catatonia.
- Signs: hypertension, tachycardia, tachypnea, hyperthermia, flushing, diaphoresis, mydriasis and blurred vision, dysarthria, slurred speech, ataxia, numbness of extremities, muscle incoordination, nystagmus, analgesia, and anesthesia.

Clinical Uses

- There are currently no approved uses of PCP in the clinical setting. Ketamine, a similar NMDA receptor antagonist also developed as a dissociative anesthetic, is still currently used in anesthesiology for this purpose. Although ketamine abuse does occur, it is still less frequent in comparison to PCP abuse.

Street Names

- Angel dust, boat, love boat, peace pill

Clinical Case Scenario #4: Phencyclidine

A 38-year-old male is brought into the emergency department with a self-inflicted stab wound to his abdomen resulting in perforation of the bowel. On preoperative evaluation, the patient appears confused, agitated, and responding to visual and auditory hallucinations. Vitals show tachycardia, hypertension, and elevated body temperature. On questioning, he admits to smoking PCP with tobacco a few hours earlier. Emergent surgery to repair the bowel continues as planned. Intraoperatively, the patient is noted to have ST segment elevations and frequent PVCs. Postoperatively, cardiac workup shows an anterior wall myocardial infarction.

Pathophysiology: The mechanism of PCP-induced myocardial infarction is not completely understood but likely involves a combination of decreased myocardial supply and increased myocardial demand. Sympathomimetic activity induces tachycardia and hypertension, which contributes to increased demand, while also inducing coronary artery vasoconstriction, which limits blood supply. Luckily, myocardial infarction is not a very common occurrence.

Treatment: Management of PCP-induced myocardial infarction is the same as treatment for any other myocardial infarction. This may include may include beta-blockers but this class of drugs should be used with caution due to the risk of unopposed alpha activity and resulting vasoconstriction.

Alcohol

Anesthetic Implications

• Acute alcohol intoxication has an increased risk of aspiration secondary to impaired laryngeal protection and vomiting. This is will significantly impair pulmonary function in addition to a number of other problems.

• Chronic alcohol abuse is often associated with resistance to the actions of CNS depressants. Additionally, adjustment to anesthetic drugs may be needed to account for hepatic dysfunction, hypoalbuminemia, and cardiac failure related to the end-organ effects of alcohol consumption.

Pharmacodynamics

• It has many effects on the activity of the brain and its cellular actions, most notably a wide variety of membrane proteins involved in the signaling pathways. This includes neurotransmitter receptors for amines and amino acids, cellular enzymes such as ATPase, adenylyl cyclase, and phospholipase C, and ion channels.

• The role of ethanol on neurotransmission by glutamate and GABA, the main excitatory and inhibitory neurotransmitters of the CNS, has been of particular interest. It potentiates the activity of GABA at the $GABA_A$ receptors, lowering the excitability of the postsynaptic neuron by increasing Cl^- influx into the neuron and increasing Cl^- efflux from axon terminals. It antagonizes the action of glutamate at the NMDA receptor, interfering with the excitability of the postsynaptic neuron by decreasing Ca^{2+} and Na^{2+} influx into the neuron. The combined action is most likely responsible for the depressant activity while the action at NDMA receptors is also implicated in the cognitive deficits, such as impaired learning and memory formation.

• Physiological effects include decreased myocardial contractility, increased left ventricle end diastolic pressure, vasodilation at lower concentration, vasoconstriction at higher concentrations, mild hypothermia, increased blood viscosity, and various effects on the endocrine system mediated by the hypothalamus. More significant and widespread effects on the body occur with chronic consumption.

Pharmacokinetics

- Ethanol is rarely ever administered by any other route than ingestion. After absorption, it is quickly distributed to the CNS, since blood flow to the brain is high and it readily crosses the blood-brain-barrier.
- Most of the ethanol is metabolized in the liver through two pathways, oxidation by alcohol dehydrogenase or oxidation by the hepatic cytochrome P450 system. Alcohol dehydrogenase is the primary pathway, although both yield acetaldehyde, which is converted by aldehyde dehydrogenase to acetate. Any remaining unchanged ethanol is generally eliminated in the urine or through the lungs.
- At a typical blood alcohol concentration (BAC), saturation of the pathways occurs and metabolism follows zero-order kinetics, a constant rate of oxidation that is independent of time or concentration. As a result, ethanol does not have a constant half-life and is instead usually identified by a rate of elimination of approximately 100 mg/kg of body weight/h.
- The BAC is the most common test rather than blood or urine detection alone. It measures the amount of alcohol in the blood expressed as weight per unit of volume or percentage and has been shown to correlate well with the changes in physiological and cognitive states. The breathalyzer test is a common method in which to extrapolate the BAC from the amount of alcohol in the expired air.

Presentation

- Ethanol presents with predictable dose-dependent symptoms closely proportional to the BAC of the intoxicated.
- At levels up to 50 mg/dL, typical effects include relaxation, talkativeness, decreased inhibition, impaired judgment, slurred speech, and incoordination.
- Between 50 and 100 mg/dL, mental and cognitive abilities are impaired, sensory-motor functioning, such as driving skills and reaction time, are attenuated, and vomiting and ataxia can occur.
- Between 100 and 300 mg/dL, sensory and cognitive functioning is significantly impaired, respiratory depression is of concern, and blackouts can occur.
- If the BAC reaches over 300 mg/dL, most individuals are stuporous or unconscious and levels greater than 400 mg/dL, ethanol can be lethal from severe respiratory or cardiovascular depression or other associated complications such as aspiration of vomit.

Clinical Uses

- One of the most important medicinal applications of ethanol is in cases of poisoning from more toxic alcohols such as methanol or ethylene glycol. In these situations, administration of ethanol interferes with the formation of significantly toxic metabolites by competing for the active site on alcohol dehydrogenase.

- Ethanol is also used as an antiseptic for its ability to disrupt the proteins and lipids of a number of microorganisms. It is very commonly found as a main component of antiseptic wipes and hand sanitizers.

Clinical Case Scenario #5: Alcohol

A 54-year-old female is brought into the emergency department following a severe motor vehicle accident resulting in several complex fractures of her extremities. Police determined that the patient had been binge drinking a few hours earlier and was driving under the influence of alcohol. Emergent surgery to repair her wounds is scheduled. Intraoperatively, the patient becomes tachycardic, tachypneic, and her oxygen saturation decreases. She is extubated at the end of the procedure. Postoperative chest radiographs reveals diffuse bilateral pulmonary infiltrates and ARDS is diagnosed.

Pathophysiology: The mechanism of ARDS in ethanol intoxication most often results from gastric aspiration secondary to vomiting. Aspiration of gastric contents causes diffuse alveolar damage and lung capillary endothelial injury resulting in accumulation of fluid in the lungs and respiratory distress.

Treatment: Management of ARDS from gastric aspiration is the same as treatment for any other cause of ARDS, requiring extensive and complex medical care.

Disulfiram

Anesthetic Implications

- Disulfiram appears to have minimal implications in regard to the administration of anesthesia. However, there have been early, infrequent reports of acute hypotension during general anesthesia in patients receiving long-term disulfiram therapy.
- The cause of such episodes has yet to be determined, but is not likely to have significant clinical effects given its rare occurrence and its response to discontinuation of the inhalation agent and fluid therapy alone or in combination with phenylephrine or ephedrine.

Pharmacodynamics

- Tetraethylthiuram disulfide, or disulfiram, is a synthetic drug that has been used in the treatment of alcoholism for more than 50 years.
- As discussed previously, ethanol is mainly metabolized by alcohol dehydrogenase to acetaldehyde, which is then converted by aldehyde dehydrogenase to acetate. Disulfiram inhibits this pathway at the intermediate stage by blocking the action of aldehyde dehydrogenase. When alcohol is consumed, acetaldehyde will accumulate in the body and the concentration in the blood and

tissues significantly multiplies, resulting in toxicity, sometimes referred to as alcohol sensitivity.

- Physiological effects in the periphery commonly include vasodilation, decreased blood pressure, increased heart rate, increased respiratory rate, bronchoconstriction, and perspiration. An important component is the stimulation of sympathomimetic activity by increasing the release of catecholamines from adrenergic nerve terminals and the adrenal glands, a likely cause of the cardiorespiratory effect. It also induces the release of histamine and bradykinin and increases prostaglandin synthesis, all factors in the vasodilation of blood vessels, notably those at the level of the skin. Histamine plays an important role in the overall allergy-type reaction that occurs with toxicity, including bronchoconstriction. In regard to effects on the brain, many studies have indicated that acetaldehyde is a CNS depressant similar to ethanol itself.

- As a treatment for alcoholism, the negative effects are most important and prominently include dizziness, nausea and vomiting, and headache, common components of the "hangover" of alcohol intoxication. The combined peripheral and central activity of acetaldehyde toxicity from disulfiram produces an overall unpleasant experience.

Pharmacokinetics

- Disulfiram is most often prescribed for oral administration, although implants are limitedly available as a possible means of circumventing adherence difficulties.

- As a prodrug, it is rapidly converted to diethyldithiocarbamate (DDC), which is metabolized in the liver to diethyldithiomethylcarbamate (Me-DDC) or degraded into dethylamine and carbon disulphide. Me-DCC undergoes oxidation to diethylthiomethylcarbamate (Me-DTC), the active metabolite acting on aldehyde dehydrogenase. The metabolites are eventually excreted in the urine.

- The half-life of Me-DTC is about 60 to 120 hours with a mean of 72 hours, but a dose and its enzymatic effect can persist in the blood up to 1 to 2 weeks after discontinuation.

Presentation

- Disulfiram does not present with symptoms until alcohol is consumed, inducing the disulfiram-alcohol reaction. The typical acetaldehyde syndrome includes tachycardia, hypertension, palpitations and chest pain, dyspnea, facial flushing, diaphoresis, throbbing headaches, blurred vision, vertigo and ataxia, nausea and vomiting, and pruritis. Large ingestion of alcohol can cause significant hypotension leading to faintness and syncope. Symptoms occur within a few minutes of consuming just one alcoholic drink and often last 30 minutes to 2 hours after the last exposure.

Clinical Use

- As noted previously, disulfiram is currently approved by the FDA for clinical use, under the trade name Antabuse, for the treatment of alcoholism. Preferably, it is prescribed in conjunction with counseling, behavioral therapy, and social support. The unpleasant central and peripheral effects of the disulfiram-alcohol reaction are intended to act as negative reinforcement to alcohol consumption. Its efficacy is one of disagreement and several extensive studies have shown mixed results.

Acamprosate

Anesthetic Implications

- The implications of administering anesthesia to patients on acamprosate therapy have not been well studied. There are few reported incidences of related complications.

Pharmacodynamics

- Calcium acetylhomotaurinate, or acamprosate, is a synthetic drug that has recently come into use in the United States for the treatment of alcoholism. It is an analogue of the amino acid taurine with a structure resembling GABA.
- Complicated interactions with the GABA, glutamate, serotonin, and catecholamine effects are involved. The best characterized actions involve stimulation of the $GABA_A$ receptor, antagonism at the glutamate NMDA receptor, and modulation of glutamate neurotransmission at the metabotropic type 5 glutamate receptor. The overall effect is decreased excitatory actions of glutamate in the brain and increased inhibitory actions through GABA. This is thought to restore the imbalance created by up-regulation of the excitatory pathway over the inhibitory pathway of the brain from chronic ethanol use.
- It has not been determined how acamprosate decreases motivation to drink and or how it prevents relapse, but it may decrease the pleasurable effects of ethanol consumption.

Pharmacokinetics

- Acamprosate is only available for oral ingestion. Once absorbed, it is widely distributed and circulates without modification or metabolism into other compounds. It is eventually excreted in the urine unchanged. The half-life is approximately 30 hours.

Presentation

- Acamprosate presents with minimal symptoms or adverse reactions and is often well tolerated by most users. There is limited data regarding toxicity, but acamprosate appears to be relatively benign in overdose.

- The most common side effects are gastrointestinal complaints such as nausea, vomiting, diarrhea, abdominal cramping, and flatulence. Less common but more serious side effects include depression and suicidal ideation.

Clinical Uses

- As noted previously, acamprosate is currently approved for clinical use, under the trade name Campral, for the treatment of alcoholism. Preferably, it is prescribed in conjunction with counseling, behavioral therapy, and social support. Its efficacy in being able to increase alcohol abstinence is one of contention with numerous studies showing contrasting results.

Carbon Monoxide

Pharmacodynamics

- Carbon monoxide (CO) is the most common cause of death by poisoning in the United States. Because it is a colorless, odorless, and nonirritating gas, it is very difficult to detect and easily missed. The most common sources include car exhaust fumes and smoke from fires.
- When inhaled, it crosses into circulation and binds reversibly to the oxygen-binding site of hemoglobin. Its affinity for hemoglobin is greater than 200 to 230 times that of oxygen, allowing it to easily displace oxygen.
- The carboxyhemoglobin that is formed cannot transport oxygen and it also interferes with the normal cooperativity of hemoglobin. Typically, the release of one oxygen molecule promotes the release of subsequent molecules from hemoglobin. Carboxyhemoglobin interferes with this dissociation, thus shifting the oxygen-hemoglobin dissociation curve to the left and decreasing the availability and release of oxygen to the tissues.
- At the cellular level, anaerobic metabolism is increased to compensate for the inability to perform aerobic metabolism. Centrally, the hypoxia is sensed, stimulating ventilatory efforts and increasing minute ventilation. This only worsens the condition because it increases inhalation of CO and leads to respiratory alkalosis, further shifting the oxygen-hemoglobin dissociation curve to the left.
- If not reversed, cell death eventually occurs. Because the heart and the brain have significant oxygen requirements, they are most susceptible to the hypoxia from CO toxicity. Prolonged hypoxia can lead to irreversible ischemia of the myocardium and brain. The prognosis of the patient is mostly dependent on the duration and severity of the hypoxia.

Pharmacokinetics

- CO ultimately dissociates from hemoglobin and is expired back into the air. Because of its high affinity for hemoglobin, it can take a significant amount of time before normal circulatory physiology resumes. This is dependent on a number of factors, which include the duration of exposure, the minute ventilation, and the fraction of inspired oxygen.

- When breathing room air, the half-life of carboxyhemoglobin is typically approximately 4 to 6 hours. This is considerably shortened to about 40 to 80 minutes when breathing 100% oxygen and to only 15 to 30 minutes when breathing hyperbaric oxygen.

Presentation

- CO toxicity presents with vague symptoms that typically vary with concentration and duration of exposure. However, a predictable sequence closely associated with the percent of carboxyhemoglobin in the blood typically occurs.
- At levels below 20%, symptoms are rarely evident, although patients occasionally experience headaches or tightness in the temporal area.
- Between 20% and 40%, dizziness, nausea and vomiting, dyspnea, and loss of visual acuity or other visual disturbances commonly manifest.
- Between 40% and 50%, depressed sensorium, confusion, and syncope often occur. After 50%, seizures and coma are of great concern, and if the concentration reaches 60% or more, cardiovascular collapse and death are highly possible.
- Since early symptoms are mild and can be easily confused with other illnesses such as the flu, CO toxicity is often ignored or missed early on. Also, the classic signs of cherry-red lips, cyanosis, and retinal hemorrhages rarely occur.

Clinical Case Scenario #6: Carbon Monoxide Poisoning

A 24-year-old female is brought into the emergency department unconscious by paramedics. Her roommate had found her in the unopened garage with the engine running. On arrival, she is tachycardic, hypotensive, tachypneic, and immediately placed on 100% face mask oxygen. Because of the high likelihood for carbon monoxide poisoning, a carboxyhemoglobin level was sent for analysis and returned a value of 30.2%.

Treatment: The management of carbon monoxide poisoning is based on administering enough oxygen to compete with the carbon monoxide. 100% oxygen therapy is essential to hasten the dissociation of carbon monoxide from carboxyhemoglobin and produce hemoglobin. Hyperbaric oxygen is also used and been shown to significantly reduce the half-life of carboxyhemoglobin.

Cyanide

Pharmacodynamics

- Cyanide is generally a rare cause of death by poisoning in comparison to CO. It most often occurs through inhalation of smoke from residential fires, specifically the smoke produced from the combustion of natural and synthetic materials. This includes polyurethane in insulation and furniture, polyacrylonitrile in plastics, melamine resins in household items, nylon, and wool that produce cyanide in its gaseous form, hydrogen cyanide (HCN). Other potential, but less common, causes include industrial or occupational exposure and overdose of cyanide-containing medications, such as amygdalin or nitroprusside.

- Once in circulation, cyanide avidly binds to the ferric iron (Fe^{3+}) of various proteins, but most importantly cytochrome oxidase, the final enzyme of the electron transport chain. This interferes with the transfer of electrons from cytochrome to oxygen, which prevents ATP production through oxidative phosphorylation. Cells are unable to utilize oxygen despite its availability, producing a hypoxic state that requires anaerobic metabolism to generate needed energy.
- Cell death eventually occurs if not reversed. As with CO poisoning, the heart and brain are most susceptible to hypoxia due to their increased oxygen requirements. If prolonged, irreversible damage to the myocardium and brain can occur.

Pharmacokinetics

- Inhalation typically causes the most rapid cellular and physiological changes, whereas ingestion has a slightly more delayed onset. Once absorbed, it is rapidly distributed in the body.
- Detoxification of cyanide occurs through a variety of mechanisms, the most significant of which is via rhodanese (thiosulphate-cyanide sulfur transferase). This is a mitochondrial enzyme that is well distributed in the body tissues but is most abundant in the liver and muscles. It is able to neutralize cyanide through catalyzing the transfer of sulfur from thiosulfate to form the thiocyanate.
- Thiocyanate is less toxic and water soluble, promoting its excretion through the urine along with small amounts of unchanged cyanide. The half-life of cyanide is approximately 20 to 60 minutes.

Presentation

- The presentation varies with the amount and duration of exposure but frequently follows a predictable sequence associated with the amount of cyanide in the blood.
- At concentrations less than 0.5 µg/mL, patients are usually asymptomatic, but when levels exceed 0.5 µg/mL, early symptoms may manifest including headaches, dizziness, confusion, anxiety, loss of visual acuity, nausea and vomiting, diaphoresis, flushing, palpitations, hyperpnea, and dyspnea.
- Between 1.0 to 3.0 µg/mL, the condition of the patient worsens, presenting with a progressively obtunded state, which can lead to significant CNS depression, seizures, unconsciousness, coma, and apnea. If the concentration exceeds 3.0 µg/mL, cardiovascular collapse and death can occur.
- Occasionally, the characteristic bitter almond smell, cherry-red skin, and cyanosis can be detected, but these are not sensitive indicators of cyanide toxicity.

Clinical Case Scenario #7: Cyanide Poisoning

A 47-year-old female is evaluated in the emergency department following a house fire. On arrival, she complains of a headache, dizziness, and nausea and vomiting that started a few hours after her house had caught on fire. She is bradycardic, hypertensive, tachypneic, and immediately placed on 100% face mask oxygen. Blood gases show metabolic acidosis combined with reduced arterial-venous oxygen saturation difference. Cyanide poisoning is strongly suspected.

Treatment: The management of cyanide poisoning is focused on oxygen administration in order to compensate for decreased aerobic activity. 100% oxygen therapy is important to increase oxygen saturation and blood content. Additionally, hydroxocobalamin (Cyanokit) and Cyanide Antidote Kit (CAK) has been approved by the FDA for treating known or suspected cases of cyanide poisoning. Hydroxocobalamin combines with cyanide to from cyano-cobalamin, which can be renally excreted. CAK contains amyl nitrite pearls, sodium nitrate, and sodium thiosulfate. Amyl and sodium nitrate induce meth-emoglobin formation in RBCs, which combines with cyanide and releases cytochrome oxidase enzymes. Thiosulfate increases conversion of cyanide to thiocyanate, which is renally excreted.

References

1. Darke S, et al. Major physical and psychological harms of methamphetamine use. *Drug Alcohol Rev.* 2008;27(3):253–262.

2. Kuczkowski KM. Anesthetic implications of drug abuse in pregnancy. *J Clin Anesth.* 2003;15:382–394.

3. Steadman JL, Birnbach DJ. Patients on party drugs undergoing anesthesia. *Curr Opin Anaesthesiol.* 2003;16:147–153.

4. Kuczkowski KM, Benumof JL. Amphetamine abuse in pregnacy: anesthetic implications. *Acta Anaesth Belg.* 2003;54:161–162.

5. Fischer SP, et al. General anesthesia in a patient on long-term amphetamine therapy: is there cause for concern? *Anesth Analg.* 2000;91(3):758–759.

6. Cruickshank CC, Dyer KR. A review of the clinical pharmacology of methamphetamine. *Addiction.* 2009;104(7):1085–1099.

7. Schepers RJ, et al. Methamphetamine and amphetamine pharmacokinetics in oral fluid and plasma after controlled oral methamphetamine administration to human volunteers. *Clin Chem.* 2003;49(1):121–132.

8. Cook CE, et al. Pharmacokinetics of methamphetamine self-administered to human subjects by smoking S-(+)-methamphetamine hydrochloride. *Drug Metab Dispos.* 1993;21(4):717–723.

9. Schep LJ, Slaughter RJ, Beasley DM. The clinical toxicology of metamfetamine. *Clin Toxicol (Phila).* 2010;48(7):675–694.

10. Verstraete AG. Detection time of drugs of abuse in blood, urine, and oral fluid. *Ther Drug Monit.* 2004;26(2):200–205.

11. National Institute on Drug Abuse. *Commonly Abused Drugs.* National Institutes of Health, ed. Bethesda, MD: US Deptartment of Health and Human Services; 2010.

12. Kuczkowski KM. Marijuana in pregnancy. *Ann Acad Med Singapore.* 2004;33:336–339.

13. Tashkin DP. Airway effects of marijuana, cocaine, and other inhaled illicit agents. *Curr Opin Pulm Med.* 2001;7(2):43–61.

14. Kumar RN, Chambers WA, Pertwee RG. Pharmacological actions and therapeutic uses of cannabis and cannabinoids. *Anaesthesia.* 2001;56(11):1059–1068.

15. Ashton CH. Pharmacology and effects of cannabis: a brief review. *Br J Psychiatry.* 2001;178:101–106.

16. Adams IB, Martin BR. Cannabis: pharmacology and toxicology in animals and humans. *Addiction.* 1996;91:1585–1614.

17. Couper FJ, Barry BK. *Drugs and Human Performance Fact Sheets*, US Department of Transportation, ed. Washington, DC: Government Printing Office; 2004.

18. Hernandez M, Birnbach DJ, Zundert AJV. Anesthetic management of the illicit-substance-using patient. *Curr Opin Anaesthesiol.* 2005;18:315–324.

19. Ellis GM, et al. Excretion patterns of cannabinoid metabolites after use in a group of chronic users. *Nature.* 1985;38(5):572–578.

20. Musshoff F, Madea B. Review of biological matrices (urine, blood, hair) as indicators of recent or ongoing cannabis use. *Ther Drug Monit.* 2006;28(2):155–163.

21. Martin BR, Wiley JL. Mechanism of action of cannabinoids: how it may lead to treatment of cachexia, emesis, and pain. *J Support Oncol.* 2004;2(4):305–316.

22. May J, White H, Leonard-White A. The patient recovering from alcohol or drug addiction: special issues for the anesthesiologist. *Anesth Analg.* 2001;92(1601–168).

23. Cami J, Farre M. Drug addiction. *N Engl J Med.* 2003;349(10):975–986.

24. Waldhoer M, Bartlett SE, Whistler JL. Opioid receptors. *Annu Rev Biochem.* 2004;73:953–990.

25. Vaughan CW, et al. How opioids inhibit GABA-mediated neurotransmission. *Nature.* 1997;390(6660):611–614.

26. Schumacher M, Basbaum A, Way W. Opioid analgesics and antagonists. In: Katzung B, ed., *Basic and Clinical Pharmacology.* New York: McGraw-Hill; 2007: 489–507.

27. Berkowitz BA. The relationship of pharmacokinetics to pharmacological activity: morphine, methadone and naloxone. *Clin Pharmacokinet.* 1976;1(3):219–230.

28. Kamendulis LM, et al. Metabolism of cocaine and heroin is catalyzed by the same liver carboxylesterases. *J Pharmacol Exp Ther.* 1996;279(2):713–717.

29. Inturrisi CE, et al. The pharmacokinetics of heroin in patients with chronic pain. *N Engl J Med.* 1984;310:1213–1217.

30. Kalant H. Hallucinogens and psychotomimetics. In Kalant H, Grant D, Mitchell J, eds., *Medical Pharmacology.* Toronto: Elsevier Canada; 2007: 334–349.

31. Baldridge EB, Bessen HA. Phencyclidine. *Emerg Med Clin North Am.* 1990;8:541–550.

32. Cook CE, Brine DR, Jeffcoat AR. Phencyclidine disposition after intravenous and oral doses. *Clin Pharmacol Ther.* 1982;31:625–634.

33. Shebley M, Jushchyshyn MI, Hollenberg PF. Selective pathways for the metabolism of phencyclidine by cytochrome P450 2B enzymes: identification of electrophilic metabolites, glutathione, and N-acetyl cystein adducts. *Drug Metab Dispos.* 2006;34(3):375–383.

34. Masters S. The alcohols. In: Katzung B, ed., *Basic and Clinical Pharmacology.* New York: McGraw-Hill; 2007: 363–373.

35. Hoffman PL, et al. Ethanol and the NMDA receptor. *Alcohol.* 1990;7:229–231.

36. Santhakumar V, Wallner M, Otis TS. Ethanol acts directly on extrasynaptic subtypes of GABAA receptors to increase tonic inhibition. *Alcohol.* 2007;41(3):211–221.

37. Pohorecky LA, Brick J. Pharmacology of ethanol. *Pharmacol Ther.* 1988;36(2–3):335–427.

38. Hawkins RD, Kalant H. The metabolism of ethanol and its metabolic effects. *Pharmacol Rev.* 1972;24(1):67–157.

39. Pawan GS. Metabolism of alcohol (ethanol) in man. *Proc Nutr Soc.* 1972;31:83–89.

40. Wecker L, et al., eds. *Brody's Human Pharmacology: Molecular to Clinical.* 5th ed. Philadelphia: Elsevier; 2010.

41. Diaz JH, Hill GE. Hypotension with anesthesia in disulfiram-treated patients. *Anesthesiology.* 1979;51(4):366–368.

42. Suh JJ, et al. The status of disulfiram: a half of a century later. *J Clin Psychopharm.* 2006;26(3):290–302.

43. Eriksson CJP. The role of acetaldehyde in the actions of alcohol. *Alcohol Clin Exp Res.* 2001;25(5):15s-32s.

44. Quertemont E, Didone V. Role of acetaldehyde in mediating the pharmacological and behavioral effects of alcohol. *Alcohol Res Health.* 2006;29(4):258–265.

45. Johansson B. A review of the pharmacokinetics and pharmacodynamics of disulfiram and its metabolites. *Acta Psychiatr Scan Suppl.* 1992;369:15–26.

46. Brewer C. Patterns of compliance and evasion in treatment programmes which include supervised disulfiram. *Alcohol Alcsm.* 1986;21(4):385–388.

47. Sadock BJ, Sadock VA. Biological therapies. In: *Concise Textbook of Clinical Psychiatry.* Philadelphia: Lippincott Williams & Wilkins; 2008: 502–503.

48. Fuller RK, et al. Disulfiram treatment of alcoholism. A Veterans Administration cooperative study. *JAMA.* 1986;256(11):1449–1455.

49. Garbutt JC, et al. Pharmacological treatment of alcohol dependence: a review of the evidence. *JAMA.* 1999;281(14):1318–1325.

50. Wilde MI, Wagstaff AJ, Acamprosate: a review of its pharmacology and clinical potential in the management of alcohol dependence after detoxification. *Drugs.* 1997;53(6):1038–1053.

51. Littleton J. Acamprosate in alcohol dependence: how does it work? *Addiction.* 1995;90(9):1179–1188.

52. Saivin S, et al. Clinical pharmacokinetics of acamprosate. *Clin Pharmacokinet.* 1998;35(5):331–345.

53. Center for Substance Abuse Treatment. Acamprosate: a new medication for alcohol use disorders. *Substance Abuse Treatment Advisory.* 2005;4(1).

54. Anton RF, et al. Combined pharmacotherapies and behavioral interventions for alcohol dependence: the COMBINE study: a randomized controlled trial. *JAMA*. 2006;296(17):2003–2017.

55. Mann K, Lehert P, Moran MY. The efficacy of acamprosate in the maintenance of abstinence of alcohol-dependent individuals: results of a meta-analysis. *Alcohol Clin Exp Res*. 2004;28(1):51–63.

56. Ernst A, Zibrak JD. Carbon monoxide poisoning. *N Engl J Med*. 1998;339:1603–1608.

57. Piantadosi CA. Carbon monoxide poisoning. *N Engl J Med*. 2002;347(14):1054–1055.

58. Varon J, et al. Carbon monoxide poisoning: a review for clinicians. *J Emerg Med*. 1999;17(1):87–93.

59. Varon J. Carbon monoxide poisoning. *Int J Tox*. 1997;1(1).

60. Holland MA, Kozlowski LM. Clinical features and management of cyanide poisoning. *Clin Pharm*. 1986;5(9):737–741.

61. Beasley DM, Glass WI. Cyanide poisoning: pathophysiology and treatment recommendations. *Occup Med*. 1998;48(7):427–431.

62. Baud FJ, et al. Elevated blood cyanide concentrations in victims of smoke inhalation. *N Engl J Med*. 1991;325:1761–1766.

63. Baskin SI, Brewer TG. Cyanide poisoning. In: Zajtchuk R, ed., *Textbook of Military Medicine*. Washington, DC: Office of the Surgeon General; 1997.

64. Hall AH, Rumack B.H. Cinical toxicology of cyanide. *Ann Emerg Med*. 1986;15(9):1067–1074.

Other Key Drugs

Chapter 27.1

1-Deamino-8-D-Arginine Vasopressin (DDAVP)

Jesse Raiten, MD

Clinical Uses/ Relevance to Anesthesiology

- Type I von Willebrand's disease perioperatively; minimizes bleeding and may permit use of neuroaxial anesthesia. Pt's factor VIII activity needs to be greater than 5%
- Platelet disorders perioperatively (secondary to renal failure or aspirin); shortens bleeding time
- Trauma patients suffering from intractable microvascular hemorrhage in the setting of platelet inhibiting drugs
- Post-CPB in bleeding pts with prolonged pump times, however data is inconsistent
- Central diabetes insipidus diagnosis and treatment

Pharmacodynamics

- DDAVP, or desmopressin, is a synthetic "analog" to the endogenous hormone vasopressin; compared to vasopressin, has greater platelet and antidiuretic effects with less BP effects
- Direct action on endothelial V_2 receptors causes a release of stored vWF with subsequent $\uparrow$ in factor VIII levels.
- By binding to V_2 receptors in the renal collecting duct, it $\uparrow$ water reabsorption in the kidney. It $\uparrow$ urine osmolality and $\downarrow$ UOP, without affecting Na^+ or K^+ reabsorption, or creatinine. Therefore, effective in central DI (impaired vasopressin production), not nephrogenic DI (collecting ducts do not respond normally to vasopressin)

Pharmacokinetics

- Bleeding disorders: onset 15–30 min, peak effect 1.5 h. Repeat doses at 12–24 h have diminished effects due to depleted endothelial vWF. At 48–72 h, after stores have been repleted, effect may be equivalent to the initial dose.
- DI: onset IV: 15–50 min; PO: 60 min; duration 5–21 h (highly variable)
- Predominantly renally excreted; renal failure will prolong actions, consider dosage adjustments

Adverse Effects

- Water intoxication, hyponatremia. Assessment of perioperative fluid administration, volume status, and electrolytes should be assessed or monitored.
- Platelet aggregation in Type IIB von Willebrand's disease. Decision to administer for von Willebrand's should be done in conjunction with hematologist and surgeon.
- Allergic reactions
- Hypertension. Although less potent than vasopressin, at high doses or when used for bleeding disorders, may be seen.

Dosages/Preparation

- PO, SQ, nasal, and IV administration are available (dependent on clinical situation and indication).
- Hemophilia A and von Willebrand's disease: 0.3 mcg/ kg IV over 30 min. Recommended that infusion should be completed 30 min prior to incision. Can ↑ factor VIII and vWF levels 2- to 20-fold.
- DI: Arrangements should be made to continue perioperatively if appropriate (nasal administration prior to surgery, IV administration intraoperatively, etc). IV dose is ~10 times more potent than nasal; adjust accordingly.

Clinical Case Scenario

A 44-year-old woman with Type I von Willebrand's disease presents for elective hysterectomy. She has a history of bleeding with dental procedures.

Background: Von Willebrand's disease is a common hereditary bleeding disorder that may cause nose bleeds, easy bruising, and increased bleeding with surgery.

Pathophysiology: Von Willebrand's disease is characterized by a deficiency of von Willebrand's factor (vWF), a protein that is necessary for proper platelet function. Patients have a tendency for easy bruising, nose and gum bleeding, and heavy menstrual periods.

Treatment: DDAVP may be administered to this patient preoperatively. DDAVP allows release of stored vWF, and may decrease her risk of bleeding with the procedure.

References

1. Ozier Y, Bellamy L. Pharmacological agents: antifibrinolytics and desmopressin. *Best Pract Res Clin Anaesthesiol.* 2010;24:107–119.

2. Hara K, Kishi N, Sata T. Considerations for epidural anesthesia in a patient with type 1 von Willebrand disease. *J Anesth.* 2009;23:597–600.

3. Rossaint R, Bouillon B, Cerny V, Coats TJ, Duranteau J, Fernández-Mondéjar E et al. Management of bleeding following major trauma: an updated European guideline. *Crit Care.* 2010;14:R52.

4. Levy J. Pharmacologic methods to reduce perioperative bleeding. *Transfusion.* 2008;48:31S-38S.

Carbidopa

Shannon Bianchi, MD and Nina Singh-Radcliff, MD

Clinical Uses/Relevance to Anesthesiology

- Possible use in combination with levodopa in the treatment of tremors associated with chronic regional pain syndrome
- Treatment of spinal myoclonus status post epidural placement when combined with levodopa
- Patients with Parkinson's disease are often treated with carbidopa in conjunction with levodopa, which is important to discover before continuing during anesthesia to prevent neuroleptic malignant-like syndrome from withdrawal of the medication (the effects are actually from the levodopa and not the carbidopa).

Pharmacodynamics

- Inhibits the decarboxylation of extracerebral levodopa to dopamine through the inhibition of aromatic L-amino-acid decarboxylase (which is also involved in the conversion of L-tryptophan to serotonin) thereby decreasing the peripheral side effects such as nausea and vomiting and the dose necessary for therapeutic action across the blood-brain-barrier by about 75%
- Prevents metabolism of 5-HTP to serotonin in the liver
- Does not readily cross the blood-brain-barrier
- Does not have any direct pharmacological effects when administered at usual dosages

Pharmacokinetics

- Half-life = 2 hours
- Peak time = 2.1 +/− 1.0
- Metabolites and unchanged carbidopa is excreted in urine and feces
- Metabolites excreted are α-methyl-3-methoxy-4-hydroxyphenyl-propionic acid and α-methyl-3,4 dihydroxyphenyl-propionic acid

Side Effects/Adverse Reactions

- In general, side effects have not been noted when carbidopa is administered alone.
- Most common side effects: Confusion, constipation, diarrhea, dizziness, drowsiness, dry mouth, headache, loss of appetite, nausea, taste changes, trouble sleeping, upset stomach, urinary tract infection, vomiting
- Severe side effects: Severe allergic reactions (rash; hives; itching; difficulty breathing; tightness in the chest; swelling of the mouth, face, lips, or tongue); black, tarry stools; blood in vomit; chest pain; confusion; depression; fast or irregular heartbeat; fever; hallucinations; increased sweating; mental or mood changes; muscle pain or unusual stiffness; severe abdominal pain; severe light-headedness or fainting; sore throat; thoughts of suicide; unusual bruising or bleeding; unusual or painful movements or spasms of the face, eyelids, mouth, tongue, arms, hands, or legs; vision changes (blurred/double vision); yellowing of the skin or eyes

Dosages/Preparation

- Tablets LODOSYN, 25 mg, are orange, round, compressed tablets, that are scored and coded 511 on one side and LODOSYN on the other
- SINEMET 10–100 (Carbidopa-Levodopa) contains 10 mg of carbidopa and 100 mg of levodopa
- SINEMET 25–250 (Carbidopa-Levodopa) contains 25 mg of carbidopa and 250 mg of levodopa
- SINEMET 25–100 (Carbidopa-Levodopa) contains 25 mg of carbidopa and 100 mg of levodopa
- Daily dosage must be determined by titration. Carbidopa should be administered in conjunction with the levodopa.
- Usually 1:10 ratio of carbidopa to levodopa with a minimum effective dose of 70 mg and a maximum dose of 200 mg

References

1. Navani A, Rusy LM, Jacobson RD, Weisman SJ. Treatment of tremors in complex regional pain syndrome. *J Pain Symptom Manage.* 2003;25(4):386–390.

2. Menezes FV, Venkat N. Spinal myoclonus following combined spinal-epidural anaesthesia for Caesarean section. *Anaesthesia.* 2006;61:597–600.

3. Brunton L, Lazo J, Parker K, eds. *Goodman & Gilman's The Pharmacological Basis of Therapeutics.* 11th ed. New York: McGraw-Hill; 2006.

Chapter 27.3

Doxapram

Shannon Bianchi, MD and Anita Gupta DO, PharmD

Role in the Practice of Anesthesiology/Relevance to Anesthesiology

- Treatment for postanesthetic shivering
- Respiratory stimulant sometimes used in postoperative respiratory depression and in acute respiratory failure in critical care medicine
- Possible use in morbidly obese patients with obstructive sleep apnea especially after gastric bypass surgery secondary to its respiratory stimulant properties
- Analeptic, central nervous system stimulant, that may hasten recovery from inhaled anesthetics
- Treatment of drug-induced CNS depression
- May slow recovery from neuromuscular transmission but effects likely minor
- Has a small pressor effect that may be utilized in anesthetic hypotension but is likely not significant enough

Pharmacodynamics

- Respiratory Stimulant: Central vs peripheral. Although controversy exists as to what extent the central versus the peripheral mechanism contributes to respiratory stimulation, various studies have shown evidence supporting each separately in a dose-dependent fashion to increase tidal volume and respiratory rate. Doxapram stimulates central respiratory centers at higher doses. Peripherally, doxapram has been shown to stimulate carotid and aortic chemoreceptors possibly through TASK tandem pore potassium channel inhibition.
- Analeptic. Doxapram is a central nervous system stimulant that increases arousal especially in patients with central nervous system depression.
- Pressor. Increases blood pressure through improved cardiac function in the form of increased cardiac contractility secondary to catecholamine release but has only a small physiological effect.

Pharmacokinetics

- Short duration of action: 8–10 minutes

- Short half-life: $T_{1/2\alpha}$ = 5.5 and $T_{1/2\beta}$ = 62 min. Doxapram is rapidly metabolized by ring hydroxylation to ketodoxapram an active metabolite in the liver and metabolites are excreted by the kidneys: 40%-50% after 24–48 hours.
- Mean volume of distribution: 1.5 l/kg
- Effective blood concentration: 2 µg/mL

Side Effects/Adverse Reactions

- Postanesthetic agitation. One study found that doxapram use and pain were the most important risk factors for emergence agitation.
- Neurologic effects: headaches, dizziness, possibly proseizure and is contraindicated for use in patients with epilepsy, head injury, or cerebral vascular accident
- Cardiovascular side effects: hypertension, tachycardia, arrhythmia, increased cardiac contractility, chest pain
- Hemolysis, gagging, mydriasis
- Respiratory side effects: laryngospasm, bronchospasm, dyspnea, tachypnea, hiccups
- Contraindicated in patients with severe cardiac impairment
- Minor side effects occurring in less than 5% of patients: Tachypnea, cough, dyspnea, phlebitis, apprehension, flushing, sweating, nausea and vomiting, diarrhea, urinary retention, fever, and muscle spasticity
- May interact with sympathomimetics or MAOIs to cause increase the pressor effect.
- May increase respiratory fatigue and therefore contraindicated in patients with mechanical pulmonary obstruction, restrictive lung diseases, pneumothorax, flail chest, acute bronchial asthma or any condition restricting the chest wall
- Contraindicated in neonates secondary to preparation containing benzyl alcohol
- Care must be taken in hypothyroidism or pheochromocytoma

Dosages/Preparation

- Doxapram Hydrochloride Injection USP, is available in 20 mL multiple dose vials containing 20 mg of doxapram hydrochloride per mL with benzyl alcohol 0.9% as the preservative
- Postanesthetic shivering: IV dosage: 0.18 mg/kg-1.5 mg/kg or 100 mg
- Postanesthetic respiratory depression:
- *IV intermittent dosage*: 0.5 to 1 mg/kg for a single injection and at 5-minute intervals with a maximum dose of 2 mg/kg
- *IV infusion dosage*: 5 mg/minute until a satisfactory respiratory response is observed, and maintained at a rate of 1 to 3 mg/minute. The maximum total dosage by infusion is 4 mg/kg, or approximately 300 mg for the average adult.
- Drug-induced CNS depression:

- *IV Intermittent dosage:* Priming dose of 1–2 mg/kg; repeat in 5 min. May repeat at 1- to 2-hour intervals until sustained consciousness or total of 3 g/24 h given.
- *IV Infusion:* Priming dose of 1–2 mg/kg by direct injection; repeat in 5 min. If no response, continue supportive measures for 1–2 h and repeat priming dose. If effective, initiate infusion at 1–3 mg/min. Discontinue infusion if patient awakens or after 2 h. Infusion may be restarted (along with priming dose) after rest interval of 30–120 min. Do not exceed 3 g/24 h.

References

1. Yost CS. A new look at the respiratory stimulant doxapram. *CNS Drug Rev.* 2006;12: 3–4, 236–249.
2. Yu D, Chai W, Sun X, Yao L. Emergence agitation in adults: risk factors in 2,000 patients. *Can J Anesth.* 2010;57:843–848.
3. Cotton J, Keshavaprasad B, Laster MJ, Eger El II, Yost CS. The ventilatory stimulant doxapram inhibits TASK tandem pore (K2P) potassium channel function but does not affect minimum alveolar anesthetic concentration. *Anesth Analg.* 2006;102:77–785.
4. Robertson GS, Macgregor DM, Jones CM. Evaluation of doxapram for arousal from general anesthesia in outpatients. *Br J Anaesth.* 1977;49:133.
5. Bamgbade OA. Advantages of doxapram for post-anaesthesia recovery and outcomes in bariatric surgery patients with obstructive sleep apnoea. *Eur J Anaesthesiol.* 2010 Dec 28. [Epub ahead of print]
6. Kranke P, Eberhart LH, Roewer N, Tramèr MR. Pharmacological treatment of post-operative shivering: a quantitative systematic review of randomized controlled trials. *Anesth Analg.* 2002;94(2):453–460.
7. Wu CC, Mok MS, Chen JY, Wu GJ, Wen YR, Lin CS. Doxapram shortens recovery following sevoflurane anesthesia. *Can J Anaesth.* 2006;53(5):456–460.
8. Singh P, Dimitriou V, Mahajan RP, Crossley AWA. Double-blind comparison between doxapram and pethidine in the treatment of postanesthetic shivering. *Br J Anaesth.* 1993;71:685–688.
9. Wrench IJ, Singh P, Dennis AR, Mahajan RP, Crossley AWA. The minimum effective doses of pethidine and doxapram in the treatment of post-anaesthetic shivering. *Can J Anaesth.* 2010;57(9):843–848. Epub 2010 Jun 5.

Chapter 27.4

Caffeine

Shannon Bianchi, MD and Anita Gupta DO, PharmD

Role in the Practice of Anesthesiology/Relevance to Anesthesiology

- Conservative treatment of postdural puncture headache
- Part of the caffeine-halothane contracture test (CHCT) performed on a muscle biopsy, which diagnoses malignant hypertension but cannot screen for susceptibility secondary to the low prevalence of malignant hyperthermia in the general population
- Prolongs duration of electroconvulsive therapy (ECT) seizures
- Treatment of apnea, reduction of the rate of bronchopulmonary dysplasia and increase in survival in preterm neonates
- Potential toxic interaction between ketamine and caffeine—street ketamine often contains caffeine
- Caffeine benzoate IV may be beneficial in decreasing reintubation of children with obstructive sleep apnea post anesthesia
- Adjuvant analgesic by antinociceptive actions possibly through antagonism of adenosine A(2A) and A(2B) receptors or inhibition of cyclo-oxygenase-2 enzyme synthesis
- May interfere with analgesic effectiveness through inhibition of antinociception likely through the A1 receptor

Pharmacodynamics

- A xanthine alkaloid that is a psychoactive stimulant
- Central nervous system and metabolic stimulant
- Prevents adenosine from slowing dopaminergic neurotransmission in the striatal spinal module both pre- and postsynaptically therefore, in effect increasing dopamine neurotransmission and psychostimulation
- It is a competitive inhibitor of adenosine as it binds directly to the G protein–coupled adenosine receptor
- Antagonism of adenosine A1, A2A, and A2B receptors, of which A1 and A2A are thought to be involved in the sleep-wake cycle, but which receptor or

to what degree each contributes to wakefulness is controversial—shown to likely be A2A in some studies

- Inhibits phosphodiesterase, promoting calcium release and inhibiting $GABA_A$ receptors
- Caffeine is thought to prevent apnea through antagonism of the A1 and A2 receptors by increasing minute ventilation, improving CO_2 sensitivity, decreasing hypoxic depression, enhancing diaphragmatic activity and decreasing periodic breathing. However, recent studies have shown a role for the A2A receptor possibly through the blockade of A_{2A} receptors on GABAergic neurons.

Pharmacokinetics

- Well absorbed from the gastrointestinal tract
- Inhalational bioavailability: 60%
- Metabolized by the liver through CYP450 and excreted by the kidney
- Normal half-life: 3–5 hours; Half-life in pregnancy: 9–11 hours
- Peak plasma concentration in healthy adults: 50–75 minutes; peak plasma concentration in neonates: 0.5–2 hours
- Readily crosses the placenta and the blood-brain-barrier
- Clearance in neonates: clearance (L/h) = $(0.00000399 \times$ current weight [grams]) + $(0.000128 \times$ postnatal age [days])
- Age >28 weeks: volume of distribution (L) = $(0.000764 \times$ weight [grams]) + $(0.0468$ postnatal age [days]); Age < or = 28 weeks, volume of distribution (L) = $(0.000755 \times$ weight [grams]) + $(0.0224 \times$ postnatal age [days])

Side Effects/Adverse Effects

- Serious reactions: hemorrhage, gastrointestinal bleed, arrhythmias, seizures, hallucinations, angina, urticaria
- Eyes: blurred vision
- Central: drowsiness, decreased or increased appetite, polydipsia, anxiety, confusion, irritability, insomnia
- Sense of balance: dizziness
- Mouth: xerostomia
- Skin: flushing, cold sweats, pallor
- Systemic: hyperglycemia, dehydration
- Respiratory: fruit-like breath odor, dyspnea
- Gastrointestinal: nausea, abdominal pain, diarrhea
- Heart: tachycardia
- Muscular: tremor, fasciculations
- Urinary: ketonuria, polyuria
- Withdrawal after chronic consumption: onset of 12–24 h, peak at 24–48 h, and lasts about 1 week

Dosing/Formulation

- Caffeine OTC: Oral tablet 200 mg: 1 tab PO every 3 to 4 hours with a maximum of 8 tablets in 24 hours (>12 years old)
- Caffeine citrate: Intravenous solution 20 mg/mL: 10–20 mg/kg IV load over 30 minutes, then 5 mg/kg PO/IV per day (neonates); 20 mg caffeine citrate = 10 mg caffeine base
- Therapeutic levels of caffeine = 5–25 mg/L (28–32 weeks gestational age)
- Caffeine/sodium benzoate solution: 125 mg/mL Intramuscular or intravenous: 500 mg caffeine/Na benzoate = 240 mg of caffeine base
- Respiratory depression: 250 mg IM or IV x 1 to 2 doses with a maximum of 1000 mg/dose and 2500 mg per 24 hours
- Headache, postdural puncture: 500 mg IV x 1 may repeat in 4 hours

References

1. Porkka-Heiskanen T, Strecker RE, Thakkar M, Bjorkum AA, Greene RW, McCarley RW. Adenosine: a mediator of the sleep-inducing effects of prolonged wakefulness. *Science.* 1997;276(5316):1265–1268.

2. Huang ZL, Qu WM, Eguchi N, Chen JF, Schwarzschild MA, Fredholm BB, Urade Y, Hayaishi O. Adenosine A2A, but not A1, receptors mediate the arousal effect of caffeine. *Nat Neurosci.* 2005;8(7):858–859.

3. Sawynok J. Caffeine and pain. *Pain.* 2010 Oct 30. [Epub ahead of print].

4. Ortweiler W, Simon HU, Splinter FK, Peiker G, Siegert C, Traeger A . Determination of caffeine and metamizole elimination in pregnancy and after delivery as an in vivo method for characterization of various cytochrome p-450 dependent biotransformation reactions. *Biomed Biochim Acta.* 1985;44 (7–8): 1189–1199.

5. Lee TC, Charles B, Steer P, Flenady V, Shearman A. Population pharmacokinetics of intravenous caffeine in neonates with apnea of prematurity. *Clin Pharmacol Ther.* 1997;61(6):628–640.

6. Fredholm BB, Battig K, Holmen J, Nehlig A, Avartau EE. Actions of caffeine in the brain with special reference to factors that contribute to its widespread use. *Pharmacol Rev.* 1999;51:83–133.

7. Ferré S. An update on the mechanisms of the psychostimulant effects of caffeine. *J Neurochem.* 2008;105(4):1067–1079. Epub 2007 Dec 18.

8. Schmidt B, Roberts RS, Davis P, Doyle LW, Barrington KJ, Ohlsson A, Solimano A, Tin W; Caffeine for Apnea of Prematurity Trial Group. Caffeine therapy for apnea of prematurity. *N Engl J Med.* 2006;354(20):2112–2121.

9. Back SA, Craig A, Luo NL, Ren J, Akundi RS, Ribeiro I, et al. Protective effects of caffeine on chronic hypoxia-induced perinatal white matter injury. *Ann Neurol.* 2006;60:696–705.

10. Mathew OP. Apnea of prematurity: pathogenesis and management strategies. *J Perinatol.* 2010 Dec 2. [Epub ahead of print]

Chapter 27.5

Nitric Oxide

Jesse Raiten, MD

Clinical Uses/Anesthetic Implications

- Pulmonary hypertension
- Right heart failure in cardiac surgery
- Hypoxemia associated with Acute Respiratory Distress Syndrome (ARDS)
- Persistent pulmonary hypertension of the newborn (PPHN)
- Lung transplantation to attenuate the response to ischemic reperfusion injury
- May be useful as a marker of inflammation; NO breath test may indicate airway inflammation

Pharmacodynamics

- Gas synthesized in the vascular endothelium from oxygen, NADPH, and L-arginine via nitric oxide synthase enzymes. NO functions as a (gas) messenger molecule that is capable of producing vascular smooth muscle relaxation (vasodilation).
- Activates soluble guanylate cyclase, which catalyzes the conversion of guanidine triphosphate (GTP) to cyclic guanidine monophosphate (cyclic GMP)

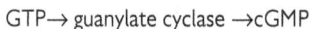

$$GTP \rightarrow \text{guanylate cyclase} \rightarrow cGMP$$

- cGMP causes relaxation of vascular smooth muscle, inhibits platelet aggregation, leukocyte adhesion, and suppresses inflammatory responses.
- Vascular pathology as seen in atherosclerosis and hypertension is associated with impaired NO pathways; additionally, increased salt intake is associated with reduced production.
- Exogenous inhaled NO provides pulmonary arterial and venous vasodilatation, with minimal effect on systemic vascular tone. Thus, PVR and mean PAP are decreased, which results in improved intrapulmonary shunting and VQ mismatch because the drug is preferentially distributed to the best ventilated alveoli (note: blood flow to atelectatic alveoli is "shunted")

- Following heart transplantation, preexisting pulmonary hypertension may predispose the transplanted heart to right ventricular failure. NO may help protect the right heart by reducing the pressure that it must pump against
- In patients with PPHN, lower pulmonary arterial pressures allow improved blood flow into the pulmonary vasculature and less right to left shunting
- In patients with ARDS, pulmonary arterial hypertension exacerbated by permissive hypercapnea may be attenuated with NO

Pharmacokinetics

- Endogenous production is increased in inhabitants of high altitudes (blunts hypoxic pulmonary vasoconstriction to alveoli with lower oxygen partial pressures)
- Rapidly inactivated in the blood by binding to intracellular heme proteins
- cGMP is converted to GMP by phosphodiesterase I and V; thus phosphodiesterase V inhibitors (sildenafil) may amplify the actions of NO

Cautions/Side Effects

- Methemoglobin is produced when NO oxidizes the iron present in heme. Uncommon when the NO dose is <20 part per million (ppm)
- NO reacts with oxygen to form NO_2, which may induce pulmonary edema, alveolar hemorrhage, and other inflammatory changes
- NO may lead to changes in DNA via formation of mutagenic nitrosamines

Adult and Pediatric Dosing

- Dosage ranges from 5 to 40 ppm for pulmonary hypertension and right heart failure
- Improvements in oxygenation may be limited to doses below 5 ppm, while doses up to 20 ppm may continue to reduce pulmonary arterial pressures
- Dosages of 5–80 ppm have been used in infants with severe PPHN

Preparation and Miscellaneous

- NO may be commercially produced by a variety of chemical reactions (sulfur dioxide with nitric acid, sodium nitrite with sulfuric acid, oxidation of ammonia over a platinum catalyst at temperatures > 500 degrees C)
- NO is stored in cylinders of aluminum alloy and are stable for two years or longer
- When employing a standard anesthesia ventilator, recirculation of expired gases may cause NO to accumulate to unsafe levels. I-NOvent is an FDA approved system capable of delivering precise concentrations of NO

Clinical Case Scenario

A 65-year-old man with a history of heart failure and severe pulmonary hypertension is in the intensive care unit one day after receiving a heart transplant. His pulmonary arterial pressures (PAP) are 65/21 and his central venous pressure (CVP) has increased from 11 to 19. On physical exam he has worsening jugular venous distention (JVD).

Background: Immediately following heart transplant in a patient with preexisting severe pulmonary hypertension, the rising CVP and worsening JVD are suggestive of acute right heart failure.

Pathophysiology: Although the transplanted heart usually has normal function, the right ventricle is not used to pumping against elevated PAP, and therefore often suffers acute failure. This is manifested by rising CVP, JVD, and other signs such as hepatic congestion and peripheral edema.

Treatment: Providing inotropic support to assist right heart contractility and using pulmonary vasodilators such as inhaled nitric oxide will improve the pulmonary hypertension and right heart function.

References

1. Cuthbertson BH, Stott S, Webster NR. Use of inhaled nitric oxide in British intensive therapy units. *Br J Anaesth.* 1997;78:696–700.

2. Adhikari NK, Burns KE, Friedrich JO, Granton JT, Cook DJ, Meade MO. Effect of nitric oxide on oxygenation and mortality in acute lung injury: systematic review and meta-analysis. *BMJ.* 2007;334(7597):779.

3. Murakami S, Bacha EA, Mazmanian GM, Détruit H, Chapelier A, Dartevelle P et al. Effects of various timings and concentrations of inhaled nitric oxide in lung ischemia-reperfusion. The Paris-Sud University Lung Transplantation Group. *Am J Respir Crit Care Med.* 1997;156:454–458.

4. George I, Xydas S, Topkara VK, Ferdinando C, Barnwell EC, Gableman L, et al. Clinical indication for use and outcomes after inhaled nitric oxide therapy. *Ann Thorac Surg.* 2006;82(6):2161–2169.

5. Puybasset L, Stewart T, Rouby JJ, Cluzel P, Mourgeon E, Belin MF, et al. Inhaled nitric oxide reverses the increase in pulmonary vascular resistance induced by permissive hypercapnia in patients with acute respiratory distress syndrome. *Anesthesiology.* 1994;80:1254–1267.

6. Steudel W, Hurford WE, Zapol WM. Inhaled nitric oxide: basic biology and clinical applications. *Anesthesiology.* 1999;91:1090–1121.

7. Branson RD, Hess DR, Campbell RS, Johannigman JA. Inhaled nitric oxide: delivery systems and monitoring. *Resp Care.* 1999;44:281–307.

Chapter 27.6

Dexmedetomidine

Shannon Bianchi, MD and Anita Gupta, DO, PharmD

Role in the Practice of Anesthesiology/Relevance to Anesthesiology

- Sedation in critically ill patients in the intensive care setting usually in mechanically ventilated patients
- Less postoperative delirium occurred in patients that were postcardiac surgery when sedated with dexmedetomidine versus morphine in the intensive care unit (ICU) while mechanically ventilated. If delirium occurred, duration was shortened comparatively. Also, increased asymptomatic bradycardia, decreased systolic hypotension and earlier extubation occurred with dexmedetomidine versus morphine.
- Sedation with dexmedetomidine versus other sedation or placebo may hasten discharge from ICU by 12 hours according to meta-analysis of 24 randomized trials in 2,419 patients. Also, showed increase in asymptomatic bradycardia with dexmedetomidine.
- Decrease in duration of mechanical ventilation and delirium
- May increase survival in septic ICU patients versus other sedation
- Sedation for pediatric MRI as a high-dose infusion
- Sedation during spinal anesthesia especially in high-risk patients such as morbidly obese, elderly, pulmonary compromise
- Pediatric sedation in combination with ketamine for procedures such as extracorporeal shock wave lithotripsy, lumbar puncture, or spinal anesthesia
- Awake fiberoptic intubation
- An adjunct in regional anesthesia: increased duration of analgesia, less rescue opioids used and decreased tourniquet pain when dexmedetomidine was added to local anesthetic during regional block for hand and forearm surgery
- May decrease postoperative agitation and analgesic usage in pediatric patients with obstructive sleep apnea syndrome undergoing tonsillectomy and adenoidectomy when infused intraoperatively.
- Awake intracranial surgery
- Has an anesthetic and analgesic sparing effect

- May improve PACU recovery time and decrease opioid usage in laparoscopic bariatric surgery
- May reduce sympathetic tone during cardiac surgery
- Palliative care and acute pain management
- Tracheal or laryngeal surgery—for example, vocal cord surgery requiring the patient to vocalize at key points

Pharmacodynamics

- Dexmedetomidine hydrochloride—S-enantiomer of medetomidine and is chemically described as (+)-4-(S)-[1-(2,3-dimethylphenyl)ethyl]-1H-imidazole monohydrochloride
- Potent selective alpha-2-adrenergic agonist with sedative and analgesic properties
- Sedative-anxiolytic class secondary to its a2 : a1 adrenoreceptor ratio of approximately 1600 : 1
- Anesthetic and analgesic sparing effects but does not appear to affect skeletal muscle dosages
- Hypnotic effect mechanism : hyperpolarization of noradrenergic neurons in the locus ceruleus: Through activation of the alpha-2-adrenergic receptor, cAMP is decreased favoring anabolic over catabolic pathways, membranes are hyperpolarized and the locus ceruleus is inhibited
- Does not cause respiratory depression
- Selectivity diminishes when given rapidly or at high doses
- Blunts sympathetic response to surgery
- Likely neuroprotective through alpha-2 activation and through cellular mechanisms not involving alpha-2
  - increases the phosphorylation of nonreceptor tyrosine kinase stimulated by alpha-2
  - increases expression of growth factors that participate in neuroprotection, inhibits neuronal sodium and potassium rectifier currents, increases extracellular phosphorylation involved in cell survival and memory and activating protein kinase C, may be effective in pre- and postconditioning against ischemia
- Appears to preserve physiological sleep
- May attenuate immunosuppression

Pharmacokinetics

- Elimination half-life = 2 hours
- Alpha half-life = 6 minutes
- Rapidly distributed
- Crosses the placenta
- Excretion = urine (95%) and feces (4%)
- Metabolism: liver—direct glucuronidation, by CYP2A6, and N-methylation

Side Effects/Adverse Reactions

- Common adverse effects: Hypotension, hypertension, nausea, bradycardia, fever, vomiting, hypoxia, tachycardia, anemia
- Cardiac Arrhythmias: Bradycardia and sinus arrest reported in young, healthy adults with high vagal tone; also associated with other methods of administration, including rapid IV administration
- Cardiovascular Precautions: hypotension and bradycardia; more pronounced in geriatric patients or those with hypovolemia, diabetes mellitus, or chronic hypertension; treatment: slowing or stopping dexmedetomidine infusion, increasing IV fluids, elevating lower extremities, and/or vasopressors; consider IV anticholinergic agents (eg, atropine sulfate, glycopyrrolate) to modify vagal tone
- Transient hypertension reported with loading dose—no treatment required
- Rare cardiac events: supraventricular and ventricular tachycardia, atrial fibrillation, extrasystoles, and cardiac arrest
- Caution in patients with advanced heart block and/or severe ventricular dysfunction
- Withdrawal Reactions: nervousness, agitation, headaches, rapid rise in blood pressure, elevated plasma catecholamine concentrations
- Adrenal Insufficiency: Cortisol response to corticotropin stimulation decreased by approximately 40% in dogs after sub-Q infusion of dexmedetomidine for one week

Dosages/Preparation

- Parenteral—for IV infusion—100 mcg per mL, Precedex® (preservative-free) by Abbott
- Must be diluted in 0.9% sodium chloride injection prior to administration to a 4 mcg/mL concentration
- Adult dosing for general sedation: IV infusion bolus of 1 mcg/kg or 0.5 mcg/kg over a 10-minute period, followed by a continuous IV infusion of 0.2 to 1.0 mcg /kg per hour—adjusted until able to obtain appropriate level of sedation
- High-dose pediatric infusion: bolus of 2 µg/kg intravenous followed by 1 µg/kg/h infusion

References

1. Shehabi Y, Grant P, Wolfenden H, Hammond N, Bass F, Campbell M, Chen J. Prevalence of delirium with dexmedetomidine compared with morphine based therapy after cardiac surgery: a randomized controlled trial (Dexmedetomidine Compared to Morphine-DEXCOM Study. *Anesthesiology.* 2009;111(5):1075–1084.

2. Tan JA, Ho KM. Use of dexmedetomidine as a sedative and analgesic agent in critically ill adult patients: a meta-analysis. *Intensive Care Med.* 2010;36(6):926–939. Epub 2010 Apr 8.

3. Memis D, Turan A, Karamanlioglu B, et al. Adding dexmedetomidine to lidocaine for intravenous regional anesthesia. *Anesth Analg.* 2004;98(3):835–840.

4. Esmaoglu A, Mizrak A, Akin A, et al. Addition of dexmedetomidine to lidocaine for intravenous regional anaesthesia. *Eur J Anaesthesiol.* 2005;22(6):447–451.

5. Pandharipande PP, Pun BT, Herr DL, et al. Effect of sedation with dexmedetomidine vs lorazepam on acute brain dysfunction in mechanically ventilated patients: the MENDS randomized controlled trial. *JAMA.* 2007;298:2644–2653.

6. Talke PO, Caldwell JE, Richardson CA et al. The effects of dexmedetomidine on neuromuscular blockade in human volunteers. *Anesth Analg.* 1999;88:633–639.

7. Abbott Laboratories. Precedex®(dexmedetomidine) injection prescribing information. North Chicago, IL; 2000 Feb.

8. Siddappa R, Riggins J, Kariyanna S, Calkins P, Rotta AT. High-dose dexmedetomidine sedation for pediatric MRI. *Paediatr Anaesth.* 2011;21(2):153–158.

9. Kunisawa T, Hanada S, Kurosawa A, Suzuki A, Takahata O, Iwasaki H. Dexmedetomidine was safely used for sedation during spinal anesthesia in a very elderly patient. *J Anesth.* 2010;24(6):938–941. Epub 2010 Oct 7.

10. Ramadhyani U, Park JL, Carollo DS, Waterman RS, Nossaman BD. Dexmedetomidine: clinical application as an adjunct for intravenous regional anesthesia. *Anesthesiol Clin.* 2010;28(4):709–722.

11. Koruk S, Mizrak A, Gul R, Kilic E, Yendi F, Oner U. Dexmedetomidine-ketamine and midazolam-ketamine combinations for sedation in pediatric patients undergoing extracorporeal shock wave lithotripsy: a randomized prospective study. *J Anesth.* 2010;24(6):858–863. Epub 2010 Oct 6.

12. Esmaoglu A, Yegenoglu F, Akin A, Turk CY. Dexmedetomidine added to levobupivacaine prolongs axillary brachial plexus block. *Anesth Analg.* 2010;111(6):1548–1551. Epub 2010 Oct 1.

13. Mantz J, Josserand J, Hamada S. Dexmedetomidine: new insights. *Eur J Anaesthesiol.* 2011;28(1):3–6.

14. Patel A, Davidson M, Tran MC, Quraishi H, Schoenberg C, Sant M, Lin A, Sun X. Dexmedetomidine infusion for analgesia and prevention of emergence agitation in children with obstructive sleep apnea syndrome undergoing tonsillectomy and adenoidectomy. *Anesth Analg.* 2010;111(4):1004–1010. Epub 2010 Aug 12.

15. Tufanogullari B, White PF, Peixoto MP, Kianpour D, Lacour T, Griffin J, Skrivanek G, Macaluso A, Shah M, Provost DA. Dexmedetomidine infusion during laparoscopic bariatric surgery: the effect on recovery outcome variables. *Anesth Analg.* 2008;106(6):1741–1748.

16. Sriganesh K, Ramesh VJ, Veena S, Chandramouli BA. Case report: dexmedetomidine for awake fibreoptic intubation and awake self-positioning in a patient with a critically located cervical lesion for surgical removal of infra-tentorial tumour. *Anaesthesia.* 2010;65(9):949–951.

17. Ohtani N, Kida K, Shoji K, Yasui Y, Masaki E. Recovery profiles from dexmedetomidine as a general anesthetic adjuvant in patients undergoing lower abdominal surgery. *Anesth Analg.* 2008;107(6):1871–1874.

18. Carollo DS, Nossaman BD, Ramadhyani U. Dexmedetomidine: a review of clinical applications. *Curr Opin Anaesthesiol.* 2008;21(4):457–461.

19. Coyne PJ, Wozencraft CP, Roberts SB, Bobb B, Smith TJ. Dexmedetomidine: exploring its potential role and dosing guideline for its use in intractable pain in the palliative care setting. *J Pain Palliat Care Pharmacother.* 2010;24(4):384–386.

20. Chan AK, Cheung CW, Chong YK. Alpha-2 agonists in acute pain management. *Expert Opin Pharmacother.* 2010;11(17):2849–2868. Epub 2010 Aug 13.

21. Shukry M, Miller JA. Update on dexmedetomidine: use in nonintubated patients requiring sedation for surgical procedures. *Ther Clin Risk Manag.* 2010;6:111–121.

22. Su F, Hammer GB. Dexmedetomidine: pediatric pharmacology, clinical uses and safety. *Expert Opin Drug Saf.* 2011;10(1):55–66. Epub 2010 Aug 18.

Chapter 27.7

Acetylcysteine

Shannon Bianchi, MD and Anita Gupta, DO, PharmD

Role in the Practice of Anesthesiology/Relevance to Anesthesiology

- Mucolytic used for multiple lung processes, tracheostomy care
- Minimizes hepatotoxicity in acetaminophen overdose through the reduction in build-up of hepatotoxic metabolite
- May protect against bupivicaine-induced myotoxicity
- Prevention of contrast nephropathy through attenuation of renal ischemia

- N-acetyl-cysteine (NAC) is known to be a powerful antioxidant that may reduce the potential oxidative damage associated with ischemia reperfusion during kidney transplant when administered as a bolus at the time of declamping of the renal artery
- May reduce renal failure after on-pump cardiac surgery
- May decrease myocardial injury when administered as part of cold-blood cardioplegia during on-pump cardiac surgery; prevent perioperative inflammation and ischemia-reperfusion injury during cardiac surgery
- May minimize hypoxic pulmonary vasoconstriction secondary to hemodilution
- Used in treatment of interstitial lung disease

Pharmacodynamics

- Antioxidant action/toxicity treatment. An antioxidant whose therapeutic action is likely due to oxygen free-radical scavenging and/or its role as a source of cysteine, which is a precursor to intracellular glutathione, a major intracellular reductant and/or by improving endothelium-dependent vasodilation.
- Mucolytic action. It lowers mucus viscosity through its free sulfhydryl group, which breaks the disulfide bonds of mucoproteins
- Modified form of the amino acid cysteine, in which the nitrogen atom of the amino group is attached to an acetyl group
- The majority of N-acetylcysteine (NAC) administered forms disulfide bonds with plasma and tissue proteins after intravenous administration leaving little in the circulation.

Pharmacokinetics

- Metabolized by the liver
- Half-life = 5.6 hours (adults), 11 hours (newborns)
- Half-life of elimination of reduced acetylcysteine = 2 hours
- Onset of action: Inhalation: 5–10 minutes
- Duration: Inhalation: >1 hour
- Distribution: 0.47 L/kg
- Time to peak, plasma: Oral: 1–2 hours
- Excretion: Kidney

Side Effects/Adverse Reactions

- Common side effects: Cold, clammy skin; drowsiness; fever; inflammation of the mouth or tongue; nausea; runny nose; vomiting
- Severe side effects: Severe allergic reactions (rash; hives; itching; difficulty breathing; tightness in the chest; swelling of the mouth, face, lips, or tongue); mouth sores; throat and lung irritation
- GI: nausea, vomiting, diarrhea, heartburn, dyspepsia, rectal bleeding, epigastric pain, stomatitis, hemoptysis, and rhinorrhea
- Neurological: dizziness, drowsiness, lightheadedness, and asthenia; headache and increased intracranial pressure rarely
- Respiratory: bronchospasm, wheezing, precipitation of asthma, and respiratory arrest; hemoptysis rarely
- Hypersensitivity: allergies with symptoms such as urticarial rash, pruritus, flushing, a warm feeling of the skin, occasional bronchospasm or hypotension, angioedema, dyspnea, a serum sickness-like reaction, and asthma
- Cardiovascular: tachycardia and hypotension
- Hematologic: increased blood loss and use of blood products when acetylcysteine was used to prevent perioperative inflammation and ischemia-reperfusion injury during cardiac surgery
- Dermatologic: transient flushing on the upper trunk, neck and face—sometimes urticarial and pruritic
- Musculoskeletal: rarely myalgia and arthralgia

Dosages/Preparation

- Preparation: 100 mg/mL (10%), 200 mg/mL (20%) sol
- Acetaminophen overdose:
- Oral: loading dose = 140 mg/kg and then 70 mg/kg every 4 hours for 17 doses
- Intravenous: loading dose = 150 mg/kg by intravenous infusion in 100 ml of 5% dextrose over 15 minutes (for those weighing less than 20 kg), followed by 50 mg/kg by intravenous infusion in 250 ml of 5% dextrose over 4 hours, then 100 mg/kg by intravenous infusion in 500 ml of 5% dextrose over 16 hours

- Mucolytic:
  - Nebulization with a face mask, mouthpiece, tracheostomy: 1 to 10 mL of the 20% solution or 2 to 20 mL of the 10% solution may be given every 2 to 6 hours; the recommended dose is 3 to 5 mL of the 20% solution or 6 to 10 mL of the 10% solution three to four times a day
  - Nebulization—Tent, croupette: requires very large volumes of the solution, occasionally as much as 300 mL during a single treatment period; the recommended dose is the volume of acetylcysteine (using 10% or 20%) that will maintain a very heavy mist in the tent or croupette for the desired period.
  - Direct instillation: 1 to 2 mL of a 10% to 20% solution may be given as often as every hour
  - Tracheostomy care: 1 to 2 mL of a 10% to 20% solution may be given every 1 to 4 hours by instillation into the tracheostomy
  - Diagnostic bronchograms: 2 or 3 administrations of 1 to 2 mL of the 20% solution or 2 to 4 mL of the 10% solution should be given by nebulization or by instillation intratracheally, prior to the procedure
- Protection against contrast-induced nephropathy: 600 mg of oral acetylcysteine twice a day 24 hr before and the day of contrast
- Renal dosing: CrCl <10: decr. dose 25%; HD/PD: not defined

References

1. Dodd S, Dean O, Copolov DL, Malhi GS, Berk M. N-acetylcysteine for antioxidant therapy: pharmacology and clinical utility. *Expert Opin Biol Ther.* 8;1955–1962:2008.

2. Atkuri KR, Mantovani JJ, Herzenberg LA. N-acetylcysteine—a safe antidote for cysteine/glutathione deficiency. *Curr Opin Pharmacol.* 2007;7:355–359.

3. Nolin T, Ouseph R, Himmelfarb J, McMenamin ME, Ward R. Multiple-dose pharmacokinetics and pharmacodynamics of N-acetylcysteine in patients with end-stage renal disease. *Clin J Am Soc Nephrol.* 2010.5:1588–1594.

4. Wijeysundera D, Karkouti K, Rao V, Granton J, Chan C, Raban R, Carroll J, Poonawala H, Beattie WS. N-acetylcysteine is associated with increased blood loss and blood product utilization during cardiac surgery. *Crit Care Med.* 2009;37(6):1929–1934.

5. Ramakrishna H, Fassl J, Sinha A, Patel P, Riha H, Andritsos M, Chung I, Augoustides J. The year in cardiothoracic and vascular anesthesia: selected highlights from 2009. *J Cardiothorac Vasc Anesth.* 2010; 24(1): 7–17.

6. Sorbello M, Morello G, Parrinello L, Molino C, Rinzivillo D, Pappalardo R, Cutuli M, Corona D, Veroux P, Veroux M. Effect of N-acetyl-cysteine (NAC) Added to fenoldopam or dopamine on end-tidal carbon dioxide and mean arterial pressure at time of renal artery declamping during cadaveric kidney transplantation. *Transplant Proc.* 2010;42:1056–1060.

7. Galbes O, Bourret A, Nouette-Gaulain K, Pillard F, Matecki S, Py G, Mercier J, Capdevila X, Philips A. N-acetylcysteine protects against bupivacaine-induced myotoxicity caused by oxidative and sarcoplasmic reticulum stress in human skeletal myotubes. *Anesthesiology.* 2010;113(3):560–569.

Chapter 27.8

Adriamycin (Doxorubicin)

Matt N. Decker, BS and Nina Singh-Radcliff, MD

Role in the Practice of Anesthesia/Relevance to Anesthesia
- Neoplastic treatment
- Cardiomyopathy, CHF, and subclinical cardiotoxicity can be compounded by the cardiodepressive effects of general anesthetics. Therefore, any pt who has taken doxorubicin must be evaluated for this possibility; manifestations may present after several years of latency following treatment.

Pharmacodynamics
- Cytotoxic effects via nucleotide base intercalation; inhibits DNA replication and the action of DNA and RNA polymerases
- Cardiotoxicity is believed to be due to free radical formation. In adults, it is believed to be due to myocardial cell loss leading to late deterioration; in children, likely due to impaired myocardium growth

Side Effects/Adverse Events
- Cardiotoxicity. Assess for clinical signs and symptoms of dysfunction (exercise tolerance, CHF), total dose (dose-dependent; significantly increased risk with dose >500 mg/m^2), risk factors (age >70 y.o. or young age, females, combination chemotherapy, mediastinal radiotherapy, HTN, liver disease, whole-body hyperthermia, and history of coronary, valvular, or myocardial disease). EKG changes include reversible arrhythmias (particularly sinus tachycardia), flattened T waves, prolongation of QT interval, and loss of R wave voltage. Echocardiograms may reveal impaired LV mass and EF and abnormal ventricular wall thickness.

References

1. Adriamycin [Package Insert]. Bedford, OH. Bedford Laboratories, 2010.
2. Singal PK, Iliskovic N. Doxorubicin-induced cardiomyopathy. *N Engl J Med*. 1998;339(13):900–905.
3. Huetteman E, Junker T, Chatzinikolaou KP, et al. The influence of anthracycline therapy on cardiac function during anesthesia. *Anesth Analg*. 2004;98:941–947.
4. Minotti G, Menna P, Salvatorelli E, Cairo G, Gianni L. Anthracyclines: molecular advances and pharmacologic developments in antitumor activity and cardiotoxicity. *Pharmacol Rev*. 2004;56(2):185–229.

Chapter 27.9

Sugammadex

Matt Decker, BS and Nina Singh-Radcliff, MD

Clinical Uses/Relevance to Anesthesiology

- Rapid and reliable reversal of muscle paralysis induced by aminosteroidal muscle relaxants (rocuronium > vecuronium >> pancuronium). Reversal efficacy does not appear to be affected by anesthetic maintenance technique (eg, volatile or propofol).
- Clinical effect is more rapid than succinylcholine's duration of action
- Reversibility is not limited by profound NMBD relaxation
- Reversibility of rocuronium can be performed as quickly as 3 min of administration
- Eliminates issue of residual blockade and recurarization

Pharmacodynamics

- A modified γ-cyclodextrin molecule that binds to NMBD in a 1:1 ratio; the water-soluble complex prevents NMBD from binding to postjunctional nicotinic receptors. Thereby, it reduces the "effective" NMBD available to compete with Ach at the AchR; muscle action potential, contraction, diaphragm, and swallowing function can resume.
- Does not complex with succinylcholine or benzylisoquinolinium NMBDs (mivacurium, atracurium, and cisatracurium).
- Unlike NMBD reversal with anticholinesterases, sugammadex does not increase Ach levels at muscarinic junctions. Therefore, coadministration with antimuscarinic drugs to offset undesirable muscarinic effects are not needed; no anticholinergic drug side effects (tachycardia, dry mouth, mydriasis)

Pharmacokinetics

- Elimination half-life = 2.2 h
- Sugammadex (not bound to NMBD) is excreted unchanged in the urine within 8 h of administration; metabolites have not been observed
- Water-soluble complexes are renally excreted
- Reversal time for rocuronium blockade is similar in both pediatric and adult patients.

Dosing

- Shallow/moderate neuromuscular blockade: 2 mg/kg
- "Deep blockade": 4.0 mg/kg
- "Immediate reversal": 16.0 mg/kg, 3 minutes after administration of rocuronium.
- Dose-response relationship at doses between 0.5–16 mg/kg in rocuronium-induced blockade.

Side Effects/Adverse Reactions

- Flushing, tachycardia, erythematous rash
- No serious adverse effects seen in doses up to 40 mg/kg
- No drug interactions reported

References

1. Rex C, Bergner UA, Pührhinger FK. Sugammadex: a selective relaxant-binding agent providing rapid reversal. *Curr Opin Anaesthesiol.* 2010;23(4):461–465.

2. Naguib M. Sugammadex: another milestone in clinical neuromuscular pharmacology. *Anesth Analg.* 2007;104(3):575–581.

3. Duvaldestin P, Kuizenga K, Saldein J, et al. A randomized, dose-response study of sugammadex given for the reversal of deep rocuronium- or vecuronium-induced neuromuscular blockade under sevoflurane anesthesia. *Anesth Analg.* 2010;110(1):74–82.

4. Bridion [Package Insert]. North Ryde, NSW, Australia. Schering-Plough Pty Limited: 2008.

5. Ploeger BA, Smeets J, Strougo A, et al. Pharmacokinetic-pharmacodynamic model for the reversal of neuromuscular blockade by sugammadex. *Anesthiology.* 2009;110(1):95–105.

Chapter 27.10

Thyroid Medications

Mona Patel, MD and Anita Gupta, DO, PharmD

Clinical Uses/ Relevance to Anesthesiology

- Hypothyroidism, goiter, pituitary TSH suppression, and myxedema coma are treated by exogenous replacement.
- Although perioperative morbidity of hypothyroidism is unknown, major complications have been reported: severe hypotension or cardiac arrest following induction, sensitivity to narcotics and anesthetics (prolonged unconsciousness), and hypothyroid coma following anesthesia and surgery.
- Chronic therapy should be continued perioperatively; long half-life allows leeway in the event of missed dose
- Chronic and acute thyroid hormone administration ↑ BMR; ↑ HR and SV (hence CO via up-regulation of beta receptors), ↑ pulse pressure (↑ SBP while ↓ DBP), ↑ blood volume. Additionally ↑ RR and TV (↑ O_2 consumption and CO_2 production).
- ↑ activity of warfarin; can enhance anticoagulation. Beta-blockers hinder T_4 conversion to T_3 (active form)

Pharmacodynamics

- Thyroid hormone functions in several capacities, including normal heart, liver, kidney, and skeletal muscle metabolism, as well as cell differentiation and growth.
- Thyroxine (T_4) and triidothyronine (T_3) are produced by follicular cells in the thyroid gland in a classic negative feedback system. TRH (from the hypothalamus) stimulates TSH release (from the anterior pituitary), which in turn stimulates the T_3 and T_4 release (from the thyroid gland). T_3 and T_4 feed back to inhibit synthesis and release of TRH and TSH; additionally, high levels of iodide ion can inhibit thyroxine synthesis and release.
- Hormone synthesis involves iodide uptake into the gland, iodination of thyroglobulin, coupling of iodotyrosines to form T_4 and T_3, and release of thyroid hormone in a 20:1 ratio. T_4 is converted to T_3 intracellularly, which binds to thyroid receptor proteins in the cell nucleus, activates DNA transcription and the rate of RNA synthesis, which ultimately affects protein synthesis.

- Hypothyroidism can ↓ the BMR by 55%, the ability to ↑ core temperature in response to cold, HR and SV (hence CO), pulse pressure, and blood volume; thereby hinders the heart's ability to respond to circulatory stress. Furthermore, it affects respiratory parameters: ↓ maximal breathing capacity, diffusing capacity for carbon monoxide, and hypoxic ventilatory drive. Can also cause hyponatremia and ↑ total body extracellular water.
- Exogenous thyroxine must be converted in vivo to T_3; triiodothyronine is in its active form

Pharmacokinetics

- Protein binding: >99% to thyroxine-binding globulin (TBG), prealbumin, and albumin. Bound hormone is not active, metabolized, or excreted.
- Onset of Action. PO thyroxine: 1 day (peak 3–5 days); IV triiodothyronine: 6–8 hrs (peak 24 hrs) in active T_3 form and does not require conversion, hence faster onset
- Bioavailability 40%-80% (small intestine). May be ↓ by age, certain foods and drugs (iron/calcium, cholestyramine, sucralfate)
- Metabolism and Degradation. Thyroxine: Elimination half-life 6–8 days if euthyroid, 9–10 days if hypothyroid, and 3–4 days if hyperthyroid. Most is metabolized via conversion to T_3 in peripheral tissues and thyroid gland (70%) and excreted unchanged in feces. Triiodothyronine: elimination half-life 2 days; excreted unchanged in feces

Side Effects/Adverse Effects

- Overdose; effects resemble hyperthyroidism. General: fatigue, ↑ appetite, weight loss, heat intolerance, fever, sweating. CNS: headache, hyperactivity, anxiety, irritability, insomnia, seizures. Cardiovascular: palpitations, tachycardia, arrhythmias, ↑ pulse pressure and BP, heart failure, angina, MI. Respiratory: dyspnea. Other effects: tremors, diarrhea, vomiting, abdominal cramps, hair loss, flushing, ↓ bone density, menstrual irregularities
- Hypersensitivity reactions: urticaria, itching, flushing, angioedema, GI symptoms (abdominal pain, nausea, vomiting, and diarrhea), fevers, arthralgia, wheezing

Dose

- PO is equivalent to ½ of IM or IV dose.
- Hypothyroidism: 12.5–25 mcg PO QD initially; ↑ dose 2–4 weeks as needed.
- Myxedema coma: 200–500 mcg IV, may repeat 100–300 mcg IV following day.

Preparation

- Thyroxine (T_4) PO tablets; Triiodothyroxine (T_3) PO tablets and powder that can be reconstituted in water solution for IV administration

References

1. Klein I, Ojamma K. Thyroid hormone and the cardiovascular system. *N Engl J Med.* 2001; 344:501–509

2. Lexi-Comp Online™, Lexi-Drugs Online™. Hudson, Ohio: Lexi-Comp, Inc.; 2010; November 28, 2007.

3. Murkin JM. Anesthesia and hypothyroidism: a review of thyroxine physiology, pharmacology, and anesthetic implications. *Anesth Analg.* 1982;61(4):371–383.

4. Wall RT. Endocrine disease. In: Hines RL, Marschall KE, eds., *Stoelting's Anesthesia and Co-Existing Disease.* 5th ed. Philadelphia: Elsevier; 2002: 378–388.

5. Roberts CG, Ladenson PW. Hypothyroidism. *Lancet.* 2004;363:793–803.

Index

449